EARLY CHILDHOOD STUDIES

AN HOLISTIC INTRODUCTION

SECOND EDITION

Edited by

Jayne Taylor RN, RHV, Dip N (Lond), Cert Ed, RNT,
BSc (Hons), PhD, MBA
Director of Quality and Learning at Hertsmere PCT and
St Albans and Harpenden PCT, UK

Margaret Woods MA, BA, Dip Ed
Formerly Dean of Quality Enhancement in the Higher
Education sector of Suffolk College, Ipswich, UK

Hodder Arnold

A MEMBER OF THE HODDER HEADLINE GROUP

First published in Great Britain in 1998 by Arnold
This second edition published in 2005 by
Hodder Arnold, an imprint of Hodder Education and
a member of the Hodder Headline Group,
338 Euston Road, London NW1 3BH

http://www.hoddereducation.co.uk

Distributed in the United States of America by
Oxford University Press Inc.,
198 Madison Avenue, New York, NY 10016
Oxford is a registered trademark of Oxford University Press

*Hodder Headline's policy is to use papers that are natural, renewable and
recyclable products and made from wood grown in sustainable forests.
The logging and manufacturing processes are expected to conform to the
environmental regulations of the country of origin.*

Whilst the advice and information in this book are believed to be true and
accurate at the date of going to press, neither the author[s] nor the publisher
can accept any legal responsibility or liability for any errors or omissions
that may be made. In particular (but without limiting the generality of the
preceding disclaimer) every effort has been made to check drug dosages;
however it is still possible that errors have been missed. Furthermore,
dosage schedules are constantly being revised and new side-effects
recognized. For these reasons the reader is strongly urged to consult the
drug companies' printed instructions before administering any of the drugs
recommended in this book.

British Library Cataloguing in Publication Data
A catalogue record for this book is available from the British Library

Library of Congress Cataloging-in-Publication Data
A catalog record for this book is available from the Library of Congress

ISBN-10   0 340 88736 2
ISBN-13   978 0 340 88736 3

1 2 3 4 5 6 7 8 9 10

Commissioning Editor: Clare Christian
Project Editor: Clare Patterson
Production Controller: Jane Lawrence
Cover Design: Amina Dudhia

Typeset in 10/12 Minion by Charon Tec Pvt. Ltd, Chennai, India
Printed and bound in Spain

What do you think about this book? Or any other Hodder Arnold title?
Please send your comments to www.hoddereducation.co.uk

19.99

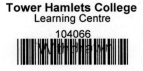

EARLY
CHILDHOOD STUDIES

CONTENTS

List of contributors   vi

Preface   vii

Introduction   Introduction to early childhood studies   viii
Margaret Woods

Chapter 1   Early childhood studies: first principles   1
Margaret Woods

Chapter 2   New beginnings: factors affecting health and well-being in the infant   23
Catherine Forsdike

Chapter 3   Physical growth and development   37
Val Thurtle

Chapter 4   Personal, social and emotional development   57
Anne Greig

Chapter 5   Children's relationships   78
David Rutherford

Chapter 6   Play, language and learning   99
Anne Greig

Chapter 7   Early childhood education and care   117
Margaret Woods

Chapter 8   The early school pathway   141
Beverley Nightingale and Sally Payne

Chapter 9   The child in society   163
Val Thurtle

Chapter 10   Social policy: the state, the family and young children   185
Erica Joslyn, Christine Such and Emma Bond

Chapter 11   Child protection, welfare and the law   203
Kevin Pettican

Chapter 12   Young children with disabilities   226
Sue Hollinrake

Chapter 13   Child health   244
Jayne Taylor and Val Thurtle

Chapter 14   The ill child   257
Val Thurtle and Jayne Taylor

Chapter 15   Children of the world   268
Jayne Taylor

Chapter 16   Perspectives on early childhood research   284
Jayne Taylor

Chapter 17   Working with young children and their families   297
Jayne Taylor

Index   305

LIST OF CONTRIBUTORS

Emma Bond BA (Hons), PGCE, ILTM
School of Education, Suffolk College, Ipswich, Suffolk, UK

Catherine Forsdike RN, SCM, ADM, PGCEA, BA, MSc
Dean of Quality (FE), Suffolk College, Ipswich, Suffolk, UK

Anne Greig Dip Ed, MA (Hons), PhD, MSc (Educational Psychology), Dip CBT
Argyll and Bute Psychological Service, Colgrain, Community Education Wing, Helensburgh, Scotland, UK

Susan Hollinrake BA (Hons), MSc, CQSW
Senior Lecturer in Social Work, Suffolk College, Ipswich, Suffolk, UK

Erica Joslyn BA (Hons), MSc, PhD
Associate Dean of Education, Suffolk College, Ipswich, Suffolk, UK

Beverley Nightingale MA, PGCE, BA (Hons)
Senior Lecturer, School of Education, Suffolk College, Ipswich, Suffolk, UK

Sally Payne BSc (Hons), MSc, PGCE
Lecturer, School of Education, Suffolk College, Ipswich, Suffolk, UK

Kevin Pettican MA, BA, CQSW
Senior Lecturer in Social Work, Suffolk College, Ipswich, Suffolk, UK

David Rutherford BA, MSc
Department of Education, Suffolk College, Ipswich, Suffolk, UK

Christine Such BSc, MA, PGCE
Faculty of Education, APU, Chelmsford, Essex, UK

Jayne Taylor RN, RHV, Dip N (Lond), Cert Ed, RNT, BSc (Hons), PhD, MBA
Director of Quality and Learning at Hertsmere PCT, and St Albans and Harpenden PCT, UK

Val Thurtle MA, BSc (Hons), RGN, RHV, Cert Ed
Senior Lecturer, London South Bank University, London, UK

Margaret Woods MA, BA, Dip Ed
Recently retired Dean of Quality Enhancement in the Higher Education Sector of Suffolk College, Ipswich, Suffolk, UK. Led development of the BA (Hons) Early Childhood Studies, MA Early Childhood Studies, and MA Special Needs in Early Childhood at Suffolk College, Ipswich, UK

PREFACE

The BA (Hons) Early Childhood Studies course was set up at Suffolk College, Ipswich in 1992. At that time it was one of only three such undergraduate degrees in the UK. Since then the programme has gone from strength to strength and, in 2005, it is now one of many early childhood/early years degree-level courses offered at universities and colleges throughout the country. Early Childhood Studies has become a respected and popular academic subject – a subject with a strong vocational orientation providing graduates who are in very great demand.

Members of the initial Early Childhood Studies team at Suffolk College were strongly committed to an holistic view of the young child and therefore to an interdisciplinary approach to early years work. They were consequently enthusiastic about developing a degree programme where the holistic philosophy underpinned the study of early childhood. To create this new discipline of Early Childhood Studies, the team brought together aspects of their traditional academic disciplines, professional expertise and research interests of relevance to the early years – for example, from education, health, psychology, sociology, social policy, child development, linguistics, social work, special needs, law, anthropology, management and research. After the Suffolk College Degree in Early Childhood Studies was established, the first edition of this textbook was written by the team primarily to introduce undergraduates and early years professionals to this holism as it relates to children's early lives.

This second edition, with some of the original and also some new authors (including two programme graduates), retains this principal goal; consequently it has preserved the elements that readers had told us were most useful. Naturally the second edition has had an overall update, recognizing significant new policies, legislation, research and terminology. There have also been changes that acknowledge the greater public and political recognition of the importance of the early years within children's lives and reflect the stronger emphasis on the holistic philosophy and interdisciplinary working among early years professionals as well as the ensuing and quite dramatic development of children's services.

As with the first edition, we hope readers will find it useful to delve into single chapters. The prime intention of the authors, however, is that readers will consider the text as a whole in order to develop or enhance their knowledge and understanding of the holistic and interdisciplinary approach to the paramount task of working with young children and their families.

Jayne Taylor
Margaret Woods

INTRODUCTION TO EARLY CHILDHOOD STUDIES

Margaret Woods

Welcome to the academic study of early childhood.

If you have taken the trouble to delve into this book, you are undoubtedly one of the many enthusiasts who enjoy the company of children and have a keen intention to increase your knowledge and understanding of childhood. Whatever your particular involvement in the early years might be – as a professional from the health, education or social services, a day-care practitioner, a member of a voluntary organization, an undergraduate student on an Honours or Foundation Degree in Early Childhood Studies, a children's nurse, health visitor, or teacher training student – our holistic introduction to early childhood may well be of interest to you and, hopefully, of use to at least some aspects of your studies or practice.

For many centuries there has been considerable academic and altruistic interest in the early childhood life-stage. As long ago as the fourth century BC, Plato (427–347 BC) claimed that children were a form of 'riches', and advocated that they be valued and nurtured because they would become the future leaders and guardians of their society. In *The Republic* (a treatise on education), Plato succinctly encapsulated his belief in the importance of the early years of childhood and the significance of children's education and environment with the statement '... *the beginning is the important part of any work, especially in the case of a young and tender thing*' (Jowett (translation), 1875, p. 376).

Nearly 350 years ago, Joan Amos Comenius (1592–1670), a Czech bishop and educationist, similarly emphasized the importance for their future citizenship within society of the right start in life for children. He envisaged this as being provided within a compulsory education system which would enable individuals to develop their natural abilities, and in which teaching would be appropriate to children's or young people's age and abilities. Comenius consequently proposed a universal education structure which should include a nursery school for children up to the age of 6 years. In this nursery, play was recommended as one of the most significant means of learning.

Another of the early years pioneers was Robert Owen (1771–1858), who was manager of his father-in-law's cotton mill in New Lanark in Scotland, as well as being a social philosopher and reformer of some repute. He limited the employment hours of young children in his mill, but is better known for opening what is regarded as the first British infant school in New Lanark in 1816 for the millworkers' children. While this reform could be open to imputations of improving his own profits, Owen does appear to have strongly believed that children's experiences in their early years are extremely influential in their later development and well-being. Much in accord with the views of Plato and Comenius, infant education was for Owen a certain way to ensure good citizens in the future.

Friedrich Froebel (1782–1852), one of the most famous and influential early years educational philosophers, also regarded early childhood as an extremely important life-stage. Froebel contributed greatly to our thinking about how children learn. He claimed that children's intellectual development begins as soon as they are born, and advocated play as an excellent medium for learning. The term 'kindergarten', which implies the 'fostering of a child's nature ... drawing on it, guarding it, tending and cultivating it like a good gardener tending a young plant' (Liebschner, 1992, p. 25) was of course one of his most illustrative and enduring concepts.

The philosophy underpinning much modern nursery-school practice has its origins in the open-air nursery of Margaret and Rachel McMillan, which was started in Deptford in London in 1911. The McMillan sisters were particularly concerned to provide a rich nurturing childhood experience which would counteract the disadvantage stemming from the impoverished and unhealthy home environments that characterized the daily existence of many children and which, if left unchecked, would undoubtedly impair their adult lives. This emphasis on promoting good health (with the setting up of clinics, open-air camps and nursery school) emanated from the McMillans' firm belief that children's learning and all-round development were unlikely to be maximized and their self-esteem and self-confidence adequate if the children remained sickly and frail. Their nursery education was planned to promote all aspects of children's development along with their good health, happiness and respect and thought for others. Such characteristics were deemed necessary by the McMillans to ensure children's well-being in adulthood and to produce a just and caring society.

More recently, the United Nations (UN) in its Convention on the Rights of the Child (UNICEF, 2003) has '... proclaimed that childhood is entitled to special care and assistance'. Recognizing the difficult conditions in which many children lived and the importance of international cooperation, the Articles were agreed in 1989 and, by 2004, had been ratified by 192 countries (see Chapters 1, 10 and 15 for more information on the Rights of the Child). At the UN Special Session on Children on 10 May 2002, the original commitments were upheld and 10 principles and objectives agreed as the basis for a plan of action to make the world fit for children, ensuring they have the '... best possible start in life' (UNICEF, 2003, p. 19). Eliminating discrimination and tackling poverty sadly had to remain within that revised vision.

Certainly in the early twenty-first century, much public attention is given to early childhood. Newspapers, professional journals, popular magazines and television programmes regularly include commentaries or debates on early years issues. A significant amount of this publicity, substantiated by the strengthening base of early childhood research and also by the increasingly numerous early years publications, reflects the growing recognition of the value of promoting children's development and well-being through high-quality early childhood services. Gratfiyingly, the United Nations Educational, Scientific and Cultural Organisation has reported that research has illustrated that investment in the early years far outperforms other public policy in terms of cost effectiveness, for example by saving on remedial actions (UNESCO, 2004). For example, we saw above that the UN fully acknowledge the pre-eminence of the early years in preventing or reducing disadvantage, realizing that: '... early childhood is the most opportune moment for preventing or breaking the poverty cycle', and '... investment in children is a key determinant of the success of anti-poverty programmes' (UNICEF, 2000, p. 39). The Organisation for Economic Cooperation and Development (OECD, 2002) has also recognized early childhood as an advantageous time for countering discrimination. Additionally, OECD has, as one of its priorities, improving the quality of, and access to, early childhood education and care (see the OECD website).

Consequently, many governments and organizations worldwide have invested in childhood (OECD, 2002). The United Kingdom is a good example – Haddad (2002,

p. 6) has noted that many UK reforms and initiatives have reversed '… a long tradition of state inattention to early childhood-related matters'. There has certainly been considerable financial investment and commitment into services to overcome inequalities in children's lives and to raise the quality of existing and new services in order to promote children's optimum development and well-being. Examples include The Children Act; SureStart; Foundation Stage Curriculum and Guidance; Framework for Effective Practice; Early Years Development and Childcare Partnerships; Ofsted's new Early Years Directorate; Together from the Start; National Service Framework for Children, Young People and Maternity Services; Investors in Children; Early Excellence Centres; and The Early Support Programme for Children 0–3 with Disabilities. There is also the appointment of the Minister for Children, and the government pledge to eradicate poverty in the UK within a generation.

Emerging from much of the recent research are two crucial principles which, when translated into practice, result in significant benefits to children and their families. These are:

1. Children's needs, development and experiences should be considered, conceptually and practically, from an holistic viewpoint.
2. There should be integration of – or, at the very least, strong coordination of/liaison between – health, education and social services. In other words, a multidisciplinary or integrated/co-ordinated approach by the early years professions.

Pleasingly, these two principles are now prominent or influential in the early years policies and priorities of the UN, UNICEF and OECD (see websites) and also of many governments, including the UK, Sweden, Norway, Denmark, Finland, Brazil, China, Senegal, Australia, New Zealand, Kenya and Spain (Haddad, 2002). Also, Bertram and Pascal (2002) note a number of countries working to integrate education and care and the increasing use of the term *early childhood education and care* (*ECEC*).

THE HOLISTIC/INTEGRATED APPROACH TO THE STUDY OF EARLY CHILDHOOD

This book offers an holistic perspective on early childhood, with the philosophies of holism and integration sustaining and unifying our text. The approach is commended or assumed in many of the books and research papers mentioned in the reference sections at the end of each chapter. A very readable account of the origin and rationale of holism is provided by Hazareesingh *et al.* (1989).

This holistic ideology values the whole child and endeavours to understand each young child as an individual within the context of his or her family, community and culture. With this approach, professionals endeavour to be sensitive and responsive to all of a child's needs and aspects of development – that is, physical, intellectual, social, emotional, cultural, moral and spiritual. Early years practitioners also realize that children's needs and developing abilities are closely inter-connected and very much intertwined with the needs and circumstances of each child's family. In addition, all aspects of a child's welfare and development are viewed as part of a co-ordinated system and are seen as growing alongside, influencing and interacting with each other. Ideally, early years professionals would strive to avoid promoting or prizing one area of development over and above, or at the expense of any of the others. Naturally, specialism in or study of one aspect of a child's development (e.g. education or health) is feasible within an holistic framework which recognizes, values and takes account of all aspects.

Professionals who adopt this holistic stance would be strongly committed to equality of opportunity for each child regardless of race, class, gender, ability, family or community. They would also recognize the many factors that are influential in a child's life, and work towards integrating the diverse and unique experiences of each child's life into a meaningful whole. Holism goes hand in hand with advocacy of greater co-operation and collaboration between early years professionals, for example teachers, nursery nurses, health visitors, social workers, playgroup supervisors and children's nurses. Indeed, UNESCO (2003) affirms that children's holistic development can only be ensured if there is close co-ordination or preferably integration of the education, social and health sectors, and they strongly urge governments to tackle this integration as part of their social and economic planning. They even offer support for this planning and implementation. Such integration needs strong political will and presents a mighty challenge for governments, communities and professionals. Consequently, many countries have not realized full or even partial integration of education and care (Bennett, 2003; Haddad, 2002).

The integrated approach requires all groups to have a shared vision and to work towards well-articulated and agreed aims and goals. It is based on a climate of close and active co-operation, communication, openness and team spirit amongst all the parties, a legitimate sharing of information about children and their families and entails each professional group recognizing, respecting and using the skills and expertise of the others. Clear government and local agency commitment, strong, supportive and sensitive leadership and sufficient and flexible resourcing are necessities. Joint training is also to be recommended.

Of course such a philosophy is very much easier to write and talk about than to put into practice. Hopefully by reading this book, which is strongly supportive of the principle of holism, some ideas for its practical implementation can be identified. While initial and in-service training and academic study with a more multidisciplinary, multiprofessional or integrated perspective will certainly help to promote realization of the tenet of holism, only by early years enthusiasts working collaboratively towards and publicly disseminating the approach can we hope to come anywhere close to such a high ideal.

WHAT DOES EARLY CHILDHOOD STUDIES ACTUALLY INVOLVE?

Very simply and obviously, Early Childhood Studies involves studying early childhood – but what exactly is the specific focus of this fairly recently evolved academic and professional subject?

As you will be well aware, children are the young of the human species, and childhood is the actual state of being a child. In contemporary Western society early childhood is usually considered to extend from birth until around 8 years of age. It is, therefore, the initial stage of life outside the womb. Human beings pass through early childhood as they progress towards and through middle childhood and adolescence and eventually into adulthood. Usually in childhood humans are viewed and treated differently to adults and in a manner deemed, in their particular culture, to befit the perceived child character, status and needs.

Early Childhood Studies as an academic discipline has drawn on the more traditional or established subjects such as psychology, sociology, education, health, social work, social policy, law as they relate to children up to the age of 8 years. Now, it is rapidly developing its own research base. In an holistic and broad-ranging study of this period of life, such as that contained within an Early Childhood Studies Degree programme or, as in this particular case, within an Early Childhood Studies textbook, intellectual attention will be focused on issues that are relevant to the familial, social and cultural realities of children's lives. The research and learning involved will be concerned with children's physical growth and development, with their personalities, cognitive abilities, health, social relationships and emotional well-being, and with some of the more significant policies, legislation and services relating to young children and their families. Strategies to develop the effectiveness of early years professionals must be considered, and the nature and possible impact of a number of the more typical experiences, problems and challenges of childhood investigated. In summary, Early Childhood Studies involves a study of the child within some form of family grouping that is in turn set within wider social and cultural contexts.

Of course we must keep firmly in our minds that childhood is what is termed a 'social construct'. It is a label that society has created for young people in the early part of their lives. Consequently, childhood can have different connotations within different cultures and in different periods of history. This leads to a variety of child-rearing practices emanating from the customs and beliefs of the particular time and place.

In 1992, for example, Agiobu-Kemmer described how in some contemporary rural African societies children were regarded as the 'essence or sap of life' and as the 'clothing and adornment for their parents' (p. 5). They were viewed very much as a status symbol in whom education and welfare should be invested in order that they may provide for their parents in old age.

It is also interesting to note the attitudes towards children of the contemporary !Kung peoples, with whom Melvin Konner lived and studied for 2 years. They apparently treated their children with considerable gentleness and generosity. They were exceedingly responsive to their children's needs, and did not advocate any form of punishment, believing that children's mental immaturity was responsible for any behaviours deemed undesirable. Education was for real life, and learning was genuinely through play and by observation and imitation of adults as they tackled their daily tasks (Konner, 1991). Interestingly, such practices have more recently been advocated for the Western world by Singer (1996) as being more effective in terms of children's learning than modern nurseries which tend to create a separate and artificially created children's world.

When we delve briefly into the history of childhood, Bryans and Wolfendale (1981) describe parents in medieval times as regarding their children in terms of the contribution they could make to the family economy and survival. In Tudor times, the children of the wealthy were well provided for educationally, while the children of the poor were often tied into harsh apprenticeships and forced to beg for money or food.

Bryans and Wolfendale (1981) also mention the high child mortality rate, the general ambivalence towards children and their exploitation by commerce and industry in previous generations. De Mause (1974) certainly presents a depressing historical picture of the considerable physical abuse to which children have been subjected from earliest times. According to his research and interpretations, many children were obviously not regarded as worthy of care, attention or respect.

In the so-called religious mortality or evangelical period of the eighteenth century, epitomized by Susanna Wesley in letters to her sons John and Charles, it is evident that the prime concern of parents was to save children's souls early in their lives because of the high expectation of death in childhood. This strongly held minority view recommended that children be brought up in an atmosphere of fear, extreme godliness and harsh physical punishment. Sangster (1963, p. 75), however, does wonder to what extent this evangelical discipline was a generally held view, and whether in practice it was quite 'as rigorous as its reputation'.

Another somewhat extreme – but again not necessarily universal – historical perspective is that of the hygienist movement of the 1920s and 1930s, when children were considered to be in need of strict discipline, and cleanliness was of prime consequence. We are already aware that the McMillan sisters, especially Rachel, who was a sanitary inspector, were justifiably concerned with the hygiene aspects of children's upbringing. We must remember, however, that this was within a caring nursery environment created to counteract the desperately impoverished and unhealthy conditions of the period. The publicly available hygienist advice to parents and practitioners was to inculcate into children, in not too kindly a fashion, the 'virtues' of self-control, strict obedience, recognition of authority and respect for elders. Recommendations were given that children were not to be picked up when they cried and not to be hugged and kissed by their parents. Newson and Newson (1974) tell us that apparently a few conscientious, well-meaning, very often intelligent and well-educated parents actually followed such guidelines explicitly, although many others felt unhappy about this somewhat harsh and regimented treatment of children. Even in 2004 the debate persists on the merits and demerits of a regimented upbringing for children against a more liberal and apparently responsive approach to child-rearing (O'Reilly and Ungoed-Thomas, 2004).

For any readers particularly interested in the history of childhood, there is a list of relevant publications at the end of this chapter. There is also a further discussion of childhood as a social construct in Chapter 9.

We must realize the importance of keeping this cultural relativism in mind when studying childhood. Since societies, cultures and indeed families differ or change over time, concepts of children, childhood and the ensuing child-rearing practices and expectations of children differ and change accordingly. Some understanding of the past and a wide range of contemporary philosophies and practices can often help us find more effective ways to work with children and families.

WHY MIGHT WE STUDY EARLY CHILDHOOD?

We have reflected briefly on what the study of early childhood might involve. Now, in the manner of the true early years professional, we should consider why we might be studying this fascinating subject. It is always a wise precept to be able to rationalize the undertaking of a particular course of action, whether it involves embarking on an Early Childhood Studies Degree programme, training to be a children's nurse, organizing a specific art and craft activity in an infant class or a children's ward, or selecting an appropriate story for a group of nursery children. Ascertaining, justifying and articulating our ultimate objectives as well as our modest, short-term aims can make our actions more confident and focused. We may, therefore, be enabled to work towards our specified goal with greater purpose and meaning. Success then becomes a more likely outcome.

Since the early 1990s, Early Childhood Studies Degrees have been running at UK higher education institutions. This was partly to support implementation of the holistic/integrated approach in early childhood provision, but these programmes were also seen as precursors to postgraduate professional courses such as Early Years PGCE and Diplomas in Social Work and also as a form of in-service training for early years professionals wishing to 'top up' their existing qualifications in order to enhance their knowledge and understanding of young children as well as improve their career opportunities. Progression for nursery nurses was also anticipated. Additionally, it was envisaged that such graduates would become articulate professionals, skilled in research methodology and able to rationalize and promote quality practice in an endeavour to enrich the experiences and improve the life chances of young children and their families. It was also anticipated that, in many instances, they would become the pioneers and leaders within the early years academic and professional arenas. Considerable research has since substantiated the very significant benefits to children and families of graduate-level early years professionals (e.g. Mooney *et al.*, 2003; Sylva *et al.*, 2003; Haddad, 2002; Siraj-Blatchford *et al.*, 2002; OECD, 2001).

Many readers will know exactly why they wish to increase their knowledge and understanding of childhood, but let us consider some of the more typical reasons – academic, philanthropic or pragmatic. Some students may wish to:

- fulfil a desire to do something worthwhile for children and their families;
- discover how children become the people they eventually will be or, as Konner (1991, p. 7) observes, '*always will be becoming*';
- establish what the main influences on children's holistic development are considered to be;
- appreciate how children might develop, and account for differences and similarities between children;
- understand how to provide the environment and experiences most conducive to promoting children's well-being and optimum all-round development; and
- become more sensitive and responsive to the diverse needs of young children and their families.

Many professionals and researchers also study early childhood because their findings can constitute a rich source of information on human beings in general. In addition, they may believe that we can improve aspects of adult life by using the results of our research to enrich the quality of childhood. We might, for example, ascertain how best to protect children against abuse, to supply a well-balanced diet, to encourage a love of learning, or to provide social and emotional stability in childhood and so create a more stable foundation for adulthood.

We must not, of course, regard childhood only as a preparation for adult life – however critical it is in terms of children's future well-being and development. Early childhood is a very significant life-stage in its own right, being a time when a great deal of learning occurs, concepts are formed, the first and all-important relationships are made and crucial attitudes develop.

Certainly for many people these are appealing and exciting reasons for studying and/or opting to work with children. They do, however, illustrate the tremendous responsibility involved in providing the optimum support and appropriate experiences necessary to promote young children's all-round development and well-being. In-depth study can undoubtedly help in this important endeavour.

REFERENCES

Agiobu-Kemmer, IS (1992): Child Survival and Child Development in Africa. *Bernard van Leer Studies and Evaluation Paper Six.* The Hague: Bernard van Leer Foundation.

Bennett, J (2003): Starting strong: The persistent division between care and education. *Journal of Early Childhood Research,* **1**(1), 21–48.

Bertram, T and Pascal, C (2002): *Early Years Education: An International Perspective.* London: QCA.

Bryans, T and Wolfendale, S (1981): Changing attitudes to children – a comparative chronicle. *Early Childhood,* **2**, 4–7.

De Mause, L (ed.) (1974): *The History of Childhood.* London: Bellen.

Haddad, L (2002): *An Integrated Approach to Early Childhood Education and Care.* Paris: UNESCO.

Hazareesingh, S, Simms, K and Anderson, P (1989): *Educating the Whole Child.* London: Building Blocks Educational.

Jowett, B (1875): *The Republic of Plato.* Oxford: Clarendon Press.

Konner, M (1991): *Childhood.* London: Little, Brown & Company.

Liebschner, J (1992): *A Child's Work.* Cambridge: Lutterworth Press.

Mooney, A, Cameron, C, Candappa, M, McQuail, S, Moss, P and Petrie, P (2003): *Early Years Childcare & International Evidence Project: Quality.* London: DfES.

Newson, J and Newson, E (1974): Cultural aspects of childrearing in the English-speaking world. In Richards, M.P.M. (ed.), *The Integration of a Child into a Social World.* Cambridge: Cambridge University Press, pp. 53–82.

OECD (2001): *Starting Strong: Early Childhood Education and Care.* Paris: OECD.

OECD (2002): *Early Childhood Education and Care for Children from Low-Income or Minority Backgrounds.* Paris: OECD.

O'Reilly, J and Ungoed-Thomas, J (2004): Queens of babycare clash over tough love. *Sunday Times,* 9 May, p. 9.

Sangster, P (1963): *Pity my Simplicity.* London: Epworth Press.

Singer, E (1996): Prisoners of the method. *International Journal of Early Years Education,* **4**, 28–40.

Siraj-Blatchford, I, Sylva, K, Muttock, S, Gilder, R and Bell, D (2002): *Researching Effective Pedagogy in the Early Years.* London: DfES.

Sylva, K, Melhuish, E, Sammons, P, Siraj-Blatchford, I, Taggart, B and Elliott, K (2003): *The Effective Provision of Pre-school Education (EPPE) project: Findings from the Pre-school Period.* London: DfES.

UNESCO (2003): *Cross-sectoral Co-ordination in Early Childhood: Some Lessons to Learn.* http://www.unesco.org/education/er/

UNESCO (2004): *Early Childhood at UNESCO.* http://www.unesco.org/education/

UNICEF (2000): *Poverty Reduction Begins with Children.* New York: UNICEF.

UNICEF (2003): *A World Fit for Children.* New York: UNICEF.

USEFUL WEBSITES

Department for Education and Science – www.dfes.gov.uk
Early Years Development and Childcare Partnerships – www.eydcp.gov.uk

National Children's Bureau – www.ncb.org.uk
Organisation for Economic & Cultural Development – www.oecd.org
Office for Standards in Education – www.ofsted.gov.uk
Qualifications & Curriculum Authority – www.qca.gov.uk
SureStart – www.surestart.gov.uk
United Nations Educational, Scientific & Cultural Organisation – www.unesco.org
United Nations Children's Fund – www.unicef.org

FURTHER READING

Aries, P (1982): *Centuries of Childhood: A Social History of Family Life*. London: Cape.

Bradburn, E (1989): *Margaret McMillan: Portrait of a Pioneer*. London: Routledge.

Hoyles, M (1979): Childhood in historical perspective: In Hoyles, M (ed.), *Changing Childhood*. London: Writers and Readers Co-operative, pp. 16–29.

King-Hall, M (1958): *The Story of the Nursery*. London: Routledge & Kegan-Paul.

Liddiard, M (1928): *The Mothercraft Manual*. London: J&A Churchill.

Sears, RR, Maccoby, E and Levin, H (1957): *Patterns of Child Rearing*. Evanston, IL: Row Peterson.

Walvin, J (1982): *A Child's World: A Social History of English Childhood*. Harmondsworth: Penguin.

Watson, JB (1928): *Psychological Care of Infant and Child*. New York: WW Norton.

EARLY CHILDHOOD STUDIES: FIRST PRINCIPLES

Margaret Woods

This chapter aims to:

- consider a set of global value principles to underpin early years practice;
- present an overview of child development perspectives;
- provide initial guidance on observing children.

INTRODUCTION

Early Childhood Studies has only relatively recently been regarded as an academic discipline in its own right. It has assimilated and built upon many of the methodologies, perspectives, theories, concepts and debates from other academic disciplines, including psychology, sociology, paediatrics, education, health, anthropology, social work and social policy. In this chapter we shall deliberate on a few of the basics or first principles of the study of early childhood since '... fine tuning our conceptions of the nature of childhood can help us to know children in greater depth' (Bloch, 2000, p. 260).

VALUE PRINCIPLES FOR STUDENTS OF EARLY CHILDHOOD

We considered in this book's introduction a little of how values and principles differ between cultures and have changed over time. Certainly we must be continually conscious of this cultural relativism and supportive of children and families from all cultures. We must also be well aware of the values and principles which constitute our own beliefs, inform our thinking and underpin our practice, recognizing that students new to the study of early childhood may still be in the process of formulating beliefs and values. To assist with this task, a global model of early childhood value principles is outlined below. It is published by UNESCO (United Nations Education, Scientific and Cultural Organisation), and its intention to '... include the child as a whole, as well as all the children in the world' (Lillemyr *et al.*, 2001, p. 19), sits comfortably with our concepts of holism and multiprofessionalism discussed in this text's introduction. A global model can help reduce ethnocentrism, encourage greater acceptance of diversity and ensure each child is viewed as a '… unique human being with societal rights' (Lillemyr *et al.*, 2000, p.19).

The value principles of Lillemyr *et al.* (2001) derive from the United Nations Convention on the Rights of the Child which was instituted to guarantee the well-being and sound development of every child. Their global model comprises six value principles:

1. The Universal Declaration of Human Rights, and in particular, the Convention on the Rights of the Child.
2. Democracy.
3. Multiculturalism.
4. Ethical responsibility and accountability.
5. The value of play.
6. A new professionalism.

Let us consider each of these value principles in turn.

The UN Convention on the Rights of the Child

This convention is a human rights treaty providing a set of universal standards and obligations relating to the rights of children and young people under 18 years of age. It was adopted by the General Assembly of the United Nations in 1989, and by 2004 it had been ratified by 192 countries. It sets out the context in which children should live – with 'peace, dignity, tolerance, freedom, equality and solidarity' (Preamble). Its four guiding principles are (UNICEF, 2003):

- **Best interests of the child** (Article 3 – 'In all actions concerning children … the best interests of the child shall be a primary consideration').
- **Non-discrimination** (Article 2 – No child should suffer discrimination 'irrespective of the child's or his parent's or legal guardian's race, colour, sex, language, religion, political, disability, birth or other status').
- **The survival and development of children** (Article 6 – 'Development should be interpreted holistically i.e. including emotional, cognitive, social, cultural and mental as well as physical aspects of development').
- **Participation** (Article 12 – 'The child's right to express an opinion, and to have that opinion taken into account, in any matter or procedure affecting the child').

In 2002, the Heads of State and government (or their representatives), in a General Assembly Special Session on children, reaffirmed and updated their commitment to the Convention through the following 10 objectives (UNICEF, 2003):

1. Put children first.
2. Eradicate poverty: invest in children.
3. Leave no child behind (equality and non-discrimination).
4. Care for every child.
5. Educate every child.
6. Protect children from harm and exploitation.
7. Protect children from war.
8. Combat HIV/AIDS.
9. Listen to children and ensure their participation.
10. Protect the Earth for children.

Democracy

As part of their overarching belief that in early childhood education and care lay the foundation for children becoming effective members of society, Lillemyr *et al.* (2001) argue that children should have first-hand experience of democracy within early childhood settings which should be 'democratic mini-societies' (p. 10) adhering to democratic values and principles and supporting children in developing the necessary competencies and appropriate personal qualities.

Multiculturalism

In order that society can learn lessons from past 'disasters, fragmentation … dissociation … and ethnocentrism' (p. 11), Lillemyr *et al.* (2001) challenge early years professionals to help children in their care to become multiculturally tolerant by developing an understanding of culture that facilitates communication and mutual understanding between people.

Ethical responsibility and accountability

This value principle is an integral element of genuine professionalism. Adults who work with children must be responsible, caring professionals whose work is based on sound, widely accepted values and who follow ethical and professional standards against which they can be held accountable.

The value of play

Play is regarded as critical in the culture of childhood and its rich possibilities must be realized.

A new professionalism

The final value principle of Lillemyr *et al.* (2001, p. 12) endorses holism by illustrating that a multiprofessional team and integrated services are the most effective ways of serving the best interests of the whole child. A three-fold approach is required from early years professionals:

- '… being professional in securing one's professional competences, as an educator, a health-worker, etc. … ;
- knowing the limits of one's competences, as well as … continuous development of these competences;
- knowledge about other relevant professionals to provide total support for the child;
- professional collaboration with other professionals and parents.'

While this is a set of value principles to which many of us might happily aspire, such a global model may seem somewhat ambitious. We should, therefore, take some time to consider each value principle in the light of our early years experience, reading and study and to discuss each with early years colleagues, tutors and/or fellow students.

OVERVIEW OF THE MAIN THEORETICAL PERSPECTIVES ON EARLY CHILDHOOD

Most developmental psychology/child development theories derive from three main stances or premises. In formal academic terminology, these three perspectives are described as rationalism, associationism, and constructivism (Richardson, 1988). Richardson argues it is necessary for students to understand these three 'poles, ideas or sets of pre-suppositions' (p. viii) before they can make sense of most of Western psychology or, in our case, early childhood studies.

It is often helpful, if a little simplistic, to imagine these three belief systems as being positioned along a spectrum. At one end is rationalism or, as it has come to be called today, nativism. This perspective is the 'nature' in the famous nature/nurture debate.

Rationalism/Nativism

Originally, rationalism entailed the belief that knowledge and concepts were innate and, in some mysterious way, present in the newborn child. Individual differences – for example in intelligence and language development – were deemed to be biologically determined or inherited, with children seen as pre-programmed to develop or mature in certain ways. This nativist stance might be considered to have been a dominant influence in early childhood practice with the practitioner providing an 'appropriate' environment but not intervening to force a child's development or learning. While research on the development of human nature (Pinker, 2003) and on the 'relative sophistication of infant cognition' have 'led to a renaissance of strong nativist views' (Goswami, 2001, p. 258), much evidence is now available to substantiate the influence of experience on children's behaviour and development and to challenge such rationalist/nativist assumptions (e.g. Ehrlich and Feldman, 2003; Horwitz *et al.*, 2003; Pinker, 2003; Ridley, 2003; Bloch, 2000; Zimiles, 2000).

Associationism/Empiricism

At the other end of the spectrum is associationism or, as is more usual nowadays, empiricism: this is the 'nurture' in the nature/nurture debate. This perspective encapsulates the view that children's knowledge and behaviour stem from their experiences and environments, with learning occurring via the formation of associations. The child is seen as somewhat passive in his/her own learning and development. Parents and early years professionals can have a powerful role in determining which experiences children ought to have; they educate and possibly mould their charges into socially conforming beings by rewarding or reinforcing learning and behaviour which they wish to develop in the child. The behaviourism of B. F. Skinner (1905–1990) was one of the most well-known theories within this perspective. Recently, however, the idea that he discounted genes has been refuted by Gaynor (2004), while the idea that behaviourism excludes feelings, emotions and thinking has also been challenged by Strain and Joseph (2004). Most of us engage in mild behaviourist practices, for example when we praise children for doing something we deem worthwhile in order to encourage repetition of that desirable behaviour.

Constructivism

With neither the rationalist nor the empiricist perspective adequately explaining children's learning, behaviour and development, the central point, constructivism, was conceived (most people believe) by Kant in his *Critique of Pure Reason* (1781). It is sometimes referred to as interactionism.

Constructivism acknowledges that children are born with cognitive capabilities and potential, and sees each child constructing knowledge and developing through cognitive activity in interaction with his/her environment. Children create their own meaning and understanding, combining what they already know and believe to be true with new experiences. The critical role of early years professionals is to support children's natural development within a suitable environment and also to be proactive in promoting development and learning with appropriate and stimulating experiences.

Understanding the interplay of internal/biological factors with external/experiential influences is unfortunately no easy task – even though it may seem a simple compromise. Implicit are the ideas of qualitative changes taking place within a child's cognitive structures and of the child being active and individual in the construction of his or her knowledge and development. Ridley (2003) provides a particularly fascinating and lightly humorous discussion on 'how genes influence behaviour and vice versa … as it becomes increasingly apparent that genes are vulnerable to experience' (p. 59). He has taken information from the decoding of the human genome and illustrated, with reference to relevant studies, that 'no longer is it nature versus nurture but (rather) nature **via** nurture' with genes as 'cogs' and 'enablers' (p. 59). Research by the renowned psychiatrist Rutter (2002) and the world-eminent behavioural geneticist Plomin (2002) also support the interactionist perspective, although they (and Ridley) articulate the need for much greater understanding of the complex causal mechanisms involved.

Constructivism has become social constructivism, with children co-constructing knowledge and understanding and making sense of their world through social learning activities. Interactions with others, especially peers, and children's socio-cultural environments are deemed extremely significant (e.g. Odom and Wolery, 2003; Plourde and Alawiye, 2003; Weisner, 2002; Dahlberg *et al.*, 1999; Bronfenbrenner, 1979).

This concept of constructivism has post-modern overtones that, according to Dahlberg *et al.* (1999), better accommodate 'human diversity, complexity and contingency' (p. 22). Knowledge is viewed as context-dependent, subjective and fluid as well as 'socially constructed and socially derived' (Zimiles, 2000, p. 6). Post-modernism, therefore, urges critical questioning of the traditional 'scientific' theories and the seeming absolute truths of, for example, the normative models of child development. It provides a more inclusive paradigm and advocates the need for multiple perspectives, cross-cultural approaches and varied interpretations of reality to achieve a deeper understanding of a subject, such as early childhood (Bloch, 2000; Dahlberg *et al.*, 1999). Most early years professionals now accept the more social nature of learning and the importance of children's social, cultural and historical contexts, though many would not be happy to go to post-modern extremes and 'deconstruct' the disciplines involved in early childhood studies. Also, post-modernism is not without its critics; for example, Bloch (2000) cautions about the possible distortions that it might induce.

Looking to the future of the study of child development, Goswami (2001) sees further development of social constructivism, and suggests there will need to be 'an increasingly interdisciplinary ... approach' with 'expertise in many (additional) disciplines' (p. 267).

OBSERVING YOUNG CHILDREN

Observing children is well-established within the early childhood tradition, being considered a fundamental aspect of the role of every early years professional (Hatch and Grieshaber, 2002). In this section, initial guidance on observing young children is provided to enable students to gain greater insight into the world of childhood and deepen their knowledge of child development.

We should regularly observe the children for whom we have responsibility. Sometimes we observe for a specific purpose – perhaps to ascertain the level of a child's language development or performance on a predetermined task. At other times we may observe in order to achieve broader knowledge and understanding of an individual child or group of children – perhaps to ascertain how they might be settling into nursery. Mostly, we shall observe children in their day-to-day activities and environments, although occasionally we may set up an activity for observation in what we term a 'controlled setting', for example in a quiet room free from the distractions of normal nursery activities.

We should always reflect on and make a reasoned analysis and interpretation of our observations. Whenever possible we should share our thoughts and discuss our assessments with respected colleagues, fellow students, tutors and/or children's parents or carers. It is this shared discussion and evaluation, as well as pooling of our joint knowledge of children, which can help to ensure conclusions are valid and reliable. Bulterman-Bos *et al.* (2002) provide helpful common-sense advice on achieving objectivity, validity and reliability in observations, for example by ensuring that the observer's judgements and interpretations can 'survive the scrutiny of fair comment' and 'reasonable criticism' (p. 1083) and are coherent, logical, well-evidenced and free from personal bias.

Why we observe young children

Through the processes of regular observation and justifiable and valid analysis, we can gain much greater insight into:

- the nature of children and childhood;
- what is unique about each child;
- what children value and care about;
- individual children's all-round development, needs, health and well-being;
- individual children's capabilities and the extent of their knowledge, skills and progress;
- ways in which individual children operate within their social and cultural environments;
- children's interaction with other children or adults;
- the interests of individuals and groups of children;
- typical patterns of all-round childhood development;
- typical childhood behaviours;
- whether children are safe or at risk;

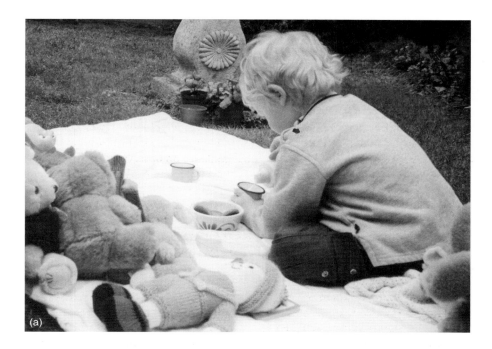

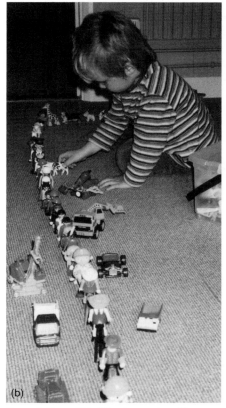

- the very different experiences and familial, social and cultural environments of individual children and groups of children;
- the possible consequences of these different backgrounds.

As professionals, it is important to act on the information gleaned and use it to inform planning and practice. With the insight from the observations and their analysis, we are better equipped to:

- know the children with whom we work;
- work in a child-focussed way;
- devise optimum environments to promote and support the holistic development of each child and respond to his or her needs;
- interact more sensitively with children and form happy relationships with them;
- monitor, evaluate and improve the provision we make for children, i.e. the care we give, the curriculum we devise, and the outcomes we achieve;

Figure 1.1 (a and b) We observe to achieve a broader knowledge and understanding of children.

■ take appropriate action if any aspect of a child's development, behaviour, health or well-being causes us concern;

■ identify and prepare individual educational plans for children with special needs;

■ work more effectively with parents/guardians;

■ reflect on and enhance our own practice.

For students, competence in observation and assessment can vividly illustrate much theory and promote the integration of theoretical knowledge of childhood with practice.

What might we observe?

Bulterman-Bos *et al.* (2002) identify four patterns of observations:

1. Triggered observation – when a child/group of children demand attention.
2. Incidental observation – where information comes incidentally from the child/children's usual activities.
3. Intentional observation – where the practitioner deliberately observes a child/children for a particular purpose.

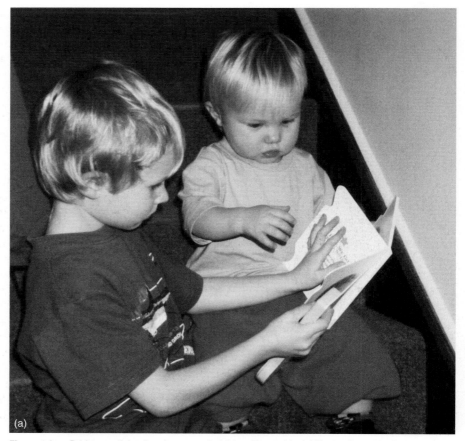

(a)

Figure 1.2a Evidence of the development of children's cognitive skills can be gained through observation.

4. Long-term observations – professionals observe a child/children over time, building up knowledge, theories and 'historical reference points' (p. 1079).

In order to increase our holistic knowledge and understanding of young children, and help us progress with our study of development in early childhood, we might usefully make observations (with analysis) of the following:

- Development of children's cognitive skills (e.g. memory; understanding; thinking; reasoning; discrimination; knowledge; formal learning skills; concentration).
- Characteristics of children's physical growth and development (e.g. appearance; height; weight; co-ordination; fine and gross motor skills; general physical activity).
- Development of children's communication skills (e.g. non-verbal; language; speech; understanding; listening; reading and writing; emergent literacy and numeracy skills).
- Evidence of emotional development and expression (e.g. general behaviour; aggression; regression; shyness; tantrum; excitement; distractibility; concentration; fear; confidence; independence; feeding and sleeping problems; obsessive tendencies; reactions to new situations).
- Behaviours revealed in different experiences (e.g. within the family; reaction to the arrival of a new baby; starting school; dad's arrival home; mum in hospital; children at risk or sick; play in the imaginative play corner; listening to a story).
- Development and different types, stages and patterns of play.
- Evidence of children's social development and relationships (e.g. social interaction in a variety of situations and with a range of people, e.g. family members; peers; appropriate adults; social skills and socialization, e.g. from different cultures; in play; in reactions to strangers; on visits; and at social events).

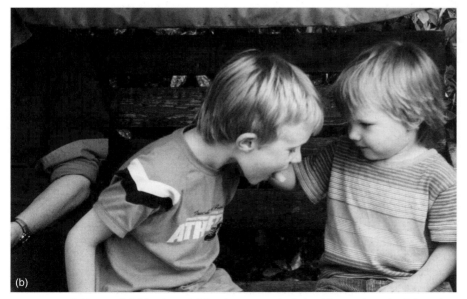

(b)

Figure 1.2b Evidence of children's social development and relationships can be gained through observation.

- Children engaged in specific activities (e.g. art and craft; music; drama; leisure activities; school work).
- Children's learning capabilities and styles (e.g. within the context of the National Curriculum or the Foundation Stage Curriculum; of the gifted child or a child experiencing difficulties).
- Behaviour of groups of children (e.g. differing abilities; varying reactions; different levels of involvement within a group).
- Identification of children with special needs (e.g. children for whom English is a second language; with physical or mental disability; or with learning difficulties).
- Children thought to be at risk of harm.
- Children in hospital or who are unwell.
- Children during screening procedures.

Embarking on the process of observation

The advice given here is for students new to the study of early childhood/childhood observations.

First, we must decide:

- What in particular we need to observe about a child or group of children (i.e. our aim).
- How we will negotiate access.
- Who will give us permission (e.g. parent, carer, educator, manager, committee, governors: we must remember to promise confidentiality/anonymity at this stage, and keep that promise).
- When and where we will undertake the observation.
- Which observation technique will be most suited to our purpose.
- Will it be participant (i.e. participate in the activity with the child/children) or non-participant (observing, listening without influencing the child/children or the activity).
- What organization and preparation we need to make.
- With whom we shall share and discuss the information obtained.
- How we shall preserve confidentiality and/or anonymity (e.g. by using a child's first name, an alternative name, or the initial of his/her first name).

The next stage of selecting the most suitable observation technique is of prime importance. To assist students in the early days of their studies, we shall consider several straightforward techniques and include a few examples of written formats. It is recognized that early years professionals will not always write up observations formally, but it is important they possess the skill, since observations can be vital documents in a child's life – for example, in child protection cases, special needs decisions, meetings with parents/guardians, reports, etc.

Narrative report

This is probably the most illuminative technique. If well done, it can vividly capture a child's behaviour, actions, stage of development, personality, mood, etc. It can be especially useful in capturing critical incidents, vignettes or situations where a child may be considered at risk.

It can be fairly time-consuming because it involves reporting in prose, in the greatest detail possible, a child's actions, utterances (verbal and non-verbal), facial expressions, head and eye movements, and use of toys, objects and play materials. Naturally, we concentrate on behaviours with particular relevance to our stated aim.

The written description should provide a valid and true representation of the child's actions and activities. Great care should be taken to record only what is seen and heard and **not** thoughts, beliefs and opinions; for example, '*John rubbed his eyes*', rather than '*John is tired*'. Within the observation report we also strive to **avoid**:

- value judgements and jumping to conclusions, e.g. '*Rukia is good at drawing*' or '*Jane is looking unhappy*';
- labelling children, e.g. '*Henry is a naughty boy*' or '*Comfort is a nice little girl*';
- generalizations, e.g. '*As always, the girls are tidying up*'.

In endeavouring to report objectively, it is often helpful to consider how a camcorder would record an incident. In the case of Rukia, drawing it would have depicted the precise movements of the hand holding the pencil, her facial expressions, any verbal or non-verbal utterances, and the development of the final product (the drawing).

Mention of a child other than the focal child or an adult should be kept to a minimum. We record only what is necessary about the actions of others to enable us to make sense of the focal child's behaviour.

It is always best to write up the full report from rough notes as soon as possible after undertaking observations, having taken rough notes during the observation if that was permitted.

Possible narrative report topics might include observing a child:

- listening to a story read by a parent or carer – alone or in a group;
- engaged in imaginative role play;
- having a tantrum.

The resulting assessments of these three observations would enable us to understand the children better, make individualized and hopefully more beneficial provision for each child or deal more effectively with the next tantrum – probable reasons for undertaking the observations in the first place.

Time sampling

With this technique, a clear focus is necessary. We note, at regular intervals, what a child is doing (or children are doing). A variety of formats is possible, and either descriptive or coded recording of data may be used. Intervals of time are selected (e.g. every minute, every 10 minutes, every half-hour) which best suit the purpose, provide maximum information, and accord with the total observation time. Obviously it would be rather impracticable to record an observation every 30 seconds for 3 hours!

Possible topics might include:

- observing a child's participation in nursery activities. He or she might be observed every 5 minutes for 1 hour when he or she is free to choose play materials and activities. (*The resulting assessment here would help us learn more about the child's interests, motivation and abilities, and enable us to plan more relevant individualized experiences.*)
- observing a child during playtime in order to note his/her level of social interaction/friendship patterns or type and stage of play, or perhaps even instances of him or her being bullied.

NAME: H		DATE: 15–19 January, 2005
AGE: 4 years, 2 months		GENDER: Male

BACKGROUND INFORMATION:	H has recently seemed to spend much time on the sidelines, not participating in nursery activities. This is not his usual behaviour. (*Here the observation is a way of verifying (or otherwise) staff's impression and concern.) This would contribute to a more informed assessment of Henry's behaviour.*
AIM:	To observe H's participation in nursery activities during the time when children have freedom of choice.
CONTENT:	Nursery playroom and outdoor play area. (*Children may move freely between these areas*)
OBSERVATION TECHNIQUE:	Time sampling – descriptive recording every 5 minutes for 1 hour over 5 days.

DAY: One   **TIME STARTED:** 9:15 AM   **TIME COMPLETED:** 10:15 AM

Time	Nursery area	H's Activity/Language/Interaction	Social group
09:15	Entrance hall doorway	Standing, looking round playroom	H and Father
09:20	Sand tray	Standing at side of tray, looking at toys in sand, listening to NN[a]	H, NN and 2 children
09:25	Sand tray	Digging in sand	Alone
09:30	Sand tray	Digging in sand	Alone
09:35	Middle of playroom	Walking across room	Alone
09:40	Outside home corner	Looking in home corner window	Alone
09:45	Book corner	Sitting on floor, listening to story read by NN, looking at NN	H, NN and 3 children
09:50	Book corner	Answered question from NN: "It's a zebra"	H, NN and 3 children
09:55	Book corner	Sitting on floor watching other children say a rhyme	H, NN and 3 children
10:00	Book corner	Standing looking at bookshelves	Alone
10:05	Outside home corner	Looking in home corner window	Alone
10:10	Outside home corner	Putting on bus driver's hat	Alone
10:15	Outside home corner	Sitting in box pretending to drive bus: "broom, broom".	Alone

[a]NN = Nursery Nurse

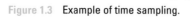

Figure 1.3   Example of time sampling.

Figure 1.3 provides an example of time sampling. Formal headings are included to aid the presentation of observations for course assignment purposes.

Event sampling

This is a convenient method of collecting frequency data. It involves recording on a check-list each time a particular behaviour occurs. As with time sampling, the data collected may provide the necessary baseline evidence to inform future action. The event sampling could also be repeated after any ameliorative programme has been completed, thus helping assess its level of success.

Possible topics might include:

- recording each time a child, for whom English is a second language, and who does not appear to be integrating into nursery, interacts with another child or

NAME: A			DATE: 3–7 June, 2005		
AGE: 3 years, 9 months			GENDER: Female		

BACKGROUND INFORMATION:	A is often considered to behave aggressively. It is necessary to verify this behaviour and note any possible provocation in order to justify and underpin any programme designed to counteract such a tendency.
AIM:	To record each instance of, and any observable provocation for, behaviours identified as aggressive.
CONTENT:	Nursery playroom.
OBSERVATION TECHNIQUE:	Event sampling.

DAY: One   **TIME STARTED: 9:15 AM**   **TIME COMPLETED: 12:00 PM**

Time	Behaviour deemed aggressive	Location	Possible provocation	Social grouping	Event number
09:23	Kicked NN[a]	Sand tray	Asked to share toys	A, NN and 2 children	1
10:15	Pushed child to floor	Home corner	Wanted child to be baby, but he did not want to	A and 2 other children	2
10:25	Threw teddy across floor and stamped feet	Home corner	Wanted a teddy which another child was cuddling	A and 2 other children	3
11:50	Pushed Lego construction from table to floor	Lego table	None evident	Alone	4

[a]NN = Nursery Nurse

Figure 1.4   Example of event sampling.

adult. (*We would distinguish between occasions when the child is initiating or responding to conversation. This would give precise information about the nature/extent/absence of interaction, and again would inform strategies for supporting the child in the future.*)

■ recording each time a child, whose behaviour is deemed aggressive, behaves aggressively and, if possible, identifying causal/related factors (see Fig. 1.4). (*By recording this information we may ascertain possible causes/triggers and, in the future, be enabled to pre-empt or deflect the aggression.*)

Check-lists

Check-lists can be a simple and reasonably quick method of collecting and presenting data from observations. A child may be observed in the course of his/her usual daily activities, or possibly in a contrived situation. Occasionally, it may not be possible to observe some aspect of the child's behaviour or development, and we may have to ask the parent or main carer to provide the information. In such instances we must beware of bias on their part (as well as our own!).

Completed check-lists can often constitute helpful baseline data for:

■ guiding future observations (e.g. suggesting a detailed focus or an aspect of behaviour causing concern);
■ planning nursery activities (perhaps to enhance an aspect of development, or which a child would particularly enjoy);
■ selecting a course of treatment (e.g. physiotherapy, speech therapy); and/or
■ assessing developmental progress (e.g. by health visitor or teacher assessment).

We must, however, always bear in mind that check-lists can miss crucial contextual information and may provide only a superficial picture of the child's behaviour and development.

When this method of observation is used to assess a child's development, data are usually collected on the basis of standardized developmental norms [e.g. Sheridan (1997) or The Denver Developmental Screening Test II (Revised 1992)]. These are deemed to give greater validity to assessment (see Fig. 1.5).

Activity/Behaviour	Yes	No	Almost	Additional information
Posture and large movements				
Can s/he raise head from pillow when lying on back?	✔			
Can s/he sit with support in cot or pram?	✔			
Does s/he hold arms up to be lifted?	✔			Only to mother
Does s/he kick strongly, with legs alternating?	✔			
Can s/he roll over from front to back?			✔	

Figure 1.5 Extract from a developmental check-list for an infant of 6 months based on the developmental norms of Sheridan (1997).

Possible topics might include:

■ collecting data on the play and interaction emanating from different nursery activities during one nursery session;

- focusing on a specific aspect of a child's development, e.g. physical development (using standardized developmental norms);
- gaining a comprehensive picture of a child's development (again using standardized developmental norms).

Figure 1.6 provides another example of a check-list. This explores the use of four nursery activities/areas during a period of free choice for the children. Coded recording is used, and a key is included to explain the codes. The results would enable us to assess the popularity of nursery activities. As a consequence, we might enhance an infrequently used corner/activity to ensure it is more often utilized by the children. If children are not experiencing all of the nursery activities, an aspect of their development may be hindered. With our holistic approach we cannot allow that to happen.

Learning areas/activities	Number of children using area/activity	Types of play observed	Interaction
Home corner/ dressing up	1111111111111111 111	ExP, IP, IP, RP, IP, RP, EP, IP, RP, RP	CC, CCC, CC, CC, CC, CCC, CA, AC, CCC, CC, CC, CCC, CC, AC, AC
Outdoor area	111111111	PP, PP, Exp, IP, PP	CC, CC, CCC, CA
Sand tray		ExP, ExP, IP, HP	CCC
Construction toys		CP, CP	

KEY

Types of play (BAECE, 1994)

ExP	*Exploratory play*	
HP	*Heuristic play*	
EP	*Epistemic play*	
IP	*Imaginative play*	
RP	*Role play*	
CP	*Constructive play*	
PP	*Physical play*	

Interaction

CC	*2 children talking*	
CCC	*3 children talking*	
CA	*Child and adult talking (child initiated)*	
AC	*Adult and child talking (adult initiated)*	

N.B. The data from this check-list would, of course, be summarized for formal presentation in an assignment or research project.

Figure 1.6 Extract from a nursery activity check-list, completed during 1 hour of free choice of activities.

Verbatim reporting

This involves recording word for word a conversation between two or more children, or between a child/children and an adult. Tape-recording and then transcribing the text provides the most accurate accounts, although being recorded can alter some participants' behaviour. Small personal radio microphones attached to the children's and adults' lapels are helpful. Transcription from a tape recording is a time-consuming but worthwhile process because it allows repeated listening which can give considerable insight into a child's language development, thinking, logic, fears or worries.

This technique has increased in significance in recent years with the recognition that 'children's voices can be powerful and possibly richer than those of adults acting on behalf of children' (Sorin, 2003, p. 31) and because of Article 12 of the Convention on Children's Rights (Participation). Even young children are now considered capable of being treated as serious participants in the research process (Fasoli, 2003; Alderson, 2000; O'Kane, 2000; Woodhead and Faulkner, 2000).

Diaries/field notes

These are notes pertinent to a long-term study/observation, written as and when appropriate, necessary or possible. They may describe children's behaviour, reactions, development, learning, social skills, aspects of health or emotional well-being. Critical incidents in early years settings and reports of visits to children in their home or in hospital can also be recorded in this manner. They are usually written as narrative descriptions, although the inclusion of codes and drawings can save time and energy. Do write up as soon as possible after the occurrence and provide sufficient detail to create a vivid memory of the event or behaviour several months later.

Diaries and field notes can provide rich illuminative data and capture the complexities of a child's nature or situation. They also constitute a fruitful basis for analytical reflections which can usefully inform and improve early years practice. Worthwhile analysis of what can be a mass of data can, of course, be daunting and requires a sound knowledge of relevant theory. Evidence for inferences and interpretations must be obvious in the notes.

A possible topic might include recording over a term any significant activities, thinking and conversations of a child whom it is believed might be gifted. Figure 1.7 provides an extract from just such a diary. By the way, it is a true incident!

Date	Significant incident	Analysis
3 May, 2005	R, after listening to a group of 7-year-olds having a lesson on multiplication, stated: "If I counted the squares down this side and along this side of the tennis racquet and if I could multiply like these big children, I could tell you how many squares there are altogether".	R has grasped the concept and function of multiplication immediately and at a very young age – evidence of advanced logico-mathematical thought.

Figure 1.7   Extract from diary/field notes: R is aged 4 years, 10 months.

Information on other observation techniques (e.g. sociograms, pie-charts, bar charts, scatter diagrams, etc.) can be found in research methodology textbooks. Readers will find Greig and Taylor's (1999) *Doing Research with Children* particularly useful.

Analysing our observations

Having completed our observation using the appropriate technique, we now come to the all-important task of analysing and utilizing those data.

In the analysis we consider the significance of our observation with particular reference to our stated aim. Whenever possible, we should discuss our observations and judgements with other (more experienced/more knowledgeable) early years professionals/tutors. Multiple perspectives can enhance the usefulness, credibility and validity of the process and the outcome. Analysis may also involve application of relevant theory; for example, we might refer to a particular theory of learning to help us to understand how a child is making sense of his or her world. Alternatively, it may be appropriate or required to refer to standardized norms for a child's age. As an example, some early years professionals might complete a check-list to assess a child's level of development against what is specified as typical for her/his age. At other times we may compare a child's present and previous performances on a task in order to ascertain whether he or she is making progress. This is called 'ipsative assessment'. Such reflective analysis within an appropriate framework of theory and research should enable us to make reasoned interpretations and assessments.

We must also avoid making tactless, discourteous, stereotypical, biased or in any way inappropriate judgements of children, the adults involved, their practices and the observation setting. We must be sensitive to children's socio-cultural contexts and needs. We are more likely to make rational and professional judgements if we ensure we have clear-cut evidence for our conclusions.

The procedure for observation analysis generally consists of three elements plus the action resulting from the process:

1. Consideration of observation evidence (mindful of the aim).
2. Identification of relevant theory, standardized norm, experience and/or knowledge (own and others).
3. Bringing together one and two to create a valid interpretation/judgement (involving professional colleagues/tutor).
4. Future planning/necessary action.

We shall consider a straightforward example of analysis. Don't worry if it seems a little mechanistic and protracted!

Example

For 15 minutes we have undertaken an observation of Aznan (aged 7 months) sitting on the carpet playing with a small piece of loofah; we have used the narrative report technique. This is part of an assessment of his overall development.

1. Refer to the aspect of observation data to be discussed. For example:

   Aznan was sitting on the floor engaged in heuristic (discovery) play – finding out about the properties of the piece of loofah. He frequently grasped hold of it using a palmar grip, peered at it and put it in his mouth.

2. Refer now to relevant theory. For example:

   Curtis and O'Hagan (2003) affirm that, when a child can sit unaided exploring objects, they can discover the properties of these objects and their senses are stimulated. This exploratory play behaviour is also noted as typical of infants around Aznan's age by Sheridan (1997) and Goldschmied and Jackson (1994). The latter theorists also confirm that 'by sucking, mouthing and handling (objects), babies are finding out about weight, size, shapes, texture, sound and smell' (p. 88), as well demonstrating considerable levels of concentration.

3. We now bring Stages 1 and 2 together to make a reasoned assessment. For example:

   We can, therefore, see that Aznan's play is typical for his age and he is learning much about objects from his environment. He is also learning to concentrate for increasing periods of time.

This three-stage process would naturally be repeated with any other aspect of the observation which it is necessary to analyse in order to achieve the holistic assessment.

4. The next important step is to consider future action to support Aznan's development. For example:

> *It would seem to be appropriate now to introduce Aznan to a wider variety of different materials and objects to maintain his interest and further stimulate his developing senses and concept formation.*

Of course an observation such as this one on Aznan would not necessarily be transmitted to paper if undertaken as part of an experienced professional's daily reflections and forward planning.

For professionals who have acquired a rich theoretical understanding of childhood and child development and gained wide experience of children, this interlinking of theory and observation becomes a very natural and indeed quintessential aspect of providing sensitive early childhood education and care. This is, of course, only so when the valid and reasoned interpretations and assessments from our observations are used to inform our planning and enrich or amend the experiences we offer in order to foster each child's all-round development, learning, health and well-being. We might, for example, devise particular activities, draw up learning programmes or consider alternative forms of support or treatment. This whole process, which is referred to as reflective practice, is the hallmark of a genuine professional (see Chapter 7, p. 134).

On some occasions we might realize that, before we can actually make any recommendations concerning a child, we need more data. We must therefore undertake further observations in order to collect specific information to improve our knowledge and understanding of the child. In addition, if we are a novice to the technique of observation, it would be wise to reflect critically on the technique we used. Was it appropriate for our purpose? Did it provide sufficient information?

Much practice in observation and assessment and discussion of the results of that practice with experienced early years professionals will greatly improve students' and practitioners' skills of observation and assessment.

ETHICAL ISSUES RELATING TO OBSERVATION OF CHILDREN (AND THE STUDY OF EARLY CHILDHOOD)

There are principles relating to professional standards of conduct which apply to all early years professionals, and are equally important to students of early childhood. These ethical issues must be clearly understood and/or addressed before any observation.

One of the first ethical issues which students will encounter is negotiating access to observe a child/children. This entails asking and gaining permission from the child's parents, guardians and/or professional carer or educator. The purpose, method, envisaged outcome and uses of observation(s) must always be explained. It is inadvisable to proceed if one parent is unhappy. Sometimes parents have genuine concerns about their child being observed, or about an aspect of his or her development or behaviour. They may, of course, simply not like the idea, or feel that they do not have the time or the appropriate home environment. Be sensitive to such feelings.

Students seek adult agreement for observations of babies and toddlers because it is felt unlikely fully informed consent can be gained from children. Fine and Sandstrom (1988), however, emphasize that the children's age should not diminish their rights (see also Fasoli, 2003; Sorin, 2003; Alderson, 2000; Woodhead and Faulkner, 2000). In line with Article 12 of the UN Convention on the Rights of the Child (participation) and the current view of the child as competent and active in making sense of his/her world, whenever possible, students should discuss with the children involved their wish/requirement to observe. It is necessary to explain in a truthful, matter-of-fact way the children will understand and to which they can easily relate; for example, 'This is my work/homework'.

It is also essential to be aware of our responsibilities as an observer. Students should not be in sole charge of a child or children, and the safety of the child or children must take precedence over the completion of observations. We may also need to consider what to do should we see or hear something an adult is not meant to and/or which causes concern – perhaps a suggestion that a child is being abused, or a plan being made to bully a child. Hopefully there will be a tutor or early years professional with whom students may discuss such worrying situations.

Confidentiality and anonymity are extremely important issues. Parents/professional carers must be assured that any data collected will be treated in the strictest confidence, and it must be treated thus. Never be tempted to disclose details gleaned professionally or under the promise of confidentiality and anonymity to anyone; this includes parents, boy-, girl- or best friends, partners, neighbours, sons or daughters. Be a true professional.

Permission to share information in a discussion, project or seminar, should be sought and agreed in advance. Within student groups, reporting of an observation should certainly be anonymous. Use a child's first name, the initial letter of his/her first name or pseudonym. Refer to professionals as 'teacher', 'nursery nurse' and 'health visitor', and to parents as 'mother' and 'father'. Omit the names of early years settings and schools, instead use terms such as playgroup, nursery class, class 1R, etc.

Our obligations as professionals or potential professionals also require us to behave in a courteous and unobtrusive manner and to be sensitive to the needs of the child or children and to the demands on practitioners and parents or carers. Students should arrange visits and observations at the convenience of the family, nursery, school or ward and fit in with the routine of the setting.

Fine and Sandstrom (1988) mention one further issue that is significant at this early stage in our text and studies – that is, consideration of the extent to which we, as adults, can truly understand and interpret a child's behaviour and viewpoint. It is often difficult for us to take ourselves back into the world of childhood and adopt a child's perspective and reasoning. We must, therefore, remain open-minded to a range of possible interpretations, explanations and influential factors.

Conclusion

In this chapter we considered a set of global value principles that might underpin the work of early years professionals. This was followed by an overview of the main theoretical perspectives underlying early childhood studies. Finally, the essential process of observation was examined and recognized as a vital tool for effective early years practitioners.

Student activity

Undertake three observations of children using a different technique for each. Follow the chapter guidance for writing up and analysing the observations. Share your observations with a fellow student or early years professional. Compare analyses and answer the following questions for each observation:

- What did you learn about the child?
- How might this affect your plans for her/him?
- How did your analysis compare with that of your colleague? Discuss possible reasons for differences.

REFERENCES

Alderson, P (2000): Children as researchers: the effects of participation rights on research methodology. In Christensen, P and James, A (eds), *Research with Children: Perspectives and Practices.* London: Falmer Press.

Bloch, MN (2000): Governing teachers, parents and children through child development knowledge. *Human Development,* **43**, 4/5, 257–266.

Bronfenbrenner, U (1979): *The Ecology of Human Development.* Cambridge, MA: Harvard University Press.

Bulterman-Bos, J, Terwell, J, Verloop, N and Wardekler, W (2002): Observation in teaching: toward a practice of objectivity. *Teachers College Record,* **104**(6), 1069–1092.

Curtis, A and O'Hagan, M (2003): *Care and Education in Early Childhood.* London: Routledge Falmer.

Dahlberg, G, Moss, P and Pence, A (1999): *Beyond Quality in Early Childhood Education and Care: Postmodern Perspectives.* London: Falmer Press.

Ehrlich, P and Feldman, M (2003): Genes and cultures: What creates our behavioral phenome? *Current Anthropology,* **44**, 1, 87–108.

Fasoli, L (2003): Reflections on doing research with young children. *Australian Journal of Early Childhood,* **28**(1), 7–12.

Fine, GA and Sandstrom, KL (1988): *Knowing Children: Participant Observation with Minors.* London: Sage Publications.

Gaynor, ST (2004): Skepticism of caricatures: B.F. Skinner turns 100. *The Skeptical Inquirer,* **28**(1), 26–31.

Goldschmied, E and Jackson, S (1994): *People Under Three: Young Children in Day Care.* London: Routledge.

Goswami, U (2001): Cognitive development: No stages please – we're British. *British Journal of Psychology,* **92**(1), 257–276.

Greig, A and Taylor, J (1999): *Doing Research with Children.* London: Sage.

Hatch, JA and Grieshaber, S (2002): Child observation and accountability: Perspectives from Australia and the United States. *Early Childhood Education Journal*, 29(4), Summer, 227–231.

Horwitz, AV, Videon, TM, Schmitz, MF and Davis, D (2003): Rethinking twins and environments: Possible social sources for assumed genetic influences in twin research. *Journal of Health and Social Behaviour*, **44**, 2, 111–128.

Lillemyr, OF, Fagerli, O and Søbstad, F (2001): *A Global Perspective on Early Childhood Care and Education: A Proposed Model*. Paris: UNESCO.

O'Kane, C (2000): The development of participatory techniques: facilitating children's views about decisions which affect them. In Christensen, P and James, A (eds), *Research with Children: Perspectives and Practices*. London: Falmer Press.

Odom, SL and Wolery, M (2003): A unified theory of practice in early intervention/early childhood special education: Evidence-based practices. *The Journal of Special Education*, 37, 3, 164–177.

Pinker, S (2003): The blank slate: The modern denial of human nature. *The Skeptical Inquirer*, 27(2), 37–42.

Plomin, R (2002): Genetics and behaviour. *Psychologist*, **14**, 3, 134–140.

Plourde, LA and Alawiye, O (2003): Constructivism and elementary preservice science teacher preparation: Knowledge to application. *College Student Journal*, 37, 3, 334–340.

Richardson, K (1988): *Understanding Psychology*. Milton Keynes: Open University Press.

Ridley, M (2003): Listen to the genome. *The American Spectator*, 36, 3, 59–65.

Rutter, M (2002): The interplay of nature, nurture and developmental influences: The challenge ahead for mental health. *Archives of General Psychiatry*, **59**(11), 996–1001.

Sheridan, M (1997): *From Birth to Five Years*. London: Routledge.

Sorin, R (2003): Research with children: A rich glimpse into the world of childhood. *Australian Journal of Early Childhood*, **28**(1), 31–36.

Strain, PS and Joseph, GE (2004): A not so good job with 'good job': A response to Kohn 2001. *Journal of Behavioral Intervention*, 6(1), 55–61.

Weisner, TS (2002): Making a good thing better: Ways to strengthen sociocultural research in human development. *Human Development*, **45**(5), 372–381.

Woodhead, M and Faulkner, D (2000): Subjects, objects or participants? Dilemmas of psychological research with children. In Christensen, P and James, A (eds), *Research with Children: Perspectives and Practices*. London: Falmer Press.

UNICEF (2003): *A World Fit for Children*. New York: UNICEF.

Zimiles, H (2000): On reassessing the relevance of the child development knowledge base to education. *Human Development*, **43**(4/5), 235–246.

FURTHER READING

Bentzen, WR (1993): *A Guide to Observing and Recording Behaviour*. New York: Delmar Publishers Inc.

Christensen, P and James, A (eds) (2000): *Research with Children: Perspectives and Practices*. London: Falmer Press.

Greig, A and Taylor, J (1999): *Doing Research with Children*. London: Sage.

Smith, PK, Cowie, H and Blades, M (2003): *Understanding Children's Development.* London: Blackwell Publishing.

UNICEF (2003): *A World Fit for Children.* New York: UNICEF.

WEBSITES

UN Convention on the Rights of the Child and the Special Session of the UN – http://www.unicef.org

Denver Developmental Screening Test II – http://www.healthscience.utas.edu.au/ medicine/teaching/kfp/kfp3/visit_8/Denver.htm

NEW BEGINNINGS: FACTORS AFFECTING HEALTH AND WELL-BEING IN THE INFANT

Catherine Forsdike

This chapter aims to:

- consider the nature and impact of early life processes and experiences which might influence the future health and well-being of children;

- describe the development of the fetus *in utero*;

- describe measures to optimize health and well-being in the newborn;

- consider the interplay between social and emotional, physical and environmental factors on pregnancy outcome;

- consider the role of the early years professional in promoting health and well-being in the newborn.

INTRODUCTION

Birth is just one stage in the development of the child. By gaining an understanding of the processes before, during and in the early period following birth we can consider the impact that these may have on future health, growth and development.

In this chapter we shall explore some of children's earliest life experiences and consider the extent to which they are beneficial or detrimental to health – not just health in the newborn, but the ongoing health of the child. The significance of early experience is reflected in the growing interest in this period of the child's life.

Consider the following dialogue, which takes place in some form at hundreds of births every day:

Midwife: It's a girl!
Mother: Thank goodness – is she all right?
Midwife: She's fine.

From this dialogue, the mother is reassured that she has given birth to a healthy baby – a reassurance that she has been seeking at various stages of her pregnancy through screening tests and the provision of antenatal care. Yet if we examine the dialogue more closely, it becomes apparent that the mother may not be aware of the complexity of her question or the superficial nature of the midwife's answer.

In effect, the mother is asking two questions. First, she is asking if the baby has suffered any ill effects from the experience of the labour and birth; and secondly she is asking whether her baby is normal and healthy.

From a superficial glance at the baby it is possible to assess his or her condition at birth and to ascertain whether there are any gross abnormalities. Although the majority of babies have no disabilities, around 2 per cent have major congenital abnormalities at birth. Some of these are immediately apparent (e.g. cleft lip), while others become apparent during the first few days or weeks of life, and yet others only become apparent later (e.g. cerebral palsy). Consequently, it is not possible to answer the mother's apparently simple question so easily.

In the first place, the question 'What is health?' raises a number of issues. Health may be considered to be the absence of disease, a state of well-being or, as the World Health Organization defined it in 1946, '… a complete state of physical, mental and emotional well-being, and not merely the absence of disease and infirmity' (in Seedhouse, 1986).

The WHO definition may be seen as an idealistic concept, but when considering the health and well-being of the newborn it is relevant to address the broader definition, rather than to concentrate solely on the absence of disease and abnormality.

This widens the scope of this chapter, which will consider preconception and prenatal influences on health, as well as factors relating to the birth and the early days and weeks of newborn life. In addition to identifying influences on the health and well-being of the child, strategies to enhance outcome and the relevance of this period to the early years professional will be considered.

Life does not begin at birth, as the individual is already 9 months old when he or she is born. It takes three to make a birth day – the mother, the father, and the newborn baby. The mother and father will each contribute to the unique genetic composition of the baby by virtue of their own genetic make-up. The whole process of embryonic and fetal development is dependent on genes, and abnormal genes can cause abnormality and disease in the newborn. The life-style of the parents before and during pregnancy will have an impact on the health and development of the fetus. In turn, social, cultural and environmental factors will influence the childbearing process. None of these factors stands alone – their integration and the interplay between them will all contribute to the early development, health and well-being of the child.

FROM CONCEPTION TO BIRTH

The development of the embryo is a unique and amazing process. Our knowledge of this complex process is increasing with advances in embryological and genetic research, yet there is still only partial understanding of the early period of human experience. To understand why the period before birth is so significant, and to appreciate the potential impact of factors such as drugs and infections on development, it is necessary to describe briefly the developmental timetable from conception to birth.

The human gestation period is approximately 38 weeks from conception, or 40 weeks from the onset of the last menstrual period. The gestation period is divided into two phases:

- The *embryonic phase* commences with conception and continues until the end of the eighth week. It is a period of rapid growth and development, and

during this phase all of the major organs of the body are formed. The first
3 weeks following conception are sometimes referred to as the pre-embryonic
period.

■ The *fetal phase* comprises the remaining 30 weeks of gestation. It is
characterized by growth and further development of the organs and systems
established in the embryonic phase.

An individual's development commences at fertilization when the sperm enters the
egg. As soon as fertilization has taken place, the new cell starts to change. Cells are the
basic unit of life, and a typical human being is composed of about 350 different types
of specialized cell, such as red blood cells and muscle cells (Wolpert, 1993). The
embryonic cells are initially less specialized, but all cells have basic characteristics and
activities. The activities which we need to consider here are cell multiplication, cell
differentiation and cell movement.

The process of cell multiplication begins about 30 minutes after fertilization,
when the egg starts to divide into two cells. The cells continue to divide, and by day 4
there is a solid ball of cells known as the morula. The morula enters the uterus and
changes into a blastocyst, which is a fluid-filled sphere, containing a group of cells
known as the inner cell mass. The inner cell mass will become the embryo, and the
trophoblastic cells will form the placenta. At approximately 7–8 days after ovulation
the blastocyst will become embedded in the wall of the uterus.

By the third week after ovulation the inner cell mass has become a disc differentiated into three different types of cells. It is from these cells that the different structures
of the body will evolve. At 4 weeks after fertilization the cells have developed to form
an embryo which is 0.5 cm long, and has curved in on itself with a head and tail fold.
Most of the body systems are now present in a rudimentary form: there is a neural
tube, which will form the brain, lung buds which will develop into a respiratory system,
and primitive eyes, nose and ears. By this stage the heart is beating. The changes have
been achieved not just by cell differentiation but also by cell movement, which trans-
forms the flat embryonic disc so that the basic body plan is laid down.

At the end of the embryonic phase of development, the embryo is covered with a
thin skin. The head has increased greatly in size and is nearly as large as the rest of the
body, and the facial features are more distinct. The embryo is making some movements, but at this stage they are not strong enough for the mother to feel them. There
is no visible difference between male and female embryos at this stage.

At 12 weeks after fertilization the fetus has eyelids which are fused. The kidneys
secrete urine, the fetus swallows amniotic fluid, and the external genitalia have
developed sufficiently for it to be possible to determine the sex of the fetus.

At 20 weeks the fetus looks distinctly human. The body is beginning to be covered
by fine hair and a thick greasy substance known as vernix caseosa, which protects the
skin from the macerating effects of the amniotic fluid. The fetal movements are now
strong enough to be felt by the mother.

By 24 weeks the fetus weighs 550–700 g. The organs have developed and matured
to such an extent that the fetus may survive with medical assistance if the birth takes
place prematurely. The fetus responds to light, sound and touch, and has developed
a sense of taste. It has also developed the ability to feel and respond to pain.

During the remaining weeks of pregnancy the fetus accumulates fat stores,
and maturation continues. The lungs, in particular, continue to develop and prepare
for function. At birth, the normal baby weighs between 3.0 and 3.5 kg. Although birth
is a stage in the developmental process, and rapid changes take place within the baby

as it adapts to life outside the uterus, birth does not represent the end of development. Many organ systems do not develop into their final form until puberty or later.

From the above description it can be seen that important milestones are reached very early in the embryonic period. At this early stage the embryo is vulnerable to harm from a variety of sources, yet many women are unaware that they are pregnant when this crucial stage of development is occurring.

FACTORS AFFECTING THE HEALTH AND WELL-BEING OF THE BABY

The factors that are likely to affect the health and well-being of the baby are complex, and involve the interplay of genetic inheritance, parental health and life-style and environmental influences. Some of these factors may be more significant at particular stages of development. For example, if the mother is infected with rubella (German measles) in early pregnancy, the effect on the baby is more profound than at a later stage of development (Department of Health, 2003). Other factors may be of ongoing significance; for example, parental smoking is known to affect growth and development in intrauterine life, and increase the risk of sudden infant death and respiratory disease and asthma in the child.

When congenital malformation or developmental defects arise this may be due to mutant genes or chromosomal abnormalities, environmental factors, or a combination of both. However, in 60 per cent of abnormalities the cause is unknown. Bearing this in mind, let us now consider some of these potential influences on the health of the baby in more detail.

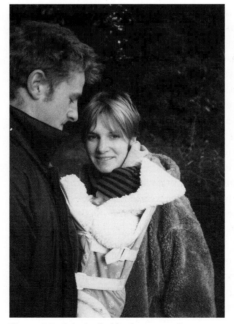

Figure 2.1   It is desirable that a couple are in optimum health before embarking on a pregnancy.

Parental influences

Parental health and well-being make an important contribution to the development of the fetus and baby. It is clearly desirable that a couple are in optimum health before embarking on a pregnancy. This is also true when there is a pre-existing medical condition. For example, diabetes mellitus in the mother may seriously complicate a pregnancy. This is particularly significant if the condition is poorly controlled, as there is an increased likelihood of congenital abnormality and problems for the newborn. However, if the condition is well managed both before and during pregnancy, the risks are decreased.

For some women, problems arise during pregnancy itself. There are many risk factors to be considered during the antenatal period, and it is important that maternal health and well-being are carefully monitored. This includes measuring the blood pressure, as pregnancy-induced hypertension may result in the baby having a low birth weight or being born prematurely. Embryonic and fetal development may also be affected by infections, which cross the placenta from the mother to the baby. In some cases the mother may not feel particularly ill, but the effects on the fetus can be considerable.

In addition to infections and complications during pregnancy, other parental factors play a part. There is increasing interest in the effects on the baby when pregnancy occurs at the extremes of maternal age. Adolescent mothers are more likely to have poorer nutritional status, smoke more, and have financial, social and emotional problems – all of which can impact on the health of the baby (Teenage Pregnancy Unit *et al.*, 2004). On the other hand, mothers aged over 35 are more prone to chromosomal abnormalities such as Down syndrome. Statistical data show that the number of women giving birth over the age of 35 almost doubled between 1991 and 2000 (Macfarlane and Moser, 2004). This could be linked to changing social phenomena, or to an increase in assisted conception.

As well as chromosomal abnormalities, there are also many genetic abnormalities, and with advancing knowledge it is becoming possible to screen couples for risk, prior to and in the early stages of pregnancy, and to make a diagnosis of some chromosomal and genetic abnormalities during pregnancy. This enables parents to make choices that were unheard of in previous generations, and to accept some responsibility in the decision-making process. These decisions involve whether to have screening in the first instance, and then deciding whether to continue with the pregnancy if an abnormality is detected or to continue and prepare for the birth of the baby. (The National Electronic Library for Health (NELH) provides up-to-date information on a range of screening tests in pregnancy.)

Down syndrome is one of the most common chromosomal abnormalities, with an incidence of 1 in 700 pregnancies. The risk increases from 1:1528 in women aged 20 years to 1:28 for women aged 45 years (Cuckle *et al.*, 1987). In recent years screening for Down syndrome has been introduced for many pregnant women, with the aim being to offer a service to all by 2004. A combination of using ultrasound to detect excess fluid at the neck in the first trimester (nuchal translucency), tests on maternal serum and maternal age are used to identify the potential risk of the baby having Down syndrome. Screening using a combination of these factors can lead to the detection of 80–90 per cent of affected babies (Wald *et al.*, 2003). Women who are shown to be at high risk are then offered invasive procedures such as amniocentesis to try to make a diagnosis.

On the one hand this may seem to be a positive step to reduce the incidence of the condition, whilst on the other hand it can be seen as a double-edged sword, with parents experiencing increased anxiety and psychological trauma. There is evidence that even with a negative diagnostic test the parents may have heightened levels of anxiety for the remainder of the pregnancy and beyond (Bryant *et al.*, 2001). The long-term effects on the family dynamics of this are still not understood. In a personal account, one mother writes, "I do not know if I am a better or different person … however it is forever etched on my mind and my heart" (Sullivan and Kirk, 2003).

Parental life-style

Parental life-style may have an impact both in the preconception period and during pregnancy itself. Many substances will cross the placental barrier. These include prescription drugs, over-the-counter drugs and illegal substances, and some of these will have a teratogenic (harmful) effect. Alcohol consumed during pregnancy also influences development as it crosses the placenta. High levels of alcohol consumption can cause a condition known as 'fetal alcohol syndrome'. Babies born with this condition may exhibit a cluster of facial features and physical abnormalities, be of low birth weight, and suffer from delayed intellectual development and behavioural problems. There has been considerable research that has increased our understanding of the impact of maternal alcohol consumption during pregnancy, and whilst there is general consensus that women should not drink excessively or binge drink, debate has continued over whether there is a safe level. The Royal College of Obstetricians and Gynaecologists advised in 1999 that there was no conclusive evidence of an effect on IQ levels or growth if a pregnant woman restricted her consumption to less than 15 units of alcohol per week. However, the confounding effects of other factors such as smoking, drug use and socio-economic status mean that the overall picture is unclear, and a more cautious approach is often advocated (Plant *et al.*, 1999).

Tobacco smoking should be discouraged during pregnancy, as there is clear evidence that it causes harm to the fetus (DoH/DfES, 2004). Birth weight decreases with an increasing number of cigarettes smoked, and pre-term labour is more likely. Smoking cessation is a key government target in the UK, with the aim of reducing the proportion of women continuing to smoke throughout pregnancy by one percentage point a year. A number of initiatives have been set up to achieve this aim, including encouraging both parents to attend smoking cessation sessions and providing support to mothers to raise their self-esteem and reduce stressors.

There is increasing interest in the role played by diet and nutrition in promoting the health of the mother and fetus prior to and during pregnancy. The effects of the mother's nutritional status on fetal growth and development are not clearly understood. Of necessity, some of the evidence is circumstantial, owing to the ethical and moral implications of manipulating the diet of pregnant women. Women who are significantly under- or over-weight do appear to place their child at greater risk (Bussell, 2000).

It has been postulated that poor nutrition in the later stages of pregnancy affects fetal growth, whilst poor nutrition in the early stages affects embryological development. This hypothesis is supported by statistical evidence from the Dutch Hunger Winter of 1944–1945. Prior to the famine conditions the mothers had been relatively well nourished, but it was found that babies exposed to the famine during the latter half of pregnancy showed the greatest reduction in birth weight. Conversely, there was a higher incidence of congenital abnormality and stillbirth in babies conceived during the course of the famine (Worthington-Roberts and Williams, 1993).

The Acheson Report (1998) refers to the effects that a mother's nutrition has on her child's health, and states that there is a need for more policies to improve the nutritional status of future mothers and their children, as poor nutrition *in utero* and during the first year of life may have long-term effects. In one study in Hertfordshire, birth records from the early part of this century were examined and a follow-up study of the adults between 59 and 70 years of age was carried out. It was discovered that low birth weight was related to an increased risk of heart disease, raised blood pressure and type 2 diabetes in adult life. It was not clear from the birth records whether the low birth weight was due to growth retardation or prematurity. However, it seems likely that the low birth weight was due to undernutrition of the fetus, since the records showed that the children who were still underweight at 1 year also showed an increased risk of developing the above conditions (Barker, 1992).

However, parental life-style cannot be isolated from the overall social context. Lower socio-economic status may, for example, affect the ability to purchase a healthy diet. The stress and strain of unemployment, poor housing and homelessness may create additional burdens for the pregnant woman. The incidence of smoking and alcohol consumption has increased among the female population, and may be a strategy employed to cope with adverse social circumstances.

It is difficult to separate the factors that affect the health and development of the fetus and newborn infant. Figure 2.2 illustrates the interrelationship between them. The characteristics of the newborn itself, in terms of sex, birth order, or whether it is a singleton or multiple birth, are also significant. For babies who are born prematurely, of low birth weight, or who are ill following delivery, advances in neonatal intensive care have increased the likelihood of survival. However, the old adage that prevention is better than cure holds true, and this will now be considered.

STRATEGIES TO OPTIMIZE HEALTH AND WELL-BEING IN THE NEWBORN

It has been demonstrated that the factors which influence health in the newborn are many and interrelated. As a result, a variety of strategies is required to reduce risk and promote health. This has been reflected in the shift of government policy from the late 1990s, which has shown increasing recognition of the complex links between social conditions and health.

Most environmental hazards are at their most dangerous when cell division in the embryo is most rapid. By the end of the embryological phase of development, most major structural anomalies that affect the fetus are already determined (Moos, 2004). A major challenge, therefore, is to provide education in the period before conception, when prospective parents can be offered a series of options that may not be available once pregnancy is confirmed. Helping people to prepare for pregnancy is a strategy known as 'preconception health promotion and care'. Preconception care is relatively new, and aims to ensure that 'the woman and her partner are in optimal state of physical and emotional health at the onset of pregnancy' (RCGP, 1995, p. 3).

Health advice is now widely available through the mass media and the World Wide Web, and these are powerful means of raising general awareness among the population. In one media campaign the importance of folic acid supplementation prior to pregnancy was promoted by advertising in the newspapers and television. Pregnant women, and those intending to become pregnant, are advised to take 400 μg of folic acid a day until the twelfth week of gestation. This reduces the risk of having a baby with a neural tube defect such as spina bifida (NICE, 2003). Despite this campaign, many women remain unaware that diet alone does not provide the level required to protect against neural tube defect, or provide protection when pregnancy is unplanned. Consequently, it has been recommended that all wheat products are fortified with folic acid (DoH, 2000).

In the United Kingdom the incidence of teenage pregnancies and young parenthood is a cause of concern, given the increased health risk to the baby and the risk of social exclusion to the parents. The government target is to reduce the incidence of teenage pregnancy by half by 2010 (Social Exclusion Unit, 1999). Good health and sex education in schools is therefore an essential part of preconception care. Teachers, health and social care professionals, parents and communities should work together

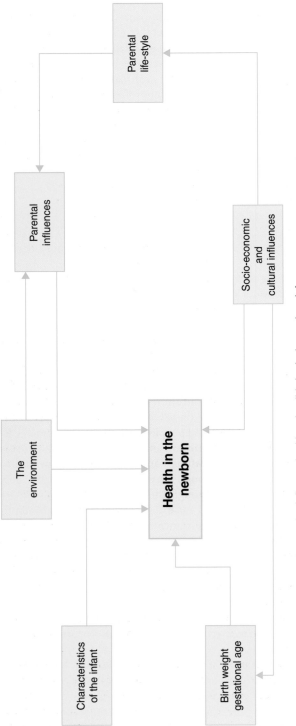

Figure 2.2 Interrelationship between factors that influence health and well-being in the newborn infant.

to provide accurate, relevant and sensitive advice with regard to conception, pregnancy and parenthood.

Family-planning clinics, well-woman and well-man clinics all provide opportunities for preconception education and raise general reproductive health awareness. In addition to raising general awareness, preconception clinics are available in some areas. They may be situated in GP surgeries or health centres, or be 'drop-in' clinics in local shopping precincts. However, they tend to be attended by motivated couples with higher socio-economic status. For preconception care to be effective, it needs to be readily accessible and sensitive to the needs of the local population and acceptable to the wide range of religious and cultural groups within contemporary society.

Preconception care consists of two elements. The majority of clients require advice on life-style and health promotion in preparation for pregnancy. A variety of approaches may be taken in the provision of preconception care, but all must start with a detailed family and obstetric history in order to determine whether any specialist referral is required. All pregnant women are offered screening for rubella, hepatitis, syphilis and HIV in pregnancy, but preconception screening can prevent or reduce problems later on (DoH, 2003). For example, although rubella immunization is offered for all children, in some cases immunity is not achieved; therefore, if the woman is not immune, then vaccination can be offered as part of preconception care. Advice on life-style may consider weight, nutritional status and the adverse effects of smoking and alcohol consumption. Opportunities should be provided for those contemplating pregnancy to talk about the implications of parenthood and to discuss their fears and anxieties.

Specialist preconception advice should be available for women with pre-existing medical conditions. Genetic counselling may be required by couples if there is a family history of genetic disorder, or if they have previously had affected children. Genetic counselling involves the provision of information about the level of risk, as well as describing the options open to the parents, and providing support for the couple through the choices they make as a result of that information. Greater recognition of the potential father's health and habits are needed, and efforts made to engage him with his partner in life-style changes. Smoking cessation and dietary changes are difficult to achieve if the partner does not make a commitment to change as well (Moos, 2004).

If preconception care is to be effective, then the needs of a local population must be identified and strategies formulated to meet local need in an acceptable form. This philosophy is reflected in schemes such as the SureStart initiative and New Deal for Communities. SureStart focuses on the importance of the early years and maternal and infant health for future health, development and well-being. A number of projects have been set up in areas of social and economic deprivation to work with all families, but the primary focus is on supporting socially disadvantaged families to attempt to break the cycle of deprivation.

Whether preconception clinics are providing a broad range of services or meeting the specific needs of couples at increased risk, the intention should be to provide sufficient information for people to make informed choices about conception. Care must be taken to ensure that all advice is non-judgemental and non-directive, so that reproductive decisions are taken by the woman or couple, and not by the healthcare professional. Equally, it should be recognized that preconception care has not failed if the clients do not act on the advice that they receive. There is evidence that schemes to improve health awareness are working, but this does not necessarily lead to a change in behaviour. What may change is the level of self-reporting. Women may say that their nicotine consumption has reduced in pregnancy, yet tests on their urine show that consumption stays constant in pregnancy (Lawrence *et al.*, 2003).

Looking forward to pregnancy, preconception clinics also provide the ideal opportunity for educating the woman about the importance of antenatal care and the decisions that she may need to make during pregnancy. Women should be offered evidence-based information to exercise choice and control during pregnancy (NICE, 2003). The mother should be able to choose whether the midwife, the General Practitioner or the obstetrician will act as the main co-ordinator of her care, and make choices relating to the type of care provided. Women are confronted with the need to make decisions about whether to have screening tests early in the pregnancy. It may be helpful to spend time considering the nature of these tests and the implications of choosing to have them before pregnancy occurs.

It has been shown that preconception care may be provided in a variety of venues by a variety of healthcare workers. It could be argued that it is especially relevant for the maternity services and in particular midwives to provide preconception care and advice. In the decade since the Changing Childbirth (DoH, 1993) report was published, midwives have been developing the concepts of woman-centred care and continuity of care and carer. If the maternity services provide preconception clinics, then the woman will be seen by the same healthcare professionals throughout the childbearing process. This can promote ongoing and consistent advice and support, which is sensitive to the needs of the woman and her partner rather than just providing a menu of options from which to choose.

The process of childbearing is a time of great psychological and physiological change. It is also a normal physiological event, and in the majority of cases the end result is a healthy mother and baby. Antenatal care was first introduced in 1915 as a means of improving the health of the mother and baby. The broad aims of antenatal care are to promote fetal and maternal well-being, to detect and treat deviations from normal, and to prepare the woman and her partner for labour and parenthood. As with preconception care, there is a significant health education element to enable informed choice during the antenatal period. The diagnostic and technical facilities used in the care of the mother and baby have become increasingly sophisticated. The maternity services have been influential in reducing infant mortality and morbidity, and it is now recommended that the pattern of care should be tailored to the needs of the individual. Identifying the at-risk cases for whom more supervision is required is a more realistic and valuable use of resources. It is also recognized that antenatal care alone is insufficient to override the problems caused by social deprivation. To make the service more flexible, accessible and appropriate for all women the National Service Framework for Children, Young People and Maternity Services sets out a 10-year development plan to improve the services to children including maternity care (DH/DfES, 2004). This complements guidelines produced by the National Institute for Clinical Excellence (NICE, 2003).

The period following birth also offers opportunities to screen the newborn for a variety of disorders, and to instigate treatment at an early stage in order to reduce or prevent the potential for harm. Again, there are opportunities to teach parents about caring for their babies, including advice on infant feeding, how to recognize when the baby is ill, and how and when to seek help.

Like pregnancy, the postnatal period may bring joy and excitement, but it is also a time of major adjustment to new roles and responsibilities. This is especially so when a baby is ill, small or premature. One important aspect of care is the emotional and psychological support offered to the mother and the family. Few women escape

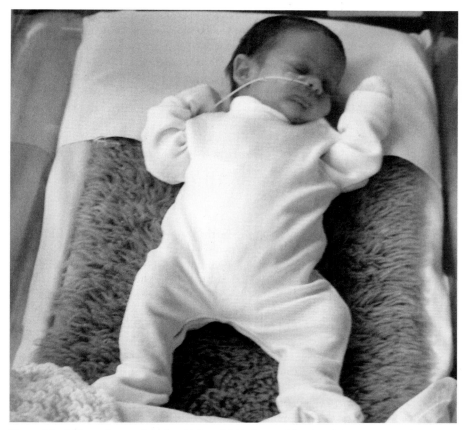

Figure 2.3   A 35-week premature, low birth weight baby receiving special care.

the transitory 'three-day blues' following delivery, but 13–25 per cent of women will go on to develop postnatal depression, which can adversely affect the ability to cope with the demands of motherhood and interfere with the developing relationship between the mother and her baby (Niven, 1992).

Womens' coping strategies in the early days following the birth may be affected by their birth experience, previous life events and social support networks. In addition to support from family and professional health and social care workers, there are a variety of groups, which enable women to share experiences and may address more issues than a one-to-one client approach. Promoting the physical, social and psychological well-being of the mother in the early months of parenthood increases her confidence in meeting the needs of her baby, and is thus more likely to ensure physical and social well-being in the child.

The aim of providing information about health is to enable women and their partners to make informed reproductive choices. The healthcare professionals seek to protect the woman and her baby throughout the childbearing process. The main protector is the woman herself, who is concerned with the physical safety of the baby and the nurturing of the new relationships (Edwards, 2004). Enabling women to make choices, based on good information, may lead the mother to make improvements in her life-style. These changes, which may be quite small, may have a significant impact on the long-term health of the mother and her child. However, it is also unrealistic to believe that improvements in pregnancy outcome can be achieved by health promotion alone. Equally, it should be recognized that problems may arise in pregnancy or the newborn period when there are no apparent risk factors and the parents have a healthy life-style. There needs to be an improvement in social conditions such as poverty, poor housing and inadequate diet. Without such an improvement, a significant proportion of the population will remain vulnerable during pregnancy.

IMPLICATIONS FOR EARLY YEARS PROFESSIONALS

As stated earlier, the period surrounding birth is important not only in relation to the health of the newborn baby, but also with regard to the presence of disease in later life. The promotion of health begins before we are born, and subsequently it is within the family that the first messages about health are given. The early years professional has the opportunity to reinforce positive health messages and to offer alternatives to negative messages. By providing information, a vital part of the preconception care of the next generation is instigated.

Whilst this may be an aspect for the early years professional to consider, it is also important that there is understanding of the early holistic influences on the children in their care. This understanding may then lead to greater insight into meeting the needs of children who have a congenital abnormality, those who have been born prematurely or of low birth weight, or have been born into poor socio-economic conditions. There are a range of opportunities for healthcare professionals, early years professionals and parents to work in collaboration to provide accessible services to optimize the health and well-being of the newborn.

Conclusion

This chapter has focussed on the factors influencing the health and well-being of the newborn baby. It has been suggested that some influences play a part before conception, whereas others arise during pregnancy and the period following birth. The factors are often interlinked, and there is a danger of blaming the victim if the wider social and environmental factors are ignored.

Health promotion and advice have been emphasized, rather than the more medical aspects of preconception and pregnancy care. This has been intentional, so that an overview of early experience can be gained. It is hoped that this chapter will act as a springboard for the reader to follow up areas of personal interest to him or her, and which are relevant to his or her particular area of early years work.

Student activity

Using Figure 2.2, identify different factors influencing health and well-being in the newborn. Complete the chart below by placing the factors into the appropriate category. Some examples have been provided for you.

Physical	Social and emotional	Environmental
Birth weight	Teenage parenthood	Pollution

Consider where there may be overlaps between categories and how this may affect strategies to optimize health and well-being in the newborn.

REFERENCES

Acheson, D (1998): *Independent Inquiry into Inequalities in Health*. London: The Stationery Office, www.archive.official-documents.co.uk/doh/ih/ih.htm

Barker, DJP (ed.) (1992): *Fetal and Infant Origins of Adult Disease*. London: British Medical Journal Publishers.

Bryant, LD, Green, JM and Hewison, J (2001): Prenatal screening for Down syndrome: some psychosocial implications of a 'screening for all' policy. *Public Health*, 15, 356–358.

Bussell, G (2000): The dietary beliefs and attitudes of women who have a low birth weight baby: a retrospective preconception study. *Journal of Human Nutrition and Dietetics*, 13(1), 29–39.

Cuckle, HS, Wald, NJ and Thompson, N (1987): Estimating a woman's risk of having a pregnancy associated with Down's syndrome using her age and serum AFP level. *British Journal of Obstetrics and Gynaecology*, 94, 387–402.

Department of Health (1993): *Changing Childbirth*. London: HMSO.

Department of Health (2000): *Folic Acid and the Prevention of Disease*. Report of the Committee of Medical Aspects of Food and Nutrition Policy. London: The Stationery Office.

Department of Health (2003): *Screening for Infectious Disease in Pregnancy*. London: HMSO.

Department of Health/Department for Education and Skills (2004): *National Service Framework for Children, Young People and Maternity Services*. London: DoH.

Edwards, N (2004): Protection – regulations and standards: enabling or disabling. *Midwives*, 7(3), 116–119.

Lawrence, T, Aveyard, P and Croghan, E (2003): What happens to women's self-reported cigarette consumption and urinary cotinine levels in pregnancy. *Addiction*, **98**(9), 1315–1320.

Macfarlane, A and Moser, K (2004): *Social Inequalities in The Health of Children and Young People*. London: Office for National Statistics.

Moos, M (2004): Preconceptual health promotion: progress in changing a prevention paradigm. *Journal of Perinatal and Neonatal Nursing*, **18**(1), 2–14.

National Institute for Clinical Excellence (2003): Antenatal care: routine care for the healthy pregnant woman. London: NICE.

Niven, C (1992): *Psychological Care for Families: Before, During and After Birth*. Oxford: Butterworth Heinemann.

Plant, ML, Abel, EL and Guerri, C (1999): Alcohol and pregnancy. In McDonald, I (ed.), *Health Ideas Related to Alcohol Consumption*, 2nd edn. Oxford: Blackwell Science.

Royal College of General Practitioners (1995): The role of general practice in maternity care. Occasional paper 72: Report of the RCGP Maternity Care Group. London: RCGP.

Royal College of Obstetricians and Gynaecologists (1999): *Alcohol Consumption in Pregnancy*. London: RCOG.

Seedhouse, D (1986): *Health – the Foundations for Achievement*. Chichester: John Wiley & Sons.

Social Exclusion Unit (1999): *Teenage Pregnancy*. London: Department of Health.

Sullivan, A and Kirk, B (2003): Specialised Fetal Investigations. In Fraser, D and Cooper, M (eds), *Myles Textbook for Midwives*. London: Churchill Livingstone, pp. 411–430.

Teenage Pregnancy Unit, Department of Health, Royal College of Midwives (2004): *Teenage Parents: Who Cares. A Guide to Commissioning and Delivering Maternity Services for Young Parents*. London: HMSO.

Wald, NJ, Rodeck, C, Hackshaw, AK, Walters, J, Chitty, L and Mackinson, AM (2003): *First and Second Trimester Antenatal Screening for Down's Syndrome; The Results of the Serum, Urine and Ultrasound Screening Study*. London: HMSO.

Wolpert, L (1993): *The Triumph of the Embryo*. Oxford: Oxford University Press.

Worthington-Roberts, B and Williams, S (1993): Prenatal nutrition – general issues. In Worthington-Roberts, B and Williams, S (eds), *Nutrition in Pregnancy and Lactation*, 5th edn. St Louis, MO: Mosby, pp. 87–172.

PHYSICAL GROWTH AND DEVELOPMENT

Val Thurtle

This chapter aims to:

- consider why early years professionals study child development;

- investigate health and growth screening in early childhood;

- reflect on ways of meeting the physical needs of young children;

- illustrate through the use of one exemplar how various factors influence growth and development.

WHY STUDY CHILD DEVELOPMENT?

Most professionals who come into contact with children are likely to have studied child development during their basic education and training. The study of the development of their prospective 'clients' is seen as a 'good' thing, and there is an understanding that there are rules and patterns in the progression of all children that can be discovered, described and perhaps understood. Reflecting on the purpose of studying child development, it can be viewed as an extremely interesting area of academic study in its own right. More practically, psychoanalytical thinking has encouraged the view that 'the child is father of the man' – what happens in childhood is seen as being influential in adulthood, and therefore must be worth exploring. Ultimately, those working with children need to have some knowledge of what a child should be doing at a particular time in his or her development – not only because of the potential to identify problems with development that might be amenable to early interventions but also to enable them to work with children in a meaningful way and better support and promote their progress.

By setting up a taxonomy of norms, milestones or stages that the majority of children are likely to reach by a certain age or point, such 'guidelines' can be used to ascertain an individual child's developmental progress. Much of the developmental screening conducted by health professionals is done in this way, and Standard Assessment Tasks and Attainment Targets within the National Curriculum set up such norms. In summary, the rationale for inclusion of child development in most programmes of study is that it underpins sound professional practice in early years provision. The study of child development facilitates the worker's understanding of the child and how he or she is likely to progress, knowledge that can be used to children's benefit.

ACQUIRING CHILD DEVELOPMENT KNOWLEDGE

Students and practitioners who come into contact with children need therefore to have some idea of what can be expected of children at particular ages, or stages. For thousands of students of children, Sheridan's From Birth to Five (Sheridan, 1997) has met, and continues to meet, this need. This slim volume sets out what large numbers of children of various ages have been found to have achieved in terms of posture and gross movement, vision and fine movement, hearing, speech, social behaviour and play. As its starting point was research carried out in the 1950s, one might question the validity of the findings and their relevance to contemporary practice. Sheridan's sample has been criticized as not being representative even at the time of data collection, with a bias toward children with a middle-class background. Child-rearing patterns have changed, as have the opportunities offered to many children.

Whilst the way in which Sheridan's schedule was constructed may have limitations, the more significant constraints of the schedule lie largely in the way it is viewed or used. If it is seen as a fixed entity it does not allow for variety in the progression of individual children. The majority are likely to follow the pattern outlined, but possibly at different rates.

The Denver Development Screening test originally developed by Frankenburg and Dodds (1967) set out to take account of this. It identifies the ages by which 25 per cent of children have achieved the developmental point in question, the point at which 50 per cent have achieved it, and so on.

Development scales of a check-list type cannot take into account the variety in the child's progression, influenced as it is by a host of factors, including genetic make-up, birth history, family background, nutritional state, socio-economic status and cultural setting, to name just a few.

Schedules would appear to be of limited value, yet there is little doubt that effective early years practice needs to be based on a sound knowledge of child development. The novice will need to learn the key developmental milestones of early childhood with at least approximate ages. A 'rough guide' is reproduced in Table 3.1 to act as a simple starting point. Any one using it – be they a novice or an experienced practitioner – will find aspects they may want to query. Children themselves and the social environment in which they live will influence so many aspects of child development. Pointing at items in a book is dependent on the child having been given books at an early age, and telling the time needs someone to have explained the whole process and given the child access to a traditional watch with hands. A child who has limited access, for example, to pencils and crayons will not have had the opportunity to draw circles or lines and may well 'fail' a traditional test. Yet what will be measured is a lack of opportunity and practice rather than a deficit in fine motor skills.

As students synthesize material from a variety of disciplines (particularly developmental psychology) with their own observations in practice, they will be able to interpret their findings by applying developmental knowledge based on their experience of many children to one child in particular. Students may well hear experienced professionals express concerns about an individual child without having undertaken any screening tests at all, but rather based on their learned knowledge of what most children can do at a particular age. In many cases, further investigation will show that their concerns are proven to be right.

Table 3.1 Developmental milestones – a rough starting point

Age	Gross motor	Fine motor	Cognition/perception	Language	Social: play
6 weeks	Holds head erect when upright	Palmar grasp	Imitates facial expressions	Coos, gurgles	Alert
3 months	When prone, lifts self on arms	Hand regard Starting to use hand to reach out to hit (and later to grab) object	Remembers specific experiences	Smiles after being talked to	Excited by familiar and pleasant situations Seems to like musical sounds
6 months	Rolls from back to front	Picks up object with palmar grasp Holds object and then drops as given another	0–2 years old: responds to sensory and motor changes in environment. No forward planning of actions	Babbles	Grasps objects Plays with own feet Handles toys and enjoys noise they make
9 months	Sits alone Stands with help May take step with support May crawl	Finger–thumb grip Points at objects Seeks dropped or hidden object	Object permanence	Da da and ma ma appropriately	Wary of strangers and separation from parents Tries to grab spoon
1 year	Crawls or bottom-shuffles	Finger-feeds Points at object		First words	Plays pat-a-cake Can drink from cup if has been given opportunity Uses spoon Co-operates with dressing Enjoys looking at books
15 months	Walks alone	Points at object to demand it		6–10 words Understands far more than he/she says	Curious and mobile Unable to perceive danger
18 months	Walking established Can stop and pick up object	Scribbles with crayon Points at items in picture book Builds three-brick tower	Up to about 18 months understands the world in terms of senses and motor actions	Knows 20 words Points to parts of body	Negative at times Domestic mimicry Enjoys sand and water

(continued)

Table 3.1 *(continued)*

Age	Gross motor	Fine motor	Cognition/perception	Language	Social: play
2 years	Runs Climbs stairs one at a time Throws or kicks a ball Jumps with two feet together	Circular scribble with crayon also dots and vertical line Simple jigsaws	Sees the world from his/her point of view Pretend play	50+ words and two-word phrases	Able to be toilet trained Wants to 'help' with adult activities Make-believe play
3 years	Pedals a tricycle Climbs apparatus	Builds bridge with bricks Draws recognizable pictures	Aware that he/she is a boy or girl Beginning to see other person's perspective	Tells what has happened to her Language comprehensible to those outside close family Grammatical system becoming established	Co-operative play Begins to take turns Some empathy with others Happy to separate from parent at playgroup or nursery Remembers nursery rhymes
4 years	Climbs up and down stairs one foot per step Hops on dominant foot Can stand on one foot	Copies X with crayon Draws house Undoes buttons	Can distinguish between reality and make-believe	Knows colours Continually asks questions	Development of individual friendships Can dress and undress self
5 years	Hops on either foot Rides two-wheeler bike Increasing skills of climbing, kicking, throwing and catching ball	Writes letters of name Hold pencil tripod style Can draw □ or △ Uses scissors	Begins to see the world in terms of rules	Rate of vocabulary varies enormously but may have 15 000 words, gaining 3000 per year	Socio-dramatic play Plays games with increasingly complicated rules Protective towards younger siblings
6 years	Skips	Uses large needle Ties bow	Tells the time Beginning to use simple logic	Some substitutions still in evidence (e.g. 'f' for 'th')	Play tends to be with children of same sex Segregates into gender groups
7 years	Confident and competent in movements	Copies ◇ Plays recorder	Able to categorize items (e.g. dinosaurs, football teams) Has simple concepts of distance, time and speed	Understands and uses conjunctions, tag questions, passive tense and infinitives	Plays in large groups or gangs

HEALTH AND GROWTH SCREENING IN EARLY CHILDHOOD

As we discuss in Chapter 13, the emphasis in child health care was traditionally focussed on the detection of abnormalities. Specific norms – competences expected by a certain age – were outlined, and children compared with this standard.

Recent good practice has seen child health in much broader terms, influenced by biological factors, life-style and the social context in which children are growing up within an overarching framework of child health promotion (DoH/DfES, 2004). A child's development may be influenced, for example, by his or her nutrition, whether family members smoke, the poverty or affluence of the family, the house in which he or she lives, the transport infrastructure in the area, and so on. The process of improving and sustaining child health encompasses activities that prevent ill health and promote good health of both the individual and of the whole community of children (see also Chapters 10 and 13).

The early detection of difficulties, seen as a key aspect of child health practice, is often referred to as 'screening', but we might want to query whether the monitoring of children's development in which all early years workers should be involved is true screening.

Hall and Elliman (2003) quote the American Commission on Chronic Illness from 1957 as saying that screening is:

> '... the presumptive identification of unrecognized disease or defect by the application of tests, examinations, and other procedures which can be applied rapidly. Screening tests sort out the apparently well persons who do have a disease from those who probably do not. A screening test is not expected to be diagnostic'.
>
> (cited in Hall and Elliman, 2003, pp. 135)

Screening, therefore, will be for a significant health problem, treatment should be available, and it will be economically worthwhile. Cochrane and Holland (cited in Hall and Elliman, 2003) describe a simple set of criteria, stating that screening should be:

- simple;
- acceptable;
- accurate;
- repeatable;
- sensitive; and
- specific.

To what extent does the traditional developmental monitoring of children's progress fit these criteria? The simple answer is 'not terribly well'. For example, the distraction test carried out on babies of approximately 8 months of age was at one time (and in some areas still is) used on all children to establish if a child was hearing adequately. Working through the criteria for screening listed above, it is a simple test and it is acceptable to the majority of parents. As we move through the list, however, it becomes more difficult to be sure that the distraction test meets the criteria (Hall and Elliman, 2003). Accuracy and repeatability hinge on the competence of the staff administering the test and the wakefulness of the child. Furthermore, there are concerns about the sensitivity of the test, as children are not able developmentally to comply with the test until they are aged 6–7 months, meaning that early intervention to deal with hearing loss is not possible. Hall and Elliman further doubt the test's sensitivity, as some children with hearing loss are missed (false negatives), while other children are diagnosed with a hearing loss when in fact they hear perfectly well, thus raising parental anxiety (false positive).

Given these difficulties, Hall and Elliman conclude that where universal neonatal hearing screening – that is, testing the hearing of all newborn babies – is in place (which it increasingly is), the universal distraction test should be abandoned. The National Service Framework for Children, Young People and Maternity Services (DoH/DfES, 2004) advocates the roll-out of such screening to all areas.

On the other hand, neonatal blood spot screening at 5–6 days of age for phenyl-ketonuria, congenital hypothyroidism and other congenital disorders is well established, appears to fit the screening criteria, and its value is both accepted and supported. The test meets all the criteria for screening. Hence the screening programme is being expanded to include more congenital anomalies that are amenable to early intervention programmes. For example, newborn blood spot screening for sickle cell disorders is part of the NHS plan, and should be implemented by the time this book is in print. Screening for cystic fibrosis (DoH/DfES, 2004) will also be implemented.

Some observations and direct questions asked of a parent by a professional might be seen as part of evaluating the child's development, but they are not true screening procedures. 'Is the child walking by a certain age?' is such an example, but with much of a child's development it is difficult to say 'yes, this child is progressing normally', or 'this child needs further investigation' on the basis of one simple test or even a set of questions. Virtually all pre-school children in the UK have access to child health programmes, but the majority of health and developmental difficulties will be picked up in the very early days or weeks of the child's life, or by parents, friends and professionals who come into contact with the child in other contexts. Their concerns may then be taken to health workers who can pursue avenues of referral, which may or may not lead to health interventions.

To be able to do this, all early years practitioners need to be working in partnership with the parents, and to have good professional relationships with each other. This is the multidisciplinary approach referred to in the Introduction of this book. Communication skills are clearly vital, as is a detailed and interpretative knowledge of children's development, behaviour and play.

PHYSICAL GROWTH AND CENTILE CHARTS

So far, we have been considering general all-round development – that is, how the child progresses through various stages. One aspect of development that is largely concerned with size and the rate of its change is physical growth. The weight and growth of the baby have assumed an importance that is perhaps out of proportion to their value in British culture, and hence their inclusion in this text. One of the first questions asked by relatives and friends after the birth of the baby concerns its weight, and regular weighing has been seen to be part of good mothering. Visiting the health centre to have the baby weighed may be of value to the parents, not only reassuring them that the child is growing but also reducing the parent's social isolation by bringing him or her into contact with others who are at a similar point in their life. Links may be developed that last many years, and such networks often foster community development. The health centre, surgery or clinic can be a way of obtaining health information on nutrition, play and safety that the parents can evaluate and apply to their family situation.

Whether it is useful or not, many health professionals spend a great deal of time each week measuring and weighing children. The actual measurement of a child's weight, length or head circumference is, however, of little value unless such measurements can be adequately interpreted and compared to the norm for children of that age. Regular weekly weighing of half-clothed children on uncalibrated scales is, in reality, of little benefit. However, accurate measurement of children with careful plotting of these measurements on an up-to-date centile chart can lead to the early detection and monitoring of conditions such as growth hormone insufficiency, coeliac disease, and organic and non-organic failure to thrive. For the majority of parents of infants, accurate measurements and plotting will be a source of reassurance that their child is growing at an appropriate rate, although there is a risk that too frequent recording of weight will lead to parental anxiety.

Measurements should be made at birth and when there is contact with health professionals, and a systematic assessment of the child's physical, emotional and social development and family needs should be undertaken by the health visiting team by the child's first birthday (DoH/DfES, 2004). Parent-held records allow measurements taken by health visitors and General Practitioners to be plotted on the same chart. The child, when measured, should be naked and weighed on regularly calibrated scales. The practice of converting from metric weight to imperial – which many parents and professionals still do – increases the chance of error and is not recommended for professionals when completing centile charts.

Weighing and measuring children over a period of time is of interest to parents, carers, grannies and health workers. If there are difficulties it will be of relevance to paediatricians and child protection conferences. It does not meet the criteria of screening as mentioned before, so Hall and Elliman (2003) refer to it as growth monitoring. Weighing needs to be done over time on regularly calibrated scales, but probably not weekly. There have been differences of opinion over the measurement of length. Fry (1993) maintains that it is of value, and that the infant should be measured in the supine position (lying on his or her back) upon a calibrated mat. He argues that growth is fastest in the first 18 months and should therefore be monitored. To do this properly requires two workers, and obviously the child should not be distressed. If done properly, it does provide reasonably accurate measurements. When the child can stand, from approximately 18 months onward, he or she should be measured in an upright position. The child's occipito-frontal head circumference should be measured at birth or when swelling or moulding has settled, and the measurement should be made again between 6–8 weeks. The data should then be plotted on the centile chart, the purpose being to identify heads that are too large or small, or which grow at an unusual rate. Serious conditions identifiable through measuring head circumference are unusual, and regular measuring of all children after this point – unless there is some concern – only raises anxiety.

Measurements are then plotted upon a centile chart (Fig. 3.1). This is a device based on a 'bell' distribution that allows for the variation in height, weight and head circumference across a population. Current charts are based on the serial and cross-sectional measurements of large groups of infants and children in the indigenous UK population, and include pre-term measurements. The most recent were published in 1996 and replaced earlier charts which had become outdated, with children in more recent years growing taller and weight gain in the early months being more rapid, probably linked to changes in feeding practice (Hall and Elliman, 2003). Measurements need to be plotted accurately, with the correct calculation of the child's age in weeks and the readings plotted at the appropriate point allowing for prematurity and post-maturity.

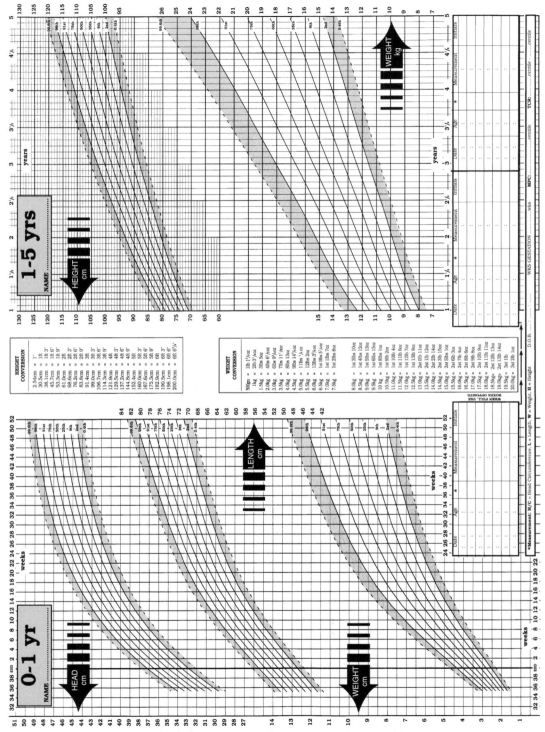

Figure 3.1 Child growth chart. © Child Growth Foundation. Reproduced with permission.

Deciding whether the measurements are of concern is where interpretation becomes significant. Little can be concluded from a single reading, and measurements should be considered over a period of time. Ideally, children's growth will be approximately along a centile line, with the head circumference and weight on a similar centile. Some infants – especially those with intra-uterine growth retardation – may take several months to settle on to 'their' line. Significant crossing of centile lines should raise concerns, although the first concern should be about the accuracy of measurement and plotting. Measurements outside the 99.6th or 0.4th centile should be queried and referred, although with a bell distribution some children will fit normally into this category. Parental stature should also be considered.

While crossing of centile lines may be the first sign of an organic problem, one of the commonest causes of failure to gain weight in the young child is underfeeding. A discussion with the carer as to what and how the child eats is likely to prove valuable. Persistent concerns about the growth of a child need to be discussed with the health visitor, General Practitioner and ultimately the paediatrician. Insufficient growth is of course a cause of concern, but with recent concern about obesity a child that appears to be putting on weight too fast should also raise queries. However, most parents regard their parent-held centile chart as a source of reassurance and a sign of their partnership in the health care of their child. Centile charts can be obtained from Harlow Printing, Maxwell St, South Shields, NE33 4PU.

MEETING THE NEEDS OF THE CHILD

In a sense, this whole volume is concerned with discovering and meeting the holistic needs of the child, and whilst identifying needs by looking at developmental milestones and physical growth (as we have done so far in this chapter) is part of the picture, developmental needs can be looked at in a much broader sense. Maslow's classic hierarchy of needs (1987) (Fig. 3.2) is a useful way of conceptualizing the needs of the child at various developmental stages.

The essence of the hierarchy is that the lower-level needs must be met before the individual can move on to the higher-level order needs. This model would therefore imply that raising a child's self-esteem will be of little value if his or her very survival is at risk, for example from hypothermia or malnutrition. Indeed, he or she is unlikely to benefit at the higher levels if the basic needs of survival, safety and security are not being met.

Using this framework, we can explore what the needs of a child will be, for example, at 6 months of age and 4 years of age. In terms of physical needs, both require adequate nutrition and hygiene, but these needs will be met in ways appropriate to each child's developmental stage. The 6-month-old needs breast milk or a modified substitute. He or she needs to move on to solid food in order to acquire the skills of chewing and to ensure an adequate iron intake, and foods will need to be puréed or at least mashed. The 4-year-old also requires a balanced diet, but has mastered the skills of chewing, is at a much reduced risk of choking, can usually handle cutlery, and will have his or her own opinions about food preferences. In terms of warmth, the 6-month-old is totally dependent upon the carer to add or subtract clothing, communicating temperature discomfort in an unspecific way. The fit 4-year-old, in contrast, can move around to generate heat, can communicate his or her perception of temperature in words, and can remove clothing as necessary. The 4-year-old still

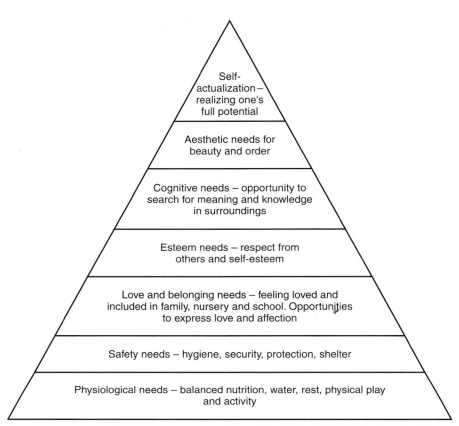

Figure 3.2   Maslow's hierarchy of needs. MASLOW, MOTIVATION & PERSONALITY, 2nd Edition, © Abraham Maslow, 1970. Adapted by permission of Pearson Education, Inc., Upper Saddle River, NJ.

requires observation and supervision, and is unlikely to be able to control the wider environment in this respect, but this child's developmental stage allows him or her to take some responsibility for his or her own warmth.

Safety and security can be discussed in terms of protection from disease, protection from accidents, and the security of loving relationships, which overflows into love and belonging. The 6-month-old requires a high standard of hygiene precautions. Feeding implements need to be sterilized, and drinking water must be boiled. Efficient and clean nappy routines are vital, but the onus is on the carer. The 4-year-old will largely be self-caring and will follow the toileting practices of the rest of the household. While able to toilet independently, he or she will need reminders about hand washing and contact with pets. Both will need protection from disease via immunization and vaccination.

The 6-month-old will gain much security from firm confident handling from a small number of caregivers. Security for the 4-year-old is grounded in relationships with the significant people in his or her life.

Both need a safe environment in which to play and explore. Many childhood accidents in the home are a result of the usual play behaviour for a particular developmental stage. Such accidents are likely to occur in a home setting, particularly in the case of children up to 5 years old. After this age, children feature more extensively in road accidents – that is, accidents outside the home. Using developmental knowledge to anticipate what skills and movements a child might acquire next can increase accident prevention for the under-fives. For example, the parent may not previously have seen the 3-month-old child roll over; however, to do so for the first time over the edge of a changing table when left unattended contributes to the high rate of falls in the under-ones. The 4-year-old will appear confident, with practised motor skills of running, jumping and riding a bicycle, albeit with stabilizers. A desire to hone these skills and to imitate or keep up with his or her siblings, particularly in outside areas, puts him or her at risk.

The love and belonging needs of each child are met by attachments to a stable group of carers. The 6-month-old is still forming such attachments, and these are likely to be limited to a small nucleus of individuals – the mother, father, and perhaps a child-minder and grandparents. The 4-year-old has wider social horizons, forming relationships outside the family group with other adults and friendships with his or her peers. Children of this age know that they belong to their nursery, finding security in established routines and practices. Both children will respond to attention, but again it needs to be developmentally specific. The 6-month-old will respond to handling, songs and speech, whereas the 4-year-old has extended his or her repertoire into conversation participation, rhymes, songs, games and a host of other activities.

It is this growth in ability and confidence that gives the developing child self-esteem. Such children need to be aware that they are valued and that their achievements are noted and appreciated. Their cognitive needs will be met by the activities with which they are presented, and by their own exploration and interaction with the environment. These will, of course, be specific to each child's developmental stage.

The aesthetic needs of children are often ignored, but are met by the beauty and order of the child's world; they may be interlinked with nature or music. With the coming of Excellence and Enjoyment, a strategy for primary schools (DfES, 2003), the curriculum should be increasingly rich, varied and exciting, encouraging creativity and the meeting of aesthetic needs.

Self-actualization is difficult to discuss for any of us. Perhaps it is a case of getting in touch with ourselves, knowing who we are and how we fit into the world around us. This is a lifetime's work which, in the early years, is facilitated by appropriate stimulation, human contact and play.

The meeting of all of these needs by any one individual or agency is probably an ideal. It may, in fact, be easier to identify situations when these needs are not met; for example, illness of the child or within the family, poverty, lack of knowledge of how to respond to a child, and outside pressures upon the family. Such situations may lead to difficulties in providing for basic needs where, for example, there is a lack of material resources or differences in priorities as carers cope with other issues. In an ideal world, all children would have a high proportion of their needs met. In reality, it may be a case of professionals such as health visitors, social workers, therapists, educationalists and family-centre personnel working with parents to meet as many needs as possible.

The developmental progress of the child and the meeting of his or her needs are influenced by a host of factors related to health, the socio-economic status of the family, culture, and child-rearing practices. It is impossible to pick out any one of these as being more significant than the others. Yet, according to Maslow's hierarchy, the contribution of the basic needs for survival must be met first. For that reason, and also because other aspects of childhood development are discussed elsewhere in this text, the remainder of this chapter will focus upon nutrition, which is itself influenced by many different factors.

INFANT FEEDING: BREAST OR BOTTLE?

Generations of midwives, health visitors, nursery nurses and mothers have been told that 'breast is best'. While they can outline the advantages of breastfeeding, in practice, Hamlyn *et al.* (2002) found that only 69 per cent of babies in England and Wales are breast-fed initially compared to 64 per cent in 1990 (White *et al.*, 1992). While there is a slight increase in mothers commencing breastfeeding, by the time the babies were 6 weeks old only 52 per cent of mothers were still breastfeeding, and by the time the babies were 6 months only 21 per cent were breast-fed (Hamlyn *et al.*, 2002). Whilst the knowledge base of mothers and professionals in terms of the benefits of breast-feeding has increased, the reality is that less than one-quarter of babies derive the maximum benefits of breastfeeding. Women express their reluctance to breastfeed, citing embarrassment, lack of privacy, distaste, a fear of under-feeding, inconveni-ence, a desire to return to work, and lack of support from partner and family members as reasons. The high number who commence breastfeeding and then cease may reflect encouragement or pressure (however it is perceived) from health profession-als in the antenatal period, but is more likely to demonstrate a lack of support, both practical and emotional, during the early weeks of motherhood.

In order to encourage health professionals to support mothers to breastfeed, Primary Care Trusts are being urged to collate data on breastfeeding rates, and such rates are increasingly being published showing comparative data across health economies. There is naturally much emphasis being placed on ensuring that midwives, health visitors, nursery nurses and others working with mothers during the perinatal period have accurate and up-to-date knowledge about breastfeeding. It is, of course, import-ant to balance this with evidence-based knowledge on bottle-feeding practice. As we can see from the data above, if only just over half of all mothers are exclusively breastfeeding at 6 weeks, then nearly half are bottle-feeding. It is important that mothers who never start, or who cease, breastfeeding are not made to feel guilty, and that they are supported and given sound advice about, for example, maintaining eye contact during feeding, using feeding time to talk to babies, and making sure that feeding time is a quiet and relaxed event. Mothers (and fathers) can also be encouraged at some (if not all) feeds to use feeding time to have skin-to-skin contact with their babies.

Long-term benefits of breastfeeding

Various long-term benefits have been claimed for breastfeeding, some of which have not stood the test of time. It seems probable that the breast-fed child is less likely to be over-fed, as the infant has more control of his or her intake. To say that the breast-fed infant cannot become an obese child is an over-generalization, although the child may have a different pattern of weight gain to his or her bottle-fed peer, gaining a sig-nificant amount of weight in the early months. Until recently, centile charts have been based on a predominantly bottle-fed population, and may not reflect the growth patterns of breast-fed infants. The Child Growth Foundation's Breast from Birth Charts are however now available. A review of many different publications concluded that breastfeeding seemed to protect children from the development of allergies or atopic disease (Odijk *et al.*, 2003), particularly if the child was breast-fed exclusively. Other benefits may include small cognitive benefits (Thompson, 2002), less chance of sudden infant death, a lower adult blood pressure and less coronary heart disease in later life (Minchin, 1985; Thompson, 2002). All of these statements are of course subject to the interaction of other factors.

Many women, and especially those who choose not to breastfeed their child, make their decision early in pregnancy or even before. This is one of the reasons why there is a move to get breastfeeding considered in personal health and social education in schools, and for breastfeeding to be facilitated and seen as an everyday ordinary way of feeding babies. There has been a huge move to make hospitals baby friendly and thus encourage and support the choice of breastfeeding and its establishment in the early days of life. Maternity units can be awarded the baby friendly standard, of which many are justifiably proud. In such a hospital full discussion on feeding the baby is encouraged in the antenatal period, including the benefits of breastfeeding, so that an informed decision can be made. Staff will ensure that immediately after delivery the baby can be held against the mother's skin for as long as she wants. A midwife will offer early help with breastfeeding, and the child is kept with the mother at all times. Ongoing and consistent help and advice are given, and no water or artificial baby milk is given except for a medical reason.

More information on the Baby Feeding Initiative can be found on their web site http://www.babyfriendly.org.uk/home.

WEANING AND THE WEANING DIET

The World Health Organization (WHO, 2002) suggests that babies should be exclusively breast-fed until 6 months of age. This idea is difficult to consider in much of the Western world, when our continuing breast-feed rates are taken into account (see above), and the early point at which solids are introduced (see later). The growth velocity of children during the first 6 months is high, and they generally double their birth weight by 5 months. Breast milk or its substitute can provide the required nutrients for such growth at first, but by 6 months the amounts of protein, energy and vitamins A and D are unlikely to be sufficient (Department of Health, 1994). Prior to 3 months, an infant cannot easily swallow a bolus of solid food. From approximately 5 months, infants hold objects and direct them to their mouths, commencing chewing by about 6 months. The development of chewing also seems to be significant in relation to the acquisition of speech. Infants who are not given the opportunity to try solids seem reluctant to accept them if they are introduced at a later stage. Significant to the carer, weaning marks a step towards family food, and is often seen as a developmental milestone in its own right.

The commencement of weaning prior to 3 months is discouraged because of the immature nature of the gut, the lack of neuromuscular co-ordination to move food from the tip of the tongue to the back of the mouth, and the poor regulation by the kidney of high load (Barker, 2002). Enzyme production changes over time, becoming increasingly more efficient at digestion. Prior to 3 months, the gut wall appears to be fairly permeable, allowing the crossing of protein molecules, which seems to increase sensitivity to foreign protein.

Iron deficiency is a recurring theme in pre-school nutrition, particularly in some minority ethnic groups and amongst children from lower socio-economic groups. Children with iron-deficiency anaemia are apathetic and subdued, and less able to make use of stimulating experiences to which they are exposed. By 6 months, the amount of iron contributed by breast milk is insufficient, and other dietary sources are necessary (Department of Health, 1994). Current recommendations in the UK are that babies should be offered a mixed diet by the age of 6 months (Department of Health, 1994). The reasons for weaning are therefore social, developmental and physiological.

Cultural and economic factors influencing weaning

Kin groups are a powerful influence on new parents. Families may live in small units, but contact is sustained with mothers and mothers-in-law, and at a time of change, such as the arrival of a new infant, their influence may be significant. By offering practical help and emotional support, they may be providing information on traditional or out-of-date weaning practices.

Professionals such as health visitors, pharmacists and doctors provide information that is valued by many, but the apparent changes in dietary advice over the past few decades have left some parents confused and disillusioned.

Health workers have tried to disassociate themselves from the manufacturers and their sponsorship, with varying degrees of success. The sponsorship of professional conferences and the provision of small gifts leave professionals open to undue bias and influence. The 'bounty bag' distributed via maternity units gives the impression that professionals back weaning foods and other baby products. While infant milks are no longer advertised directly to mothers and samples are not given, it may be that manufacturers can access parents via their professional advisers.

Religious practices and the families' own eating practices may also be significant. Cordon *et al.* (2003) found that Bangladeshi mothers knew of a weaning ceremony that took place in Bangladesh but was not practised in Britain. The Bangladeshi and other ethnic groups were not stimulated by discussion about weaning in the way they had been about breastfeeding, indicating that it was not as culturally defined, or that the research method was unsuitable for collecting such data. Nevertheless, a vegetarian family will not offer a child meat, and certain foods may be unacceptable for particular groups. It is important for health professionals to discuss with the family what is significant to them, and to remember that culture changes over time and some will observe religious practices more than others.

The economic status of the family is important in both weaning and the feeding of pre-school children. Home-produced food may be cheaper if the rest of the family is eating food appropriate for the infant. If the mother feels that family food is unsuitable, buying a jar may be preferable in her eyes, especially if she knows that the infant will eat it and the packaging claims that the contents provide a balanced meal. The time involved in preparation and the lack of confidence that she can produce a baby meal as nutritious as that provided by a manufacturer may all be part of her decision-making process. Many years ago, Blackburn (1991) argued that parents living in poverty largely know what is considered to be good for their children's health in terms of nutrition, but are frustrated that they cannot meet their own goals. They may be more inclined to follow short-term goals, for example adding cereals to the bottle in order to quieten a fractious child and so maintain family harmony, rather than following the professionals' long-term goals of promoting speech development and a healthy diet. With the continuation of child poverty (especially in London), there is no reason to believe this is not still the case.

In many cultures food is caught up with love and nurturing, and the carer feels that she is doing the right thing if the child accepts the food happily. That in itself may influence the types of foods a child is given.

Weaning: what really happens?

Having outlined government recommendations and factors that may influence weaning, it is worth looking at what really happens. *Infant Feeding 2000* (Hamlyn *et al.*, 2002) showed that, compared to 1995, mothers were introducing solids later. However, by the time the child was aged 3 months, one-quarter of UK mothers (24%) had introduced solid foods; this represented a substantial decrease over the rates in 1995, when 56 per cent of children were weaned by this age. Most mothers (85%) had introduced solids by 6 months. Solid food tended to be introduced at an earlier age in Northern Ireland, by mothers with heavier babies, by mothers in lower social classes, and by those with lower education levels. White mothers tended to introduce solids earlier than mothers of black, Asian or mixed ethnic origins. Mills and Taylor (1992), some 10 years previously, studied 488 infants aged 6–12 months, in whom solids had been introduced even earlier, probably indicating that there has been a change in infant nutrition. They found that commercial foods were important in the diets of the 6- to 9-month-old infants, but less so in the diet of the 9- to 12-month-olds. Commercial foods were a major source of the children's iron intake, and of those that ate no commercial feeds, only 62 per cent had the recommended nutritional intake. Not surprisingly, those with siblings were more likely to eat family foods.

By the age of 9–12 months, 50 per cent of the children had eaten chocolate (albeit in small amounts), and one-third had eaten crisps – again in contrast to recommendations to omit salt.

Mills and Taylor (1992) concluded that the diets were, on average, nutritionally adequate, although possibly short of zinc, iron and vitamin D. Clearly, parents did not do everything according to Department of Health recommendations in the early 1990s, but we need to ask if they do now – and if not, why this might be the case.

FEEDING THE PRE-SCHOOL CHILD

Nutrition in the early years is likely to impact on later life, with coronary heart disease, diabetes, some types of cancer and some bowel disorders and certainly obesity being linked to poor diet in early childhood. Good practices need to be established from weaning onwards, with children seeing good role models. As the child moves on to family food it may seem that recommendations for an adult diet become relevant. Recommendations aimed at the adult population need to be modified for the child. High-fibre, low-fat diets are not suitable for toddlers, who have a higher metabolic rate than adults and higher energy requirements per unit of body mass. In addition, a child's higher body surface area means that they lose more body heat. Attention needs to be paid to calorific intake, ensuring that the child has sufficient energy intake. The child who consistently fails to ingest sufficient calories, for whatever reason, will fail to thrive. Fat, particularly from whole milk, is an important source of calories in the early years. Although fibre in the form of fruit, vegetables and whole grains needs to be encouraged, care must be taken that the diet is not so bulky that the child is unable to obtain sufficient calories.

Iron deficiency is the most commonly reported nutritional disorder in early childhood (Department of Health, 1994). Although widespread among children in the UK, it is particularly common in families with low income, those of Asian origin and vegetarians. Children's dislike of meat, or a reluctance to chew it, exacerbates iron deficiency. Children so affected are likely to be apathetic, with reduced exercise capacity and possible psychomotor delay. However, some appear happy and healthy and remain undiagnosed (Department of Health, 1994). Iron can be supplied through meat and well-cooked eggs. Eating green leafy vegetables, grains and legumes can increase the iron intake of the vegetarian, and eating foods rich in vitamin C, such as oranges and kiwi fruit, can enhance the uptake of iron.

Vitamin D deficiency leads to rickets, a deficiency disease that affects the bones, with most cases being found among the Asian community. The number of cases has decreased in recent years, although children on a strict vegan diet or from Rastafarian families are also recognized as being at risk (Department of Health, 1994). Vitamin D is synthesized by the skin when exposed to sunlight, which may explain why communities from the Indian subcontinent are more at risk in the less sunny UK. Vitamin D can be obtained from commercially manufactured formula and follow-on milks. It is present in fatty fish such as sardines and herrings. These may not be acceptable to some families, nor palatable to many children. Eggs provide a minor source, and vitamin D is added to many margarines and spreads. Vitamin supplements including vitamin D are recommended from 1 to 5 years of age (Department of Health, 1994). However, these are not necessary if the child is breast-fed or is drinking formula or follow-on milk.

In some instances not enough thought is given to what pre-school children drink, and liquid, therefore, may only be given incidentally. Consequently some children do not receive sufficient fluid, while others are exposed to high levels of sugar which can impact adversely on their teeth, especially if taken via a bottle which directs the sweet drink to the back of their new teeth. Others receive large amounts of artificial sweeteners and colours, which may affect behaviour. Even apparently 'healthy' drinks may contain a limited proportion of fruit juice and a high degree of sugar. Tea is given to some young children, but this needs to be kept to a small amount as tannin reduces the absorption of minerals from food. Encouraging children to drink (and like) water is good practice – and it is of course free!

As with the weaning diet, the diet of pre-school children is subject to many influences. Toddlers have a small appetite, but their growth velocity is slowing down so they may need little more than a 1-year-old. The small size of the stomach means that he or she needs small frequent meals, but snacking – particularly on sugar-laden foods – should be avoided. Food refusal and definite food preferences are common, and are often used as a way of asserting personality. Clashes of will with the parent need to be separated from meal times where possible, with a calm approach being taken. Outside influences begin to bear directly on the child; for example, television advertising is increasingly difficult to withstand, but imitation of sound role models can be encouraged.

The diet of the family remains highly significant, with the child's diet being based on the cultural and religious norms of the family. The desire to do the 'right thing' by young children may be an opportunity to 'upgrade' the nutrition of the whole family, increasing the quantity of fruit, vegetables and whole grains, as well as decreasing the amount of refined carbohydrates and salt in the diet.

Vegetarians may be seen to be at risk of poor nutrition, but well-informed vegetarians are likely to have a well-balanced diet. Early years workers need to establish the type of vegetarian diet that is being followed. Some vegetarians may eat fish and dairy products, whereas others (vegans) exclude anything derived from animal origins from their diets. Depending upon the type of vegetarian diet followed, there may be difficulty in obtaining sufficient vitamin B_{12}, which can be given in a supplement, fortified soya milks or spreads. To ensure an adequate supply of amino acids to build protein, a mixture of vegetable proteins, beans, nuts and grains needs to be eaten each day. Vegetarian children will not have access to haem iron, but iron can be obtained from peas, beans, lentils and wholemeal grains, with vitamin C improving uptake. Calcium intake can be a problem for those who do not consume milk, but the mineral can be found in fortified soya milk, sesame seeds and some nuts.

Poverty is probably a more significant factor in limited pre-school nutrition. Families on low incomes are likely to eat only small amounts of fruit and vegetables, white bread rather than wholemeal bread, cheaper fatty meats rather than lean meats, and food that is fried and has a higher content of sugar and preservatives. These foods are eaten because they are usually cheaper and their familiarity means that they are less likely to be wasted. The very familiarity means that the eating habits of one generation form the basis of the eating habits of the next. However, these foods are contrary to virtually all dietary recommendations of recent years.

We know that parents appreciate what they should be doing (Blackburn, 1991). When parents were asked 'If you had an extra £10 to spend on food for your children, what foods would you like to buy?', the majority of 350 respondents in the National Children's Home (1991) survey said that they would buy fresh meat and poultry (60%), fruit (54%) and vegetables (38%). Only a minority said that they would buy 'unhealthy' luxuries such as cakes, biscuits and ice-cream. Parents in the same survey had often gone hungry in order to feed their children. Exhortations to use cheap markets and budget carefully are thwarted by poor transport, the lack of inclination of those caught up in long-term poverty, a general lack of choice in life, and the knowledge that the children must eat something, even if it is unhealthy.

The preceding discussion has demonstrated that feeding children the 'right' diet can become a complex issue. In summary, children should be offered foods from each of the following four main food groups:

- starch foods, such as potatoes, bread and rice;
- protein foods, such as meat, fish and pulses;
- fatty foods, such as milk, cheese and eggs;
- fruit and vegetables.

Foods with a high sugar content should be taken in small amounts, and hidden fats in fried and commercially prepared foods should be kept to a minimum. Attention also needs to be paid to the possibility of iron deficiency.

Children in the UK are rarely malnourished, but it seems that many are suffering from sub-nutrition. These are likely to be children who are already disadvantaged in other ways. With poorer nutrition than some of their peers, it may be that they are less likely to benefit from care and education programmes to which they have access.

SCHOOLCHILDREN'S DIET AND BEYOND

In recent years, children have become taller and heavier – sometimes too heavy. A national study on the nutrition of school-aged children (Gregory and Lowe, 2000) indicated that some things had improved in comparison to earlier studies. These authors concluded that children and young people generally were consuming less fat, but worryingly one child in five ate no fruit at all in a typical week. They also identified that 8.5% of 6-year-olds are obese, and many more are overweight.

Obesity has had a high profile in the popular press in recent years, and it appears that a high proportion of adults and increasingly children are either overweight or obese

(Reilly *et al.*, 1999; Chinn and Rona, 2001). Obesity from poor nutrition may have an impact on their future health, in turn contributing to coronary heart disease and joint problems, yet even in childhood it may well affect the self-esteem, giving them a negative self-image and increasing their risk of taunting or bullying by other children. Children, even those under the age of 8, need to be involved in the strategies to prevent and deal with obesity. This needs to be done in partnership with parents, carers, school, and their local community. Preventing obesity and generally improving nutrition is part of the Food in Schools Programme (Department of Health, 2004), a joint venture between the Department for Education and Skills and the Department of Health. The programme is worked out differently in different schools, but includes breakfast clubs, tuck shops, work on lunch boxes as well as water provision.

Work with children and parents on child nutrition may involve the giving of information on what should be eaten, albeit in a friendly, non-threatening and fun way, although as noted earlier many know what is the healthy choice. Structural change may contribute towards an alteration of what children eat. It may be a case of changing what is available at snack time; for example, the government fruit scheme (Department of Health, 2002) now available in all schools should help here. School meals – particularly with young children – have the potential to give them a hot, nutritionally sound meal, thereby exposing them to foods that are not part of the family diet. The government guidelines (DfES, 2000) for school lunches are having a positive effect. Fruit and vegetables must be available every day, and fruit-based desserts should be available twice a week. Food from the starch group, or foods cooked in fat or oil should not be offered more than three days each week, while red meat should be served at least twice a week and fish at least weekly.

While nutrition is important and has formed a major part of this chapter, a reduction in the sedentary behaviour of all is part of reducing obesity and promoting the physical well-being of us all. Those working with school-aged children need to ensure that there is physical activity during the school day (there is a government target to increase the number of children (aged 5–16 years) who have 2 hours of physical education and sports each week) and to encourage after-school games, dancing or similar. Walking children to school may be part of this regime, and a 'walking bus', where volunteers or paid escorts walk children to school via a set route, will facilitate this.

Conclusion

Knowledge of growth and development is an important part of the competency requirements for working with children, so that professionals are able to maximize the potential of each child and detect when a child is not developing normally. The routine monitoring of growth and development is currently a crucial part of the work of many early years professionals, but it needs to be done sensitively and without rigidity. Over the next decade, as the proposals of Hall and Elliman (2003) are fully adopted, such monitoring will become more focussed upon only those screening activities that meet certain criteria (DH/DfES, 2004).

Optimum growth and development needs can be viewed much more broadly than physical growth and the attainment of motor skills. One view, outlined in this chapter, is dependent upon a variety of components that may be seen as a hierarchy of needs, with the most basic needs requiring to be met before those of a higher order. The meeting of a basic survival need of nutrition, which initially seems simple and concrete, is itself influenced by a variety of social, economic and physiological factors.

Overall, however, growth and development are influenced by the early experiences of the child. We took nutrition as an exemplar of this, looking at how parental choices related to feeding can influence development from birth through to school age. There are many more examples that we could have used, and suggest that you take a further example for the student activity below.

Student activity

In this chapter we have taken one factor – nutrition – and looked at how it affects growth and development. Select a different factor – for example, exercise, exposure to tobacco smoke or other pollutants, geographic location (rural versus urban living), or think of a factor of your own – and identify the impact of your chosen factor on the growth and development of infants, pre-school and school-age children.

REFERENCES

Barker, H (2002): *Nutrition and Dietetics for Health Care*, 10th edn. Edinburgh: Churchill Livingstone.

Blackburn, C (1991): *Poverty and Health*. Buckingham: Open University Press.

Chinn, S and Rona, RJ (2001): Prevalence and trends in overweight and obesity in three cross-sectional studies of British children 1974–94. *British Medical Journal*, **322**, 24–26.

Cordon, L, Ingram, J, Hamid, N and Hussein, A (2003): Cultural influences on breast feeding and weaning. *Community Practitioner*, **76**(9), 344–349.

Department for Education and Skills (2000): *Summary of the Education (Nutritional Standards for School Lunches) (England) Regulations*. Nottinghamshire: DfES.

Department for Education and Skills (2003): *Excellence and Enjoyment – a Strategy for Primary Schools*. Nottinghamshire: DfES.

Department of Health (1994): *Weaning and the Weaning Diet*. London: HMSO.

Department of Health (2002): *National School Fruit Scheme*. Information for schools. London: Department of Health.

Department of Health (2004): *Food in Schools Programmes*. www.dh.gov.uk

Department of Health/Department for Education and Skills (2004): *National Service Framework for Children, Young People and Maternity Services*. London: DoH.

Frankenburg, WK and Dodds, JB (1967): Denver developmental screening test. *Journal of Paediatrics*, **71**, 181–191.

Fry, T (1993): Charting growth: developments in the assessment and measurement of child growth. *Child Health*, **1**, 104–109.

Gregory, J and Lowe, S (2000): *National Diet and Nutrition Survey: Young Children Aged 4 to 18 years. Vol. 1: Report of the Diet and Nutrition Survey*. London: Stationery Office.

Hall, DBM and Elliman D (2003): *Health for all Children*, 4th edn. Oxford: Oxford University Press.

Hamlyn, B, Brooker, S, Oleinikova, K and Wands, S (2002): *Infant Feeding 2000*. London: The Stationery Office.

Maslow, AH (1987): *Motivation and Personality*, 3rd edn. New York: Harper and Row.

Mills, A and Taylor, H (1992): *Food and Nutritional Intakes of British Infants 6–12 Months*. London: Ministry of Agriculture, Food and Fisheries.

Minchin, M (1985): *Breastfeeding Matters*. Victoria, Australia: Alma Publications.

National Children's Home (1991): *Poverty and Nutrition Survey*. London: National Children's Home.

Odijk, J van, Kull, I, Borres, MP, *et al.* (2003): Breastfeeding and allergic disease: a multidisciplinary review of the literature (1966–2001) on the mode of early feeding in infancy and its impact on later atopic manifestations. *Allergy*, **58**(9), 833–843.

Reilly, JJ, Dorosty, AR and Emmett, PM (1999): Prevalence of overweight and obesity in British children: cohort study. *British Medical Journal*, **319**, 1039.

Sheridan, M (1997): *From Birth to Five: Children's Developmental Progress*. London: Routledge.

Thompson, J (2002): The benefits of breastfeeding and current controversies: part 1. *Community Practitioner*, **75**(2), 64–65.

White, A, Freeth, S and O'Brien, M (1992): *Infant Feeding 1990*. London: HMSO.

World Health Organization (2002): *Infant and Young Child Nutrition: Global Strategy on Infant and Young Children Feeding: Report by the Secretariat*. 55th World Health Assembly. WHO A55/15.

FURTHER READING

Barker, H (2002): Diet in infancy, childhood and adolescence. In Barker, H., *Nutrition and Dietetics for Health Care*, 10th edn. Edinburgh: Churchill Livingstone, pp. 129–146.

Bee, H and Boyd, D (2002): *Lifespan Development*, 3rd edn. New York: Allyn and Baker.

Berk, L (2003): *Child Development*, 6th edn. New York: Allyn and Baker.

Coad, J and Tunstall, M (2001): *Anatomy and Physiology for Midwives*. London: Mosby.

Department of Health (1994): *Weaning and the Weaning Diet*. London: HMSO.

Hall, DBM and Elliman D (2003): *Health for all Children*, 4th edn. Oxford: Oxford University Press.

Polnay, L (ed.) (2003): *Community Paediatrics*, 3rd edn. Edinburgh: Churchill Livingstone.

Sheridan, M (1997): *From Birth to Five: Children's Developmental Progress*. Windsor: NFER-Nelson.

PERSONAL, SOCIAL AND EMOTIONAL DEVELOPMENT

Anne Greig

This chapter aims to:

- examine the holistic aspects of personal, social and emotional development within individuals and in reference to the social and cultural systems in which children develop;

- introduce and critically evaluate the latest theories on personal, social and emotional development.

INTRODUCTION

> *Often, that sunny autumn, when the weather permitted, the small girls took their lessons seated on three benches arranged around the elm. 'Hold up your books,' said Miss Brodie quite often that autumn, 'prop them up in your hands, in case of intruders. If there are any intruders, we are doing our history lesson … or our poetry … English grammar.' The small girls held up their books with their eyes not on them, but on Miss Brodie. 'In the meantime I will tell you about my last summer holiday in Egypt … I will tell you about the care of the skin, and of the hands … about the Frenchman I met on the train to Biarritz … and I must tell you about the Italian paintings I saw. Who is the greatest Italian painter?'*
> *'Leonardo da Vinci, Miss Brodie'.*
> *'That is incorrect. The answer is Giotto, he is my favourite.'*
> (*The Prime of Miss Jean Brodie*, Muriel Spark, pp. 10–11, 1961/1980)

The fabulous Miss Brodie, above, so obviously 'in her prime' but also, perhaps, a little ahead of her time! Her subversive lessons on matters personal, social and emotional suggested that, in her classroom, the likes of history, poetry and grammar were not everything. Today's reality is that leading authors and researchers are producing convincing evidence that IQ is not, indeed, everything, and that other forms of intelligence, including personal, social and emotional intelligences, are just as important for successful life outcomes (Block, 1995; Gardner, 1993; Goleman, 1996). These other intelligences are now finding their way on to the curriculum, albeit in less significant ways than the traditionally valued intelligences of literacy and numeracy.

In this respect, early years professionals have always been ahead of the times with the established view that early childhood is a period of rapid development of all psychological functions (language, social interaction, physical growth, moral and spiritual intelligences) that are interdependent and best fostered by an holistic approach that is sensitive to the whole child (Hughes and Kleinberg, 1999; see Introduction of this book). Children have to learn to cope with people and settings outwith the family, become increasingly independent, and form positive social relationships, particularly with other children (Howes, 1988; Hartup, 1992; Hay, 1994). To support children through this significant step, we are advised that providing secure, warm and caring relationships, giving praise appropriately, encouraging humour and helping children to feel good about themselves is necessary if children are to have good mental health and to be able to take advantage of the learning environment (e.g. Sylva, 1994; Ladd *et al.*, 1999; SCCC, 1999; Trevarthen, 1997).

Nevertheless, there is considerable evidence of society failing children in exactly this way. Political priorities for raising academic achievement often seemed to render personal, social and emotional (PSE) education the 'Cinderella' of educational and welfare reform, although for several years there has been increased reporting of PSE-related problems in even the youngest children. For example, Campbell (1991) reported that 25 per cent of pre-schoolers and early primary children met the criteria for oppositional defiant disorder or early-onset conduct problems. More recently, Greig (2004) reviewed the evidence and nature of depression in school children, noting that an estimated eight in every 400 primary school pupils could be depressed at any one time, and two in 100 children aged under 12 years needed psychiatric help (see also Meltzer *et al.*, 2000). Figures for poor areas, difficult social circumstances and during adolescence can be double this (MIND, 2001). Those children with emotional problems were observed to be the least likely to be in contact with services. Thus, Goodyer (2001) suggested that early years professionals have a key role to play in early detection and intervention. Getting off to a good start does appear to be critical for many children. There is certainly some evidence that criminal actions are carried out to a greater extent by persons who have a history of early childhood aggression (Kazdin, 1995), and many antisocial children remain involved with mental health agencies throughout their lives. Indeed, risk factors identified for youth crime often overlap with mental health and school failure problems (Rutter *et al.*, 1998). As the antisocial acts of a 5-year-old may be prototypic of the acts of the delinquent adolescent, the younger the child is at the time of the intervention beginning, the more positive the subsequent adjustment to home and school (Estrada and Pinsof, 1995; Kovacs, 1997).

It is in consideration of these serious consequences of the neglect of the development of the PSE competencies, especially in the early years, that the view is taken here that we ignore them at our peril. It has been noted by Orbach (1997) that:

'... *(society needs to) create an emotionally literate culture, where the facility to handle the complexities of emotional life is as widespread as the capacity to read, write and do Arithmetic'.*

This chapter is an exploration of the other 'literacies': personal, social and emotional (PSE). This includes an examination of the theoretical basis that defines the PSE competencies and a contextual analysis of PSE development in the early years.

A THEORETICAL REVIEW OF PERSONAL, SOCIAL AND EMOTIONAL (PSE) COMPETENCE

Although the PSE competencies have been extensively addressed in the literature to date, it has not yet resulted in a single, integrated theory (Guralnick, 1997). Nevertheless, in a research field that is constantly evolving, considerable insights have been gained in recent times. There are several different theories that could be presented, in their own right, as organizing constructs for the interactive competencies of early childhood. These include:

- emotional and multiple intelligences or competencies theories (Gardner, 1984, 1993; Goleman, 1996);
- social competence theory (including self/other, autonomy/connectedness dimensions; Rose-Krasnor, 1997);
- the theory of the development of pro-social competence (Hay, 1994; Hay *et al.*, 1999);
- attachment theory (e.g. Bowlby, 1980, 1991; Crittenden, 1992);
- theory of mind or social understanding (Baron-Cohen, 1993; Dunn, 1988, 1994);
- transactional theories and theories on the influences of systems, ecology, and dialectical relationships (e.g. Bronfenbrenner, 1986, 1992; Hinde, 1992, 1997).

The first two theories are not specifically directed at young children or the developmental precursors of competence. They do however, potentially inform about the nature of the 'skills' associated with competence. The theories of mind, attachment and pro-social behaviour, are developmental and reflect on early socialization systems, but, until fairly recently, the overlaps in skills, processes and mechanisms common amongst them have been relatively unexplored. Each theory contains significant elements of the others. Hence, the complex and interacting nature of social, emotional and cognitive functions makes it difficult to ascertain where one theory ends and another begins. The approach taken within this chapter, therefore, is to use the concept of multiple intelligence (Gardner, 1983), and in particular the interpersonal and intrapersonal intelligences (Gardner, 1993), as an organizing construct within which to explore the development of the personal, social and emotional competencies which contribute to it.

Defining emotional intelligence and emotional literacy

According to Gardner (1993, p. 9), emotional intelligence is both inter- and intra-personal:

> 'Interpersonal intelligence is the ability to understand other people: what motivates them, how they work, how to work co-operatively with them. Intrapersonal intelligence is a correlative ability, turned inward. It is a capacity to form an accurate, veridical model of oneself and to be able to use that model to operate effectively in life.'

The meaning of this for early childhood was described by Saarni (1990, p. 116), who noted that this competency enables children to '... respond emotionally, yet simultaneously and strategically apply their knowledge about emotions and their expression to relationships with others, so that they can negotiate interpersonal exchanges and regulate their emotional experiences.' Nevertheless, in his ancient wisdom in *The Nicomachean Ethics*, Aristotle (cited in Goleman, 1996, p. 6), lets us know what a tall order this is for anyone, let alone children:

> '*Anyone can become angry – that is easy. But to be angry with the right person, to the right degree, at the right time, for the right purpose, and in the right way – that is not easy.*'

In an early childhood context, an 'emotional literacy' interpretation of Aristotle's observations allows us to consider emotional intelligence as a matter of a type of care and education that facilitates the young child's needs to be:

- emotionally reflective about himself/herself and others;
- able to regulate emotions;
- able to use emotion positively;
- responsible for emotional mistakes.

('Antidote', 2003; Steiner and Perry, 1997).

Just as there is evidence of the damage caused by emotional illiteracy, there is growing evidence about the resilience features of emotional competence from longitudinal studies. Children who have good emotion recognition skills at age 5 are more likely to have good social skills and academic ability at age 9 (Izard *et al.*, 2001). As observed by Damasio (1996), a loss of contact with emotions breaks down rationality which (with learning) requires the support of our emotions (Goleman, 1996). Even in the early pre-school period, the positive contributions of emotional competence to social competence over the longer term mean that teaching about feelings is important even before the age of 4 years. Those children who are especially emotional may benefit from learning a means to avoid dysregulated coping and how to respond to the emotions of others pro-socially instead of antisocially (Denham *et al.*, 2003).

This brief emotional literacy review illustrates the interdependence of the PSE competencies. This is a broad interpretation of 'intelligence' that presents a useful framework for the exploration of the themes of this chapter:

1. Skills approaches.
2. Theoretical approaches – interacting processes (or systems).
3. The developmental progression of personal, social and emotional competences.

Initially, evidence will be drawn from a variety of programmes that mainly targeted older children and teenagers in order to extract skill-based definitions of each competency in isolation from an early childhood developmental model. The general limitations of these approaches will be explored. A brief exploration of the relevant theories will follow. Finally, the personal, social and emotional development of the child in the early years will be mapped out, together with a contextual examination of mediating factors.

SKILLS APPROACHES

Stone and Dillehunt (1978) chose to emphasize *personal* skills or '*self-science*'. This was broadly defined as 'a sense of self in relations to others', a theme which will presently be seen to recur in other approaches. These *skills* could be summarized into a few main headings: awareness of self and others; understanding and insight into the thoughts and emotions of self and others; empathy; and co-operation. Although this theory predates the emergence of the theory of mind literature and the theory of pro-social development (see below), it is, in effect, the importance of these that researchers had recognized.

Salovey and Mayer (1990) emphasized the emotional domain skills which can be summarized as including the recognition of emotion, its regulation and management in both self and in relationships with others. As before, the importance of perspective taking regarding emotional awareness is relevant to the theory of mind literature and implicit is attachment theory (see below) in its recognition of the importance of the emotional quality of relationships.

The Grant Consortium project on the school-based promotion of social competence was both a skill and multi-domain approach (CPPRG, 2002a,b; Greenberg and Kusche, 1998). The authors took care to find appropriate skills for the psychological domains of cognition, emotion and behaviour. The skills of *emotion* could be summarized as the recognition, gauging and management (or regulation) of emotional states. The *cognitive* skills could be summarized as ways of processing information (or ways of going about understanding the social world and oneself within it). It could be argued here then, that the cognitive dimension includes the understanding and integration of the self and others as already noted in other approaches. Appropriate social *behaviours* included pro-social responses, positive peer relationships and the skills of verbal and non-verbal communication. Again, the overlaps between many of the skills are apparent; for instance, to what extent is the ability to interpret social cues a cognitive skill or a social skill? The themes of self in relation to others, perspective taking, empathy and quality of relationships are also again evident.

The final skills approach to be considered at this stage is that of Rose-Krasnor (1997). In defining social competence as 'effectiveness in interaction', Rose-Krasnor begins with the two major domains of the 'self' and 'other' (or autonomy or connectedness). Whilst other approaches have noted the importance of these two domains, they have not been given the same construct status. Hence, the personal *systems* that support inter- and intra-personal intelligence could be construed here as the 'self system' and the 'other system'. Social skills within the 'self system' could be summarized as a sense of self-efficacy, agency and success in achieving one's own goals. Social skills within the 'other system' could be summarized as quality and status in peer relationships, social responsibility and good social network supports. Behavioural and motivational skills supporting these systems include integration of self and other perspectives, emotional security and regulation, empathy and communicative and problem-solving abilities.

Consistent with all approaches reviewed above, a number of key processes or mechanisms emerge as playing a crucial role in the skills for inter/intra-personal intelligences. These are understanding of self and others' perspectives and feelings, attachment security including quality of relationships and relating, and pro-social action. These appear to be significant 'within-system (self/other)' skills for the PSE competencies alongside other cognitive skills linked to communication and problem solving. An undue emphasis, however, on skills and specific skill domains may be over-simplifying what is meant by a 'skill', describing each as if they were individually and separately attainable with little attention to developmental processes and interacting mechanisms. Simple lists of underlying social competence 'skills', even if located within a specific 'system', do not address the fact that both skills and systems interact with each other in complex and important ways throughout the course of early childhood development. It also tends to mask the fact that these 'skills' are largely the products of early socialization (e.g. Hay *et al.*, 1999; Dunn, 1996;

Fonagy *et al.*, 1997; Saarni, 1990). These observations serve to illustrate the complex and interdependent nature of these skills (and systems) and suggest that a purely skills-based approach may be of limited help in assisting assessment and intervention.

In general, the 'skills' authors did not seek to address the overlapping nature of skills, systems and developmental progression. Indeed, the above lists of competencies read as a daunting prospect of achievement even for many adults. There is a need to interpret 'skills' in a developmentally appropriate way and in the context of the more recent research on the emergence of children's social understanding, on attachment theory, on the nature of pro-social development and on how these 'domains' actually interact (Greig and Howe, 2001; Harris, 1999; Meins, 1999; Hay, 1994; Hay *et al.*, 1999). In order, therefore, to address the inherent weaknesses of the predominantly 'skills'-based approaches, it is necessary to review other relevant theories in some detail and to consider potential contributions to the bigger picture of personal, social and emotional intelligences. This includes theories of developmental psychopathology; humanism; attachment; social understanding; and pro-social development.

THEORETICAL APPROACHES: INTERACTING DEVELOPMENTAL PROCESSES AND MECHANISMS

Cicchetti (1992) addressed the development of socio-emotional problems within an integrated, multi-causal, developmental and systemic framework. The three principal elements to Cicchetti's theory were causes, developmental tasks and systems. *Causes*, he argued, are not unidimensional. For instance, depression in childhood has a variety of symptom patterns and sources and it is not always possible to determine exact causes. Rather, it is more a matter of contributing factors. This is arguably true of many early childhood personal, social and emotional disorders. *Developmental tasks* refers to the successful completion or attainment of a number of regulatory functions. These include physiological regulation, affect differentiation, self–other awareness and attachment to caretakers. *Systems* refers to the fact that the successful attainment of these tasks may become thwarted by dysfunctional systems such as the family, school and society. So, for example, in the case of childhood depression as described by Cicchetti, a dysfunctional family environment (or system) is likely to involve poor parenting, parental mental health problems, low socio-economic status and income, and higher proportions of significant life events, stresses and difficulties such as unemployment, divorce, single-parenthood, etc. A dysfunctional school environment (or system) is likely to have features that increase emotional risks at transition times and to be lacking a caring, nurturing environment that can, in turn, trigger mental health problems. The school is also thought to play a key role in accessing the wider ecology of support services and helping children and families to take advantage of working alongside other service providers. The final, and potentially thwarting, system is that of political forces such as the availability of government resources to prevent or improve children's social and emotional problems.

Humanism, self-concept and self-esteem

The importance of the healthy development of the self-concept and self-esteem has been established for quite some time by seminal works in social and humanistic psychology. Baldwin's (1906/1894) self-discrepancy theory was an important early Vygotskian reference to self-esteem as being social in origin, and defined as the discrepancy between the perception of an actual self (attributes persons believe they possess) and an ideal self (attributes persons believe they would like to possess). There is, in addition, an 'ought-self' that refers to attributes persons think they ought to possess. The suffering caused by such discrepancies that result in a low self-esteem has been noted to be associated with specific patterns, for example, an actual-ideal discrepancy leads to dejection, disappointment and sadness and an actual-ought discrepancy leads to agitation, apprehension and nervousness (Higgins, 1989). The self-esteem needs of children are therefore crucial for good mental health. Maslow (1954/1970) pointed out that, without healthy self-esteem, children would have impairments in cognitive exploration and aesthetic aspirations that would result in a failure to develop their full individual potential. According to Maslow, an individual child will achieve 'self-actualization' in all developmental tasks or competencies only if certain successive foundations are successfully laid in early development (see also Chapter 3, p. 46). In his *hierarchy of needs*, the most basic foundation (level 1) is for physiological or survival needs such as sufficient food and water. Once this is in place, the child needs to feel secure and safe, both physically and emotionally (level 2). Successful attainment in these needs will nurture the needs of love, affection and belonging (level 3). Once these are in place for a child, the need of self-esteem (level 4) can be achieved. Once the conditions of levels 1 to 4 have been met, the child can become self-actualized by an ability to access play and learning opportunities, engaging in the learning process, and having experiences of success and control (level 5). Within a PSE framework, educators have accepted this pivotal, developmental role of self-esteem and are seeking to better assess (Davis-Kean and Sandler, 2001) and promote it in young children (Lawrence, 1987; Emler, 2001; Mosley, 1996, 2001; Dalgleish, 2002; Roberts, 2002; Donnellan, 2003). For a recent socio-cultural extension of Baldwin's theory, see Bizman and Yinon (2004) and Dweck (1999).

Attachment theory

The seminal work of Ainsworth *et al.* (1978) identified three patterns of child behaviour in unfamiliar or fearful situations (which includes learning situations): the secure pattern and two types of insecure patterns, avoidant and ambivalent. Insecure children have developed an insecure, avoidant and coercive strategy using threats, bribes and inappropriate emotional displays. Secure children are better able to use the mother as a secure zone in order to explore and play in the surrounding environment. According to Crittenden (1992), however, the new pre-school developmental task associated with attachment involves the adjustment of the partnership towards the potentially differing goals of the child and mother and includes aspects of reciprocity, perspective taking, management of relationships and empathy. Crittenden (1992) identified three strategies and one combination strategy relevant to pre-schoolers based on studies of children including maltreated and emotionally abused children: secure, insecure-defended, insecure-coercive, and insecure defended/coercive (or disorganized). These attachment behaviours are typically manifested during situations of perceived stress or danger.

Whilst the most severely affected children with respect to attachment security will require a multi-agency support system in the way of a planned intervention, other researchers are now beginning to 'take attachment theory to school', documenting the role that teachers and schools play at stressful periods for children, notably transition, and how they can help children to feel more secure (Dunn, 1994). Others have been looking at attachments to daycare workers and teachers as a means of compensating for difficulties elsewhere and at the links between the home and school environments with respect to attachment behaviours and supports (De Mulder *et al.*, 2000; Mitchell-Copeland *et al.*, 1997; Cabello and Terrell, 1999). Early childhood professionals interested in supporting the educational and social interests of vulnerable children, such as children in care or those with emotional disorders, can find the theoretical, assessment and intervention models of attachment in Howe (1995) and Howe *et al.* (1999), and in two of a series of three books by Daniel and Wassell (2002/2004a,b). See also Chapter 5, pp. 85–87, for more information about attachment.

Social understanding: theory of mind and emotion

In the extensive body of literature now existing, 'theory of mind' refers to the ability to infer other people's mental states such as their thoughts, intentions, desires, feelings and beliefs. The skill is an ability to use this understanding to interpret and make sense of people's actions and predict what they will do next (Dennett, 1978). More recent practical formulations now refer to theory of mind as 'mind-reading' or 'social understanding' (Howlin *et al.*, 1999; Dunn, 1994; Greig and Howe, 2001). Indeed, Howlin *et al.* noted the valuable contribution that the ability to mind-read makes to understanding subtle aspects of communicative intent (including the figurative aspects of humour, irony, sarcasm and metaphor); in deception; in appreciating emotion in others; in self-reflection (thinking about one's own thinking); and in attempting to change the minds of others. Those who are afflicted by the 'mind-blindness' characteristic of autism will suffer from a formidable list of interpersonal problems including insensitivity to the feelings of other people; the inability to read and respond to what others know, intend, or perceive; failure to understand misunderstandings, unwritten rules or conventions, deception, and reasons for others' actions. Children progress from the ability to understand what others see, through how things look to others to the significant achievement around three years of age that 'seeing-leads-to-knowing' (the understanding that the child who has seen inside a container will know the contents and the child who touched the container will not know). It is not until about 4 years of age that children are able to pass the 'theory of mind' test: the false-belief task. In this test, the child is presented with a puppet-play scenario involving Anne who has a box and Sally who has a basket. The child sees how puppet Sally puts a marble into her basket in front of puppet Anne, and then Sally goes away for a walk. When Sally has gone, the child sees Anne take the marble from the basket and put it into her box. Sally comes back and wants to play with her marble. The child is then asked where Sally will look for the marble (in the basket or in the box). By 4 years of age, most children are able to appreciate that Sally will have a false belief about where the marble is now located (Wimmer and Perner, 1983).

The ability to pass the false-belief task is now known to be influenced by certain socialization experiences such as attachment security; symbolic mentalizing ability; number of siblings and quality of relationships and pretend play with mothers and siblings (e.g. Perner *et al.*, 1994; see development section below). Researchers are now considering that mind and emotion understanding may be distinct but nonetheless overlapping (Greig and Howe, 2001; Denham *et al.*, 1994), demonstrating that the ability to read the minds and emotions of others is related in complex ways to other psychological processes and mechanisms such as attachment and self-awareness. Indeed, Goodyer (2001) described the development of emotional

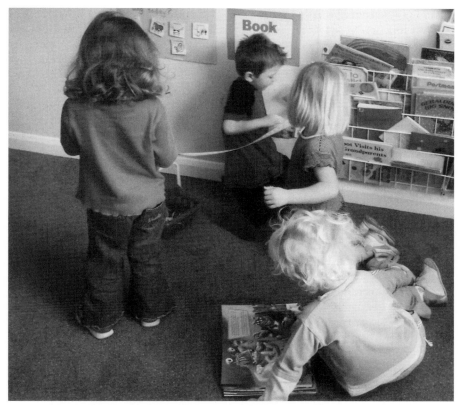

Figure 4.1   Co-operation is an important developmental milestone.

intelligence as occurring within the development of a theory of mind, and how thinking affects both emotion and behaviour. He advocates a cognitive-behavioural approach (teaching about the links between thinking, feeling and behaving) to early interventions for children encountering early problems in understanding the minds and emotions of self and others. Other researchers believe it is possible to teach children emotion and mind-reading abilities (Howlin *et al.*, 1999; Dunn, 1994; Baron-Cohen, 2004).

Pro-social development

Being social, getting along with others, co-operating with them and helping them is an important developmental milestone. According to Hobson (2002), thought itself emerges through social relationships! Mind- and emotion-reading abilities are indeed prerequisites for pro-social action, enabling us to 'empathize' with others and form healthy relationships. Empathy has been defined as 'an affective response more appropriate to someone else's situation than to one's own' (Hoffman, 1987), and is therefore an ability that has the potential to ensure adaptive responses to distress in others. The fact that individuals can vary considerably in their pro-social tendencies has also been linked to experiences of socialization such as levels of parental affection, attachment security, parental mental health, family discussion and explanations of feelings of self and of others (e.g. see Hay, 1994; Hay *et al.*, 1999 for reviews; Denham, 1986). Hay recommends that the emergence of pro-social competence should not be conceived as a linear, developmental progression but rather as being partly a function of self–other perspective taking, attachment mechanisms and the socialization experiences that mediate them. Individual difference could be said to be operating with some individuals (and genders) being clearly more caring and sharing than others. Developmentally (see also below), the important, early pro-social milestones include the diminishing of the initial pro-social reflex; the emergence of gender differentiation in pro-social action as a result of socialization experiences; and the emergence of increasing social understanding. It is Hay's contention that the failure to regulate early pro-social action may lead to later psychopathy. Expanding somewhat on the ideas of both Rose-Krasnor and Cicchetti, Hay recommended the study of long-term, developmental, pro-social changes that span time and consider particular relationships, social contexts and family characteristics such as parental mental health and numbers of siblings.

Friendship in the early years is crucially important to young children (Howes, 1988; Hartup, 1992), and the ability in the early years to co-operate with others and to form positive peer relationships is known to contribute to emotional, social and academic competence in later childhood; it also serves as a protective factor against externalizing problems (Hay and Pawlby, 2003). There can be longer-term mental health problems however for children who are highly pro-social and those who consistently fail to establish mutual, positive peer relationships (Hay *et al.*, 2004).

To summarize the various theories reviewed, it would appear to be essential for professionals to be aware of the systems that potentially help or hinder the child's successful attainment of the developmental tasks that are required for effective personal, social and emotional competencies. Also required is the appreciation that failure to attain developmental tasks means that certain child needs will simply not be met, thereby increasing the likelihood that the child will fail to thrive personally, socially, emotionally and educationally. Furthermore, what has been repeatedly described are several 'nominally different but clearly overlapping children's abilities, namely, to interpret the mental states of others, to empathize with their feelings, and to adopt their differing social perspectives' (Warden and Christie, 1997). These, in turn, are affected by early socialization experiences such as early attachment relationships. In order to better understand such competencies, theorists advocate both a developmental and systemic approach. This chapter will therefore conclude with a systemic overview of the development of these personal, social and emotional competencies in the early years.

THE DEVELOPMENT OF PERSONAL, SOCIAL AND EMOTIONAL (PSE) COMPETENCE

Below is a summary of the main developmental milestones and precursors to personal, social and emotional competences in the early years, according to recent research accounts. Each developmental 'stage' description is followed by a brief consideration of the evidence indicating how systems can hinder the development of crucial developmental tasks known to mediate the inter- and intra-personal intelligences.

First 8 months

The first 6–8 months of a child's life is a period of early preverbal communication sequences between infant and carer when they become 'attuned' to each other. This is a basic form of empathic exchanges, during which the child's feelings, such as smiling, are sensed by the parent, played back to the child by the parent in a manner demonstrating that the child's feelings are understood, and reciprocated by the carer (Stern, 1987). Prototypical conversational exchanges occur in the babbling exchanges between infant and carer as the child learns to co-operate in collaborative exchanges and turn-taking with others. This occurs during feeding, caring and playing routines (e.g. Hubley and Trevarthen, 1979; Hay, 1979). Infants also show a form of early empathic reactions by crying when they hear the distress of others, feeling it as if it were their own (Zahn-Waxler and Radke-Yarrow, 1990). An infant this young does not yet have a sense of self-separate-from-others, but nevertheless shows a preference for same-sex faces (Lewis and Brooks, 1974).

Impact of socialization by 8 months

Early socialization experiences with carers can disrupt these early, formative, interactive processes. For example, infants of mentally ill, rejecting or neglectful carers may fail to bond or to become attuned. Infants can also 'catch' depression from carers. Thus early interactive experiences may put a child at a greater risk of later emotional and social disorders (Murray, 1992; Cummings and Davies, 1994).

12 months

Between 8 and 12 months, the child attains the awareness of object permanence and an associated sense of self as separate from others. Empathically, this means that they begin to understand that others' distress is not their own, yet may react inappropriately (e.g. by wiping their own eyes upon observing another's tears) (Dunn and Brown, 1991). This 'motor mimicry' lasts until the second year. The infant also develops a fear of strangers as a result of the newly developed 'object permanence' of the mother (e.g. Ainsworth *et al.*, 1978).

Impact of socialization by 12 months

Early socialization experiences with the carer can lead to the formation of either a secure or insecure attachment to the carer. A parent who is not attuned to the child's fear, who does not return to the child in times of distress and anxiety, creates the possibility of an internal working model of expectations of responses from others (Murray, 1992; Stern, 1987; Bowlby, 1980). Hence, either a secure or insecure behavioural pattern of responding to situations involving the unfamiliar, change, stress or anxiety is established and continued in interactions with others, with pathological outcomes for disorganized infants perhaps even into adulthood (Crittenden, 1992).

18 to 36 months

At around 18 months the child develops a sense of pretence that enables simple pretend or symbolic play (e.g. a rope is a snake) (Leslie, 1987). A growing vocabulary during the second year creates a new medium for the continuation of attuned (or indeed not attuned) interactive sequences with carers and, by 2 years, the beginning of the ability to negotiate to achieve self-interests. Children become more self-assertive and begin to develop a sense of guilt or conscience together with self-regulatory capacities (Kagan, 1989; Kochanska, 1993). Gender-appropriate toy preferences and play styles emerge, with boys being notably more aggressive than girls and having a general preference for same-sex playmates (Maccoby and Jacklin, 1980). They may also begin to spend more time with peers and form their first friendships – a social context in which they learn to co-operate with others and jointly solve problems (Howes, 1988). There is an increasing ability to demonstrate actual care or comfort for others in distress and by about 3 years, it becomes apparent that some

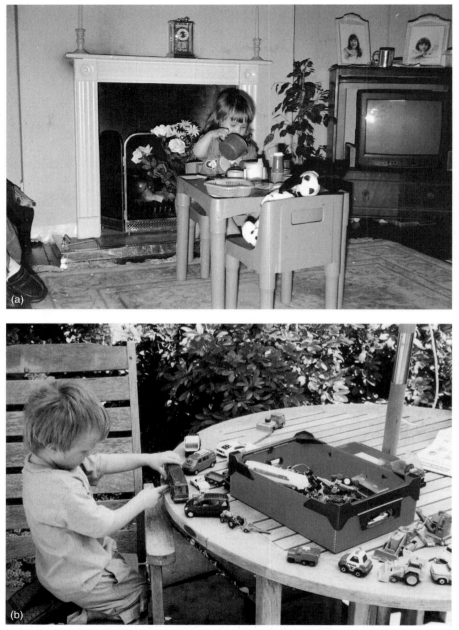

Figure 4.2 (a and b)   Gender-appropriate toy preferences and play styles emerge between 18 and 36 months.

children are becoming more caring (Dunn and Munn, 1986) and sharing than others (Hay *et al.*, 1993). Most children of this age are able to co-operate with carers in simple household duties (Hay, 1994) and are becoming aware of the norms in their families and communities that regulate their behaviour, such as teatime rules and moral imperatives (such as no hitting or violence) (Dunn and Munn, 1987).

Impact of socialization at this stage

Early problems of socialization, including day care experiences, mean that some children may, due to insecurity, unregulated fear or anxiety, fail to access and form successful peer relationships. Children whose carers have failed to become attuned to them may lack the interactive skills to positively access others and the strategies to defend themselves from bullies. This is important because there is evidence indicating that the patterns of interaction at pre-school associated with later conduct problems, depression and withdrawal may have originated in these very early relationships (Denham *et al.*, 1990; Rose-Krasnor, 1997). Children who do attend day care will be experiencing their first home–care transitions, a potentially fearful encounter for most toddlers (Dunn, 1994). Children whose guilt over their own misdemeanours is mismanaged by carers can develop further emotional and behavioural difficulties later on (Hoffman, 1976; Bugental *et al.*, 1992; Chapman *et al.*, 1987). Fortunately, it has been noted that day care can bring positive experiences to children by facilitating the formation of early friendships and moral reasoning. It is also possible to socially mediate these difficulties because increasing verbal skills mean that children are better able to talk about emotional experiences with parents and other carers (Denham and Auerbach, 1995). Hence, everyday conversations can be used as a means of scaffolding the emotional experiences of the child (Dunn and Brown, 1991).

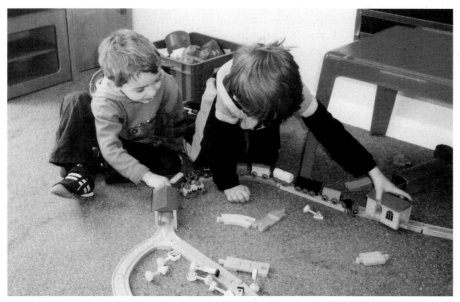

Figure 4.3   Day care can facilitate the formation of early friendships.

36 months to 48 months plus

Between 3 and 4 years of age, pretend play becomes increasingly sophisticated with the emergence of role or socio-dramatic play, and perspective taking begins to emerge. That is, the child begins to understand that others have their own thoughts, intentions and beliefs that may be different from their own and that these beliefs may be wrong. They also begin to appreciate that others think and act on the basis of these beliefs, false or otherwise. This is referred to as a 'theory of mind' in the literature (Baron-Cohen, 1993; Lewis *et al.*, 1989). Affectively, at 3 and 4 years, spontaneous pro-social action begins to be replaced by 'the respectable pursuit of self-interest', and this may be linked to gender (Hay *et al.*, 1999). Children should be becoming better able to understand the perspectives of others with respect to feelings and emotions. Most recent findings, however, suggest that an appreciation of the thoughts or beliefs of others need not mean a sound appreciation of another's feelings or of empathic reactions. This is perhaps because the development of the child's understanding of emotions of others is more sensitive to early socialization experiences than the development of the understanding of logically-based beliefs and intentions of others. In this way, children may be more inclined to show developmental lags in understanding emotions rather than intentions (Greig and Howe, 2001). Patterns of secure or insecure-defended or insecure-coercive behaviour are established in the pre-school years, as disorganized pre-schoolers manifest a lack of coherence and positive resolution in their play and interactions (Crittenden, 1992; Bretherton *et al.*, 1990). Also on the increase over this period is the awareness of family and community norms and that transgressions have consequences (Smetana and Braeges, 1990). The appreciation that one is either male or female emerges between the ages of 4 and 7, which is also a period during which girls develop pro-social and acceptable means of resolving peer disputes, being better able to pursue self-interests in a more quiet and covert way than boys (Hay *et al.*, 1992).

Impact of socialization between 36 and 48 months

The impact of early socialization on the development of social understanding is considerable. Research studies often refer to the skill as 'mentalizing ability', and competence in it has been linked to attachment security (Meins, 1999); abilities to reflect about oneself (Fonagy *et al.*, 1991, 1997); number of siblings at home; extent of conversational exchanges at home (Bartsch and Wellman, 1989; Dunn and Brown, 1991); pretend play in the family (Youngblade and Dunn, 1995); and the carer's tendency to treat the child as a 'mentalizing' agent (Meins *et al.*, 1998). The early socialization of emotion understanding is often reported alongside studies on theory of mind (Harris, 1989), but others report emotion understanding as a separate 'skill' (Denham *et al.*, 1990, 1994) that has also been linked to attachment conversational exchanges with carers about conflicts and emotional experiences and parental mental health (Denham and Auerbach, 1995; Denham *et al.*, 1994; Dunn and Munn, 1987). The above review also indicates that children are being exposed to gender socialization from a very early age. Girls begin to take a more nurturing and pro-social role than boys, and this may put them at risk of later emotional psychopathy (Hay *et al.*, 1999). Socialization experiences of maternal mental ill-health and insecure attachments may predispose some children to pathological pro-social behaviour and/or more aggression than other children. Furthermore, the manifestations of difficulties associated with early relating may be different for boys and girls. Whilst boys may become more aggressive, girls may be internalizing guilt (Hay *et al.*, 1999; DeMulder and Radke-Yarrow, 1991; Zahn-Waxler *et al.*, 1990).

This chapter has considered a range of skill-based definitions of the personal, social and emotional competencies that contribute to a broadly defined personal, social and emotional intelligence. The complex and interdependent nature of the developing personal, social and emotional competencies was also explored. There were several recurring themes that included perspective-taking, or theory of mind, and its associated sense of self and others (autonomy and connectedness), attachment, and pro-social competence. These could be described as mechanisms or processes that underlie most of these competencies and interact in complex ways with early experiences of socialization. Nevertheless, the fact that the development of these interactional intelligences is so dependent upon the types of experiences children have with significant others, that is, socially mediated, implies that it may possible to socially remedy many of the difficulties.

Conclusion

To conclude, it may be interesting to return to Miss Brodie and her subversive curriculum, for despite her enlightened views on the need to teach about matters that are personal, social and emotional, the character also famously quipped the Watsonian 'blank-slate' phrase '… give me a girl at an impressionable age, and she is mine for life'. This chapter has considered how the children we work with do not come to our attention as blank slates. But to what extent can we remedy difficulties that have been socially mediated in the developmental process at impressionable ages? This chapter shows that we are only beginning to really understand the complex nature of personal, social and emotional development and intelligence. How to best teach, support it and to remedy the damage is quite another matter. It is a complex process, and those of us familiar with the fate of Miss Brodie will consider the possibility that even well-meaning, enlightened, middle-class school teachers could get it wrong! But at least she tried. Can any of the rest of us really say the same?

Student activity

Identify three children of different ages under 8 years. By observation of the children or discussion with parents/carers, elicit examples of these children's: (i) perspective taking; (ii) attachment to a significant other; and (iii) pro-social competence. Discuss your findings with a fellow student, colleague or tutor.

REFERENCES

Ainsworth, MDS, Blehar, M, Walters, E and Wall, S (1978): *Patterns of Attachment: A Psychological Study of the Strange Situation*. Hillsdale, NJ: Erlbaum.

Antidote (2003): *The Emotional Literacy Handbook: Promoting Whole-School Strategies*. London: David Fulton Publishers.

Baldwin, JM (1906): *Mental Development in the Child and Race: Methods and Processes* (3rd revised edn; original 1894). New York: Macmillan.

Baron-Cohen, S (1993): Children's theories of mind: where would we be without the intentional stance? In Rutter, ML and Hay, DF (eds), *Development Through Life: A Handbook for Clinicians*. Oxford: Blackwell.

Baron-Cohen, S (2004) *Mind Reading: The Interactive Guide to Emotions*. Basingstoke: Taylor & Francis.

Bartsch, K and Wellman, H (1989): Young children's attribution of action to beliefs and desires. *Child Development*, **57**, 194–201.

Bizman, A and Yinon, J (2004): Social self-discrepancies from own and other standpoints and collective self-esteem. *Journal of Social Psychology*, **144**(2), 101–113.

Block, J (1995): On the relation between IQ, impulsivity and delinquency. *Journal of Abnormal Psychology*, **104**, 395–398.

Bowlby, J (1980): *Attachment and Loss, Volume 3: Loss, Sadness and Depression*. New York: Basic Books.

Bowlby, J (1991): *The Making and Breaking of Affectional Bonds*. Oxford: Penguin.

Bretherton, I, Ridgeway, D and Cassidy, J (1990): The role of internal working models in the attachment relationship. In Greenberg, M, Cicchetti, D and Cummings, EM (eds), *Attachment in the Preschool Years: Theory, Research and Intervention*. Chicago IL: University of Chicago Press, pp. 273–308.

Bronfenbrenner, U (1986): Ecology of the family as a context for human development: research perspectives. *Developmental Psychology*, **22**, 723–742.

Bronfenbrenner, U (1992): Ecological systems theory. In Vasta R (ed.), *Six Theories of Child Development: Revised Formulation and Current Issues*. London: Jessica Kingsley, pp. 187–249.

Bugental, DB, Blue, J, Cortez, V, Fleck, K and Rodriguez, A (1992): Influences of witnessed affect on information processing in children. *Child Development*, **63**, 774–786.

Cabello, B and Terrell, R (1999): Making students feel like family: how teachers create warm and caring classroom climates. *Journal of Classroom Interaction*, **29**(1), 17–23.

Campbell, SB (1991): Longitudinal studies of active and aggressive preschoolers: individual differences in early behaviour and outcome. In Cicchetti, D and Toth, SL (eds), *Rochester Symposium on Developmental Psychopathology*. Hillsdale, NJ: Erlbaum, pp. 957–990.

Chapman, M, Zahn-Waxler, C, Iannotti, R and Cooperman, G (1987): Empathy and responsibility in the motivation of children's helping. *Developmental Psychology*, **23**, 140–145.

Cicchetti, D (1992): *Developmental Perspectives on Depression*. Rochester, NY: University of Rochester Press.

Conduct Problems Prevention Research Group (CPPRG) (2000a): The Implementation of the fast track program: an example of a large-scale efficacy trial. *Journal of Abnormal Psychology*, **30**(1), 1–18.

Conduct Problems Prevention Research Group (CPPRG) (2002b): Evaluation of the first three years of the fast track prevention trial with children at high risk for adolescent conduct problems. *Journal of Abnormal Psychology*, **30**(1), 19–35.

Crittenden, PM (1992): Quality of attachment in the preschool years. *Development and Psychopathology*, **4**, 209–241.

Cummings, EM and Davies, PT (1994): Maternal depression and child development. *Journal of Child Psychology and Psychiatry*, **35**(1), 73–112.

Dalgleish, T (2002): *Self-Esteem: Ages 6–8: Activities to Develop Children's Self-Esteem, Across the Curriculum*. London: A. & C. Black.

Damasio, AR (1996): *Descartes' Error: Emotion, Reason and the Human Brain*. London: Papermac.

Daniel, B and Wassell, S (2002/2004a): *The Early Years: Assessing and Promoting Resilience in Vulnerable Children 1*. London: Jessica Kingsley.

Daniel, B and Wassell, S (2002/2004b): *The School Years: Assessing and Promoting Resilience in Vulnerable Children 2*. London: Jessica Kingsley.

Davis-Kean, PE and Sandler, HM (2001): A meta-analysis of measures of self-esteem for young children: a framework for future measures. *Child Development*, **72**(3), 887–906.

De Mulder, E and Radke-Yarrow, M (1991): Attachment with affectively ill and well mothers: concurrent behavioural correlates. *Development and Psychopathology*, **3**, 227–242.

De Mulder, EK, Denham, S, Schmidt, M and Mitchell, J (2000): Q-sort assessment of attachment security during the preschool years: links from home to school. *Developmental Psychology*, **36**(2), 274–282.

Denham, SA (1986): Social cognition, pro-social behaviour, and emotion in preschoolers. *Child Development*, **57**, 194–201.

Denham, S and Auerbach, S (1995): Mother–child dialogue about emotions and preschoolers' emotional competence. *Genetic, Social and General Psychology Monographs*, **121**(3), 311–337.

Denham, SA, McKinley, M, Couchoud, EA and Holt, R (1990): Emotional and behavioural predictors of preschool peer ratings. *Child Development*, **57**, 194–201.

Denham, SA, Zoller, D and Couchoud, EA (1994): Socialisation of preschoolers' emotion understanding. *Developmental Psychology*, **30**(6), 928–936.

Denham, SA, Blair, KA, De Mulder, E, Levitas, J, Sawyer, K, Auerbach-Major, S and Queenan, P (2003): Preschool emotional competence: pathway to social competence? *Child Development*, **74**(1), 238–256.

Dennett, D (1978): Beliefs about beliefs. *Behavioural and Brain Sciences*, **4**, 759–770.

Donnellan, C (2003): *Self-Esteem*. Cambridge: Independence.

Dunn, J (1988): *The Beginnings of Social Understanding*. Cambridge, MA: Harvard University Press.

Dunn, J (1994): Understanding others and the social world: current issues in developmental research and their relation to preschool experiences and practice. *Journal of Applied Developmental Psychology*, **15**, 571–583.

Dunn, J (1996): The Emanuel Miller Memorial Lecture 1995. Children's relationships: bridging the divide between cognitive and social development. *Journal of Child Psychology and Psychiatry*, **37**(5), 507–518.

Dunn, J and Brown, J (1991): Relationships, talk about feelings and the development of affect regulation in early childhood. In Garber, J and Dodge, KA (eds), *The Development of Emotion Regulation and Dysregulation*. Cambridge, MA: Cambridge University Press.

Dunn, J and Munn, P (1986): Siblings and the development of pro-social behaviour. *International Journal of Behavioural Development*, **9**, 265–284.

Dunn, J and Munn, P (1987): The development of justification in disputes with mother and sibling. *Developmental Psychology*, **23**, 791–798.

Dweck, CS (1999): *Self-Theories: Their Role in Motivation, Personality and Development*. Philadelphia, PA: Psychological Press.

Emler, N (2001): *Self-Esteem: The Costs and Causes of Low Self-Worth*. Layerthorpe: Joseph Rowntree Foundation by York Publishing Services.

Estrada, AU and Pinsof, WM (1995): The effectiveness of family therapies for selected behavioural disorders in childhood. *Journal of Marital and Family Therapy*, **21**(4), 403–440.

Fonagy, P, Steele, H, Steele, M and Holder, J (1997): Attachment and theory of mind: overlapping constructs? *Bonding and Attachment: Association of Child Psychology and Psychiatry Occasional Papers No. 14*.

Fonagy, P, Steele, M, Steele, H, Moran, GS and Higgitt, AC (1991): The capacity for understanding mental states: the reflective self in parent and child and its significance for security of attachment. *Infant Mental Health Journal*, **12**, 201–218.

Gardner, H (1983): *Frames of Mind: The Theory of Multiple Intelligences*. New York: Basic Books.

Gardner, H (1993): *Multiple Intelligences: The Theory in Practice*. New York: Basic Books.

Goleman, D (1996): *Emotional Intelligence: Why it can Matter More than IQ*. London: Bloomsbury Publishing.

Goodyer, IM (2001): The development of emotional intelligence. In Goodyer, IM, *The Depressed Child and Adolescent*. Cambridge: Cambridge University Press, pp. 24–45.

Greenberg, MT and Kusche, C (1998): *Promoting Alternative Thinking Strategies (PATHS)*. From Elliott, DS (Series Editor) Blueprints for Violence Prevention. Colorado: C&M Press.

Greig, A. (2004): Childhood depression – Part 1: Does it need to be dealt with only by health professionals? *Educational and Child Psychology*, **21**(4), 43–54.

Greig, A and Howe, D (2001): Social understanding, attachment security of preschool children and maternal mental health. *British Journal of Developmental Psychology*, **19**(3), 381–393.

Guralnick, M (ed.) (1997): *The Effectiveness of Early Intervention*. Baltimore, MD: Paul H. Brookes.

Harris, P (1989): *Children and Emotion: The Development of Psychological Understanding*. Oxford: Blackwell.

Harris, P (1999): Individual differences in understanding emotion: the role of attachment status and psychological assessment. *Attachment and Human Development*, **1**(3), 307–324.

Hartup, WW (1992): Friendships and their developmental significance. In McGurk, H (ed.), *Childhood Social Development: Contemporary Perspectives*. Hove: Erlbaum.

Hay, DF (1979): Cooperative interactions and sharing between very young children and their parents. *Developmental Psychology*, **15**, 647–653.

Hay, DF (1994): Pro-social development. *Journal of Child Psychology and Psychiatry*, **35**(1), 29–71.

Hay, DF and Pawlby, S (2003): Pro-social development in relation to children's and mothers' psychological problems. *Child Development*, **74**(5), 1314–1327.

Hay, D, Payne, A and Chadwick, A (2004): Peer relations in childhood. *Journal of Child Psychology and Psychiatry and Allied Disciplines*, **45**(1), 84–108.

Hay, DF, Castle, J, Davies, L, Demetriou, H and Stimson, CA (1999): Pro-social action in very early childhood. *Journal of Child Psychology and Psychiatry*, **40**(6), 905–916.

Hay, DF, Stimson, CA, Castle, J and Davies, L (1993): The construction of character in toddlerhood. In Killen, M and Hart, D (eds), *Morality in Everyday Life*. Cambridge: Cambridge University Press.

Hay, DF, Zahn-Waxler, C, Cummings, EM and Iannotti, R (1992): Young children's views about conflict with peers: a comparison of the sons and daughters of depressed and well women. *Journal of Child Psychology and Psychiatry*, **33**, 669–683.

Higgins, ET (1989): Self-discrepancy theory: what patterns of self-belief cause people to suffer. In Berkowitz, L (ed.), *Advances in Experimental Social Psychology*. New York: Academic Press, **22**, pp. 93–136.

Hinde, RA (1992): Human social development: an ethological/relationship perspective. In McGurk, H (ed.), *Childhood Social Development: Contemporary Perspectives*. London: Erlbaum.

Hinde, RA (1997): *Relationships: A Dialectical Perspective*. Hove, UK: Psychology Press.

Hobson, P (2002): *Cradle of Thought*. London: Macmillan.

Hoffman, M (1987): The contribution of empathy to justice and moral judgment. In Eisenberg, N and Strayer, J (eds), *Empathy and its Development*. Cambridge: Cambridge University Press.

Hoffman, M (1976): Empathy, role taking, guilt, and the development of altruistic motives. In Lickona, T (ed.), *Moral Development and Behaviour*. New York: Holt, Rinehart and Winston.

Howe, D (1995): *Attachment Theory for Social Work Practice*. London: Macmillan.

Howe, D, Brandon, M, Hining, D and Schofield, G (1999): *Attachment Theory, Child Maltreatment and Family Support*. London: Macmillan.

Howes, C (1988): Peer interaction and young children. *Monographs of the Society for Research in Child Development*, **53**(1), 94.

Howlin, P, Baron-Cohen, S and Hadwin, J (1999): *Teaching Children with Autism to Mind-Read: A Practical Guide for Teachers and Parents*. Chichester: John Wiley & Sons Ltd.

Hubley, P and Trevarthen, C (1979): Sharing a task in infancy. In Usgiris, IC (ed.), *Social Interaction During Infancy*. San Francisco: Jossey-Bass.

Hughes, A and Kleinberg, S (1999): Organisation and management in nursery and infant schooling. In Bryce, TGK and Humes, WM (eds), *Scottish Education*. Edinburgh: Edinburgh University Press.

Kagan, J (1989): *Unstable Ideas: Temperament, Cognition and Self*. Cambridge, MA: Harvard University Press.

Kazdin, A (1995): Child, parent and family dysfunction as predictors of outcome in cognitive-behavioural treatment of antisocial children. *Behaviour Research and Therapy*, **3**, 271–281.

Kochanska, G (1993): Towards a synthesis of parental socialisation and child temperament in early development of conscience. *Child Development*, **64**, 325–347.

Kovacs, M (1997): The Emmanuel Miller Memorial Lecture 1994. Depressive disorders in childhood: an impressionistic landscape. *Journal of Child Psychology and Psychiatry*, **38**(3), 287–298.

Ladd, GW, Birch, SH and Buhs, ES (1999): Children's social and scholastic lives in kindergarten: related spheres of influence? *Child Development*, **70**(6), 1373–1400.

Lawrence, D (1987): *Enhancing Self-Esteem in the Classroom*. London: Paul Chapman Publishing.

Leslie, AM (1987): Pretence and theory of mind: the origins of theory of mind. *Psychological Review*, **94**, 412–426.

Lewis, M and Brooks, J (1974): Self, other and fear: infants' reactions to people. In Lewis, M and Rosenblum, M (eds), *Fear: The Origins of Behaviour*, 2. New York: Wiley.

Lewis, M, Stranger, C and Sullivan, MW (1989): Deception in 3-year-olds. *Developmental Psychology*, **25**, 439–443.

Maccoby, EE and Jacklin, CN (1980): Sex differences in aggression: a rejoinder and reprise. *Child Development*, **5**, 964–980.

Maslow, AH (1954/1970): *Motivation and the Personality*, 2nd edn. New York: Harper & Row.

Meins, E (1999): Sensitivity, security and internal working models: bridging the transmission gap. *Attachment and Human Development*, **1**(3), 325–342.

Meins, E, Fernyhough, C, Russell, J and Clark-Carter, D (1998): Security of attachment as a predictor of symbolic and mentalizing abilities: a longitudinal study. *Social Development*, **7**, 1–24.

Meltzer, H, Gartward, R, Goodman, R and Ford, T (2000): *Mental Health of Children and Adolescents in Great Britain*. London: The Stationery Office.

MIND (2001): *Children and Young People in Mental Distress*. London: MIND.

Mitchell–Copeland, J, Denham, S and De Mulder, EK (1997): Q-sort assessment of child–teacher attachment relationships and social competence in the preschool. *Early Education and Development*, **8**(1), 27–39.

Mosley, J (1996): *Quality Circle Time in the Primary Classroom: Your Essential Guide to Enhancing Self-Esteem, Self-Discipline and Positive Relationships*. Wisbech, Cambridge: LDA.

Mosley, J (2001): *More Quality Circle Time*. Wisbech, Cambridge: LDA.

Murray, L (1992): The impact of postnatal depression on infant development. *Journal of Child Psychology*, **33**, 543–561.

Orbach, S (1997): Quoted in the pamphlet *Realising the Potential: Emotional Education for All: An Antidote Report*.

Perner, J, Ruffman, T and Leekham, S (1994): Theory of mind is contagious: you catch it from your sibs. *Child Development*, **65**, 1224–1234.

Rose-Krasnor, L (1997): The nature of social competence: a theoretical review. *Social Development*, **6**(1), 111–129.

Rutter, M, Giller, H and Hagell, A (1998): *Antisocial Behaviour by Young People: A Major New Review of the Research*. Cambridge: Cambridge University Press.

Saarni, C (1990): Emotional competence: how emotions and relationships become integrated. In Thompson, RA (ed.), *Socioemotional Development/Nebraska Symposium on Motivation*, 36.

Salovey, P and Mayer, JD (1990): Emotional intelligence. *Imagination, Cognition and Personality*, **9**, 185–211.

SCCC (1999): *A Curriculum Framework for Children 3 to 5*. Scottish Consultative Council on the Curriculum. Edinburgh: The Scottish Office.

Smetana, JG and Braeges, JL (1990): The development of toddlers' moral and conventional judgements. *Merrill-Palmer Quarterly*, **36**, 329–346.

Steiner, C and Perry, P (1997): *Achieving Emotional Literacy*. London: Bloomsbury.

Stern, D (1987): *The Interpersonal World of the Infant*. New York: Basic Books.

Stone, KF and Dillehunt, HQ (1978): *Self-Science: The Subject is Me*. Santa Monica: Goodyear Publishing Co.

Sylva, K (1994): The impact of early learning on children's development. In Ball, C (ed.), *Start Right: The Importance of Early Learning*. Royal Society for the Arts, Manufacturers & Commerce, pp. 84–96.

Trevarthen, C (1997): The curricular conundrum. In Dunlop, AW and Hughes, A (eds), *Preschool Curriculum Policy Practice and Proposals: A Forum for Policy Makers and Practitioners in Scotland*. Strathclyde University.

Warden, D and Christie, D (1997): *Teaching Social Behaviour: Classroom Activities to Foster Children's Interpersonal Awareness*. London: David Fulton Publishers.

Wimmer, H and Perner, J (1983): Beliefs about beliefs: representation and constraining function of wrong beliefs in young children's understanding of deception. *Cognition*, 21, 103–128.

Youngblade, LM and Dunn, J (1995): Individual differences in young children's pretend play with mother and sibling: links to relationships and understanding of other people's feelings and beliefs. *Child Development*, 66, 1472–1492.

Zahn-Waxler, C and Radke-Yarrow, M (1990): Origins of empathic concern. *Motivation and Emotion*, 14, 107–130.

Zahn-Waxler, C, Kochanska, G, Krupnick, J and McKnew, D (1990): Patterns of guilt in children of depressed and well mothers. *Developmental Psychology*, 28, 126–136.

FURTHER READING

Barnes, P (ed.) (1995): *Personal, Social and Emotional Development of Children*. Milton Keynes: Open University Press.

Cooper, P (ed.) (1999): *Understanding and Supporting Children with Emotional and Behavioural Difficulties*. London: Jessica Kingsley.

Roberts, R (2002): *Self-Esteem and Early Learning*, 2nd edn. London: Sage.

Schaffer, R (1996): *Social Development*. Oxford: Blackwell.

Spence, SH (2003): Social skills training with children and young people: theory, evidence and practice. *Child and Adolescent Mental Health*, 8(2), 84–96.

5

CHILDREN'S RELATIONSHIPS

David Rutherford

> This chapter aims to:
>
> ■ study the development, nature and impact of the more significant relationships in the lives of young children.

INTRODUCTION

Some years ago I asked our 5-year-old son, Nat, who his important relationships were with. He immediately listed his parents, sister, brothers, grandmothers, cousins, aunts and uncles, friends, friends' parents and the cats (but not the goldfish!). Recently, I asked him again (he is now 14), and his answer was much the same, although the cats had dropped out and his dog, his sister's husband and new baby had replaced them. Most psychologists would agree that these individuals are likely to play a significant part in the emotional, social and cognitive development of children in Western societies. In all cultures the survival, health, behaviour and development of skills in children are dependent upon the nurturance, training and control offered by the people with whom they have close relationships (Whiting and Edwards, 1988). The process of socialization, whereby children are shaped to fit their own particular culture, has traditionally portrayed children as passive recipients of adult influence but, as any parent knows, it is not as simple as that, and children are clearly and determinedly active participants in their own socialization, constantly modifying and challenging intended influences in pursuit of their own goals and personalities.

The study of relationships is central to social psychology, and in the past few years there has been considerable growth in our knowledge about children's relationships. Currently, theorists from social psychology, ethology, social anthropology and sociology – as well as from developmental psychology and psychiatry – are making significant contributions to our understanding of children's relationships. From the early work of John Bowlby (1953) and Sigmund Freud, where the emphasis was almost entirely on the mother–child relationship, there have been some important developments in recent years. First, the whole area has become much more complex, and the multiple interactive nature of children's relationships is being explored. Second, pivotal concepts such as attachment, the family, and temperament have been refined and elaborated to reflect the subtlety of relationships. Third, a multicultural perspective has evolved which enables us to examine possible universals of relationships, as well as cultural diversity. Fourth, the significance of a child's relationships with father, siblings, grandparents, other caregivers and, most recently, friends and peers, is increasingly recognized as being important for that child's future development. Fifth, it is recognized that children's relationships always occur within a social context of already existing relationships which may exert a powerful influence upon the child. Finally, our understanding of the impact upon a child of relationship disturbance, such as parental discord or sexual abuse, encourages intervention strategies and ways of improving relationships.

FAMILY RELATIONSHIPS

Most children are born into a family. Although there are many problems about defining precisely what comprises a family – ranging from the relatively straightforward conjugal nuclear family to the non-conjugal/reconstituted/extended family – members of families are likely to have persistent relationships involving emotional bonds. That is to say, they belong to a group of interconnected and interdependent people who have psychologically meaningful social interactions (Richards, 1995). In the twenty-first century, blood ties, common residence or legal connections are not considered necessary for the recognition of a family unit. What is important is that there is *mutual recognition* of family membership. This allows for the diversity of family units which have developed over the past 50 years. Although the traditional nuclear family with both biological parents and two children still exists, the majority of children today are being brought up in families with variable and often changing members. It is possible for some children to have as many as five or six 'parents' (work that out!), several step-parents and siblings, half-brothers and half-sisters and numerous grandparents, whereas others live in lone-parent families with no siblings and little contact with relatives.

Whatever a child's family type, psychologists and lay people all acknowledge the significance of family relationships as sources of socialization, nurturance, happiness and comfort (as well as irritation, anxiety and frustration). Life-events studies, from the initial work of Holmes and Rahe (1967) onwards, demonstrate that many significant aspects of a person's well-being are related to changes in family relationships. Both major changes (such as the birth of a child into an existing set of family relationships) and minor changes (uplifts and hassles such as birthdays or tonsillitis) have direct and indirect influences on family members. There is currently a large body of research showing that, in general, our physical and mental health, recovery from illness, and even the number of accidents we have are related to the quality of our close relationships. However, although relationships often provide a buffer against adversity, they can also be sources of severe injury, distress and life-long psychological damage. For example, it is now several years since the details of the complex destructive family relationships of Fred and Rosemary West emerged and showed the world that, even in a proper nuclear family with its own house and mortgage, the most appalling acts of abuse could go undetected for many years. Also, Lord Laming's report in 2003 on the inquiry into the death of Victoria Climbié has generated more than a hundred recommendations for ensuring the care and protection of children in families and institutions throughout the UK.

Parenting

Early research into the ways in which families affect children identified two main dimensions of parental behaviour that were thought to affect a child's subsequent development:

1. The dimension *warmth–coldness* referred to the amount of affection and playfulness shown towards children.

2. The dimension *permissiveness–restrictiveness* referred to parental toleration of aggressiveness and control of a child's behaviour.

Few associations between parenting styles and children's development were found, but this research paved the way for the influential work of Diana Baumrind (1971), who examined the ways in which different types of relationships between parents and children affect a child's behaviour. Baumrind argues that normal parenting is mainly concerned with influencing and controlling children. Parental *demandingness* refers to '... the claims parents make on children to become integrated into the family whole, by their maturity demands, supervision, disciplinary efforts and willingness to confront the child who disobeys'. Parental *responsiveness* is '... the extent to which parents intentionally foster individuality, self-regulation and self-assertion by being attuned, supportive, and acquiescent to children's special needs and demands' (Baumrind, 1991, p. 62). Following a research tradition in the study of leadership, she identified three parental styles related to three patterns of children's behaviour (Fig. 5.1).

Parental style	Child's behaviour
Permissive	Impulsive – aggressive
Authoritarian	Conflicted – irritable
Authoritative	Energetic – friendly

Figure 5.1   Parental styles and children's behaviour.

- *Permissive* parents tend to have very relaxed relationships with their children and, because they do not believe in restricting their child's independence, they exercise less control and accept lower levels of performance, both cognitively and behaviourally. Often their discipline is inconsistent and a child's freedom of expression is valued highly.

The children of permissive parents are often found to be aggressive in their relationships with parents, other adults and other children, unable to control their own feelings of anger, impulsive in their actions and to have low levels of goal-directed achievement orientation.

- *Authoritarian* parents have very controlling relationships with their children. They tend to restrict a child's activities, set strict rules for the child and use harsh, punitive discipline for transgressions. They show low levels of affection and are uninvolved in family and cultural events.

The children of authoritarian parents are often very vulnerable to stress, fearful and anxious about their relationships, and appear moody and unhappy. They react irritably, are rather deceitful, and tend to alternate between sulky, passive withdrawal and overt aggression.

- *Authoritative* parents achieve a workable balance between setting high and clear standards for a child's behaviour and encouraging independence. Discipline is firm but fair, with the child's viewpoint being taken into consideration and control achieved by reasoning and explaining from an early age. Such parents are warm and committed to the child's cognitive, social and moral development.

The children of these (ideal!) parents were found to be energetic and cheerful, to have good relationships with peers and other adults, and purposefully to pursue high levels of achievement. The authoritative style is consistently associated with cognitive and social competence in children at all developmental stages and there are low levels of problem behaviour in girls and boys from infancy to adolescence. Several independent studies have confirmed Baumrind's findings, and recent work shows that the association between parental styles and children's behaviour persists over the longer term.

- A fourth style – the *Uninvolved* – has been identified by other researchers (Maccoby and Martin, 1983). Here, the parents give the minimum of care to maintain the child, and are indifferent to the child's needs. In extreme cases, uninvolved parenting becomes *neglect,* and the child's social, cognitive and emotional development is very likely to be impaired.

It is important to note that this research is mostly *correlational*, and that we cannot conclude that parental style *causes* patterns of children's behaviour (although that is what Baumrind argues). As any parent knows, it is easy to be warmly involved with a child who cheerfully co-operates with parental wishes. The child's characteristics influence the parenting styles as much as the parent affects the child, and it may be that parents use the authoritative style because their children are temperamentally co-operative and conforming. Disobedient or disruptive children test the strength and endurance of even the most rational, patient parents.

Critiques of Baumrind's classification of parental styles suggest that identifying only three styles greatly over-simplifies the real situation. Not only do most parents use a mixture of styles, rather than just one, but styles may change over time as children develop. Parents know how impossible it is to achieve absolute consistency with different children at different ages in different situations.

Parent education

The concept of parent education has existed for many years, and new parents have always received help and guidance from their own kin, passing child-rearing skills from generation to generation, possibly without much deliberation. Indeed, for the whole history of humanity this has worked pretty successfully, and there is evidence that all over the world different societies have found for themselves that responsive and moderately demanding parenting is linked to the healthy psychological development of children. However, from the early years of the twentieth century the growth of systematic scientific knowledge has led to a continued, but ever-changing, programme of formal parent education, and there are currently many schemes aiming to help parents to improve their skills in bringing up their children. In both the United States and increasingly in the UK, the changing nature of families, and concern about the growing numbers of absent fathers, single mothers, teenage pregnancies, women in employment and children in child care, has led to many attempts to develop programmes and guidelines for effective parenting. Research has frequently shown that parent education can significantly improve mothers' sensitivity and skills in interacting with their children and therefore enhance the development of their cognitive abilities.

The STEP (Systematic Training for Effective Parenting) is one programme that was developed to produce socially responsible children, and has been used widely in the USA. It includes topics such as understanding yourself and your child, listening and talking to your child, and helping your child to co-operate. Responsible parents give their children choices and allow them to experience the result of their decisions (Dinkmeyer and McKay, 1996). Other programmes emphasize different strategies, including democratic relationships, warmth and acceptance, communication, explicit reward and punishment and use of praise. Although parental education has been shown to be effective in a variety of settings, some critics have argued that rather than teaching specific skills to parents a greater benefit would be achieved by educating them to understand the broad area of child development psychology. At the moment there is little evidence on the long-term effects of parental training in any single strategy, and we await the necessary research with interest.

There has been great progress in our understanding of the factors affecting parenting, and below are some major areas of current interest:

- **Social class**: the different life and working conditions, value systems, educational levels and economic security of middle- and working-class parents are associated with various differences in child-rearing behaviours.
- **Poverty**: the charity organization End Child Poverty claims that, in 2004, there were 3.8 million children living in poverty in the UK. Both here and in the USA the proportion of children living in poverty has increased steadily since 1975, and has only recently begun to level off with 20–30 per cent of dependent children living in families below the poverty line. These children are at significantly greater risk of illness and accidents, mental health problems, limited language and cognitive development, and future unemployment. Poverty is obviously very stressful for the parents, and may have a negative affect upon their behaviour. The likelihood of punitive, non-nurturing parenting, withholding affection, and corporal punishment is increased, although there are many other factors to be taken into account (Evans, 2004).
- **Ethnicity**: different ethnic and cultural groups have distinct parenting beliefs and practices, although all cultures are similar in their valuing and respecting children. Variations in demandingness occur in different groups. For example, Chinese parents in the USA emphasize discipline, control and respect for elders, whereas in Hispanic families respect for the father's authority is combined with strong maternal warmth. The extended family of African-Americans has for many years been a buffer against the negative forces of racism and poverty, and parents in these families rely on the support and knowledge of grandparents and other kin to enhance authoritative parenting (Barbarin and McCandies, 2002).
- **Single parents**: although single parents are not a homogeneous group, about three-quarters of single-parent households are run by mothers. There are a number of problems for mothers raising children on their own, and many areas of stress. About half of single mothers are poor, and for many families the main source of income is the mother's earnings, which are typically low. Child care costs are high, so even if a mother can work to support her family, much of her income is absorbed by day care costs. It is commonly acknowledged that many single mothers suffer from anxiety, feelings of despair, depression and various health problems, as well as having to cope with low social status, poor-quality housing and education, and chronic fatigue, all of which make good-quality parenting very difficult. When single parents have adequate income, parenting problems

appear to diminish considerably. Single fathers, divorced parents, step-parents, or gay and lesbian parents affect smaller numbers of children, but there is significant growth in the understanding of the parenting issues in these areas.

Family structures

Research conducted over the past 30 years has identified two main dimensions on which families can be differentiated (Olson *et al.*, 1989). The first of these, namely *adaptability*, refers to the ability of a family to change in response to external or internal demands. The second dimension, *cohesion*, refers to the strength of emotional bonding between family members. On each of the dimensions a family can be classified into one of four different types, and therefore located on a space on a four-by-four grid (see Fig. 5.2).

		Cohesion			
		Disengaged	**Separated**	**Connected**	**Enmeshed**
Adaptability	**Rigid**	Extreme	Mid-range	Mid-range	Extreme
	Structured	Mid-range	Balanced	Balanced	Mid-range
	Flexible	Mid-range	Balanced	Balanced	Mid-range
	Chaotic	Extreme	Mid-range	Mid-range	Extreme

Figure 5.2 Cohesion in family structures.

Families located at the extremes of either dimension are postulated to function less well than those that fall in the mid-range or balanced categories. A *chaotic* family has few clear rules or roles, the children receive little guidance and inconsistent discipline, and they consequently are uncertain about appropriate behaviour and difficult to control. On the other hand, a *rigid* family has rules and roles strictly defined with power exercised by inflexible authoritarian control. In *structured* and *flexible* families, the rules and roles are negotiated by parents and children democratically, and discipline is firm but fair.

Extremely cohesive families are described as *enmeshed*. Here, family members are so strongly identified and bonded with each other that the outside world is of little significance. *Disengaged* families have little sense of family identity, and each member functions separately with little reference to the others. Between the two extremes the members of *connected* and *separated* families are bound together by emotional ties at the same time as maintaining their own individual identity and activity.

Empirical evidence in relation to this model offers clear support for the hypothesis that balanced families function better than other types. They cope with the changing needs of developing children more effectively, with fewer disruptions and less unhappiness than either the mid-range or extreme families (McCubbin *et al.*, 1996).

Balanced, optimal, healthy, energized, well-functioning families

Despite concern expressed by political parties and the tabloid press about the 'breakdown of the family', many families continue to function very well, the members caring for each other with little conflict, and producing responsible, well-adjusted, contributing members of society (Anderson and Sabatelli, 2003).

The following characteristics have been identified by a number of different researchers, and although the list is not exhaustive, it indicates the range of desirable attributes:

- relationships – close and warm;
- communication – clear, supportive and empathic; ability to listen;
- power – shared, but with parental control and parental coalitions;
- roles – clearly defined, but not rigid or stereotyped;
- rules – negotiated and modifiable and related to strong value system;
- conflict – regulated and resolved by discussion and negotiation;
- world view – collectively agreed and continually reviewed; connected with other social systems;
- autonomy – encouraged and accepted (Olson and DeFrain, 2000).

As anybody who lives within a family knows, these counsels of perfection are easier to state than they are to achieve. Nevertheless, many families do strive to reach the ideals with relatively good success. Some families, however, seem to fail more often than they succeed, and these are identified as dysfunctional families.

Dysfunctional families

Leo Tolstoy wrote in *Anna Karenina*, 'All happy families resemble each other; each unhappy family is unhappy in its own way.' Although the foregoing discussion suggests that he was probably right about happy families, he was clearly mistaken about unhappy families in that they, too, share common characteristics. Whether they are rigid or chaotic, enmeshed or disengaged, they are incapable of consistently dealing successfully with ordinary everyday life, and are very likely to do significant harm to the psychological well-being of their members. As can be seen from the model of Olson *et al.* (1989), dysfunctional families are characterized by their extremity. They are extremely rigid or extremely chaotic, extremely disengaged or extremely enmeshed. In terms of the desirable attributes of healthy families, dysfunctional families seem to operate differently, and the following characteristics have been identified:

- relationships – either distant and cold or engulfing, may be abusive;
- communication – inadequate, unclear, ambiguous, double-binding;
- power – rigid hierarchy, cross-generation alliances;
- roles – either inflexibly or poorly defined;
- rules – rigidly enforced or very inconsistent;
- conflict – frequent destructive clashes without resolution;
- world view – idiosyncratic and distorted;
- autonomy – either strongly inhibited or irrelevant.

Any family with many of these characteristics is unlikely to provide an adequate environment for its members, particularly for children, and it is likely that at times of stress in particular, one or more of the family members will come to a community's attention as being in need of help in coping with adversity.

MOTHERS

More has probably been written about a child's first relationship, usually with his or her mother, than all of the child's other relationships put together. Following the work of John Bowlby in the first edition of his popular classic *Child Care and the Growth of Love* in 1953, there has been a massive development of theory and research evidence in the area, much of it within the framework of two major theoretical positions. *Ethology* adopts an evolutionary, biological perspective and takes the view that the survival of an infant depends upon the inborn behaviour and characteristics of infants (crying, smiling, chuckling, large eyes, round faces) which elicit caregiving behaviour from the mother such as feeding and comforting. Recent developments in the new discipline of Evolutionary Psychology suggest that maternal care has evolved to ensure the continuity of her genes (Buss, 1999), and although it is argued that the caregiving behaviours of mothers have a biological basis in humans, they are very significantly modified by cultural learning. The *social learning* approach takes the view that the interaction between biological bases and social environment is best accounted for by principles of reward, punishment, imitation and observation in the relationship between a child and his or her primary caregiver.

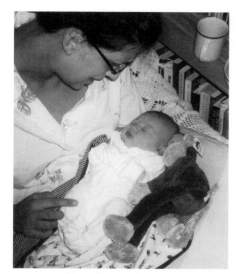

Figure 5.3 Mutually rewarding encounters between mother and child begin the process by which an enduring bond is formed.

Mutually rewarding encounters between mother and child begin the process by which an enduring emotional bond is formed, the quality of which is thought by many theorists to be the foundation for all other relationships that the child will develop.

The concept of *attachment* is central to an understanding of the mother–child relationship. Originally, the term was used to denote an emotional bond of affection for one individual, not interchangeable – an intense driving force towards seeking closeness with another person. This view sees attachment as residing in the individual, whereas more recent researchers have taken the position that attachment refers to a dynamic set of behaviours in the relationship between two people, a transaction in which both child and mother play crucial parts.

Although the newborn baby shows no evidence of attachment, it soon shows preferences – for other people to be nearby, for human faces, for social stimuli, and for human voices – which permit the development of attachments. By 6 weeks the infant is using its limited repertoire of behaviour to attract attention (smiling or crying), and by 3 months infants are reacting more positively to their usual caretakers than to strangers. At between 6 months and 8 months the infant begins to show clear evidence of primary attachment, usually – but not always – to the mother. Several factors seem to be important at this stage. First, *object permanence* emerges as part of the child's cognitive development, and the infant realizes that someone out of sight still exists. The mother's absence is noticed, and *separation protest* occurs. *Fear* begins to emerge as a strong emotion, and wariness of strangers often causes crying and searching behaviour in the child. Mobility also increases at this stage, and the infant now begins to be able to crawl towards the primary caregiver when anxious. After about

9 months, attachments begin to be formed with others in the child's environment, such as siblings, the father and grandparents.

Maternal bonding, which is the mother's emotional attachment to the child, begins before the baby is born and continues through the first hours and days of the baby's life. Early contact with the baby, with skin-to-skin touching, is thought by some researchers to be important but not necessary for good bonding to occur (Rode *et al.*, 1981).

Ainsworth *et al.* (1978), using the *Strange Situation Procedure*, have identified three main categories of attachment.

Type B: Secure attachment

This was found in 50–70 per cent of the children studied.

- The child:
  – shows a clear preference for the mother;
  – is outgoing with strangers while the mother is present;
  – uses the mother as a base for active exploration of the environment;
  – maintains periodic eye contact with the mother;
  – shows distress on separation from the mother;
  – is comforted and warmly greets the mother's return.
- The mother:
  – is sensitive and responsive to the baby's needs;
  – encourages exploration and communication;
  – is warm and emotionally expressive.

Type A: Anxious – avoidant attachment

This was found in 20–25 per cent of the children studied.

- The child:
  – ignores the mother;
  – is not especially wary of strangers, and ignores them;
  – shows little exploration when with the mother;
  – is not distressed upon separation;
  – avoids the mother upon her return.
- The mother:
  – is rigid and self-centred;
  – is cold and uninvolved with the baby;
  – avoids physical contact;
  – tends to be intolerant and irritable;
  – is unresponsive to the baby's needs.

Type C: Insecure – ambivalent attachment

This was found in 10 per cent of the children studied.

- The child:
  – is sometimes clinging and sometimes rejecting;
  – is reluctant to explore;
  – is very wary of strangers;
  – becomes very distressed at the mother leaving;
  – both seeks and rejects comfort upon reunion.

- The mother:
  - – is inconsistent in her caregiving;
  - – has difficulty in interpreting the child's needs;
  - – attempts close physical contact;
  - – has difficulty synchronizing with the baby.

Subsequent studies have found a fourth pattern, namely *disorganized* attachment, which occurs in high-risk families and where the child appears confused and apprehensive about his or her relationship with the mother (Main and Solomon, 1986).

There is some clear evidence that the quality of the primary attachment has significance for a child's subsequent relationships in childhood, and even later. Securely attached infants are likely to become more confident, skilful, socially orientated, co-operative and outgoing, and to be more popular and to have more friends (La Freniere and Sroufe, 1985). There is also evidence that poor-quality attachment between mother and child is linked to the mother's own insecure attachment as a child. Both security and insecurity may be transmitted from one generation to the next. The Adult Attachment Interview was developed by Mary Main, and is seen as a major breakthrough in attachment research in recent years (Cassidy and Shaver, 1999). It is suggested that *autonomous* parents who have a positive view about their own childhood attachments are better able to respond to their children's needs than are *dismissive* or *preoccupied* parents who, because of unresolved attachment issues and memories, are unable to focus on their own infant.

FATHERS

As a sensitive, 'New Age' father of five children, maximally involved in responsibility for the care of the children from birth onwards ('I wish', says my wife!), I have long been frustrated by the lack of knowledge about the nature of the father–child relationship and the impact of the father on the development of the child. Although most writers assert the father's importance, the mother–child relationship has been predominant in research until recently. Now, however, with growing numbers of women bringing up children on their own, with increasing numbers of women in the work-force, and with higher levels of male unemployment, both the presence of fathers and their absence have been studied. In the past few years, research into fathers has increased considerably in both the USA and Europe, led by the influential work of Michael Lamb and his colleagues in 1987.

These authors identified three main dimensions of parental involvement as:

1. Engagement – the time spent interacting with a child on a one-to-one basis, for example while reading a story.
2. Accessibility – the parent is occupied, but available to respond to the child if necessary, for example while reading the paper.
3. Responsibility – the parent is accountable for the everyday care and welfare of the child, for example feeding and clothing.

Fathers appear to spend about 20 per cent of the time that mothers do *engaged* with their children, 30 per cent of the time that mothers are *accessible* to their children, and take only 10 per cent of the *responsibility* for child care. For example, it is almost always mothers who stay at home with ill children or take them to the doctor. Thus, although there is undoubtedly a culture advocating the significance of the father's role, the

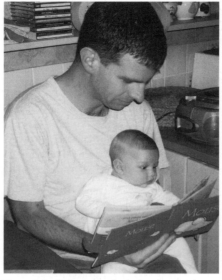

Figure 5.4 **Fathers can be just as involved as mothers in interaction with their babies.**

reality has probably not changed greatly in recent years. Mothers still do the majority of the work associated with children. In families where the mother goes out to work, fathers spend a slightly higher proportion of time with their children, but this is not because fathers are doing more – it is because employed mothers do less (Lamb, 1997).

Research by Parke and his co-workers (Parke, 1981) has shown that, with new-born infants, fathers were just as involved as mothers in interaction with their babies, and nurtured, touched, looked at, kissed, talked to and held them equally. In only one behaviour – smiling – did mothers surpass the fathers. However, in the earliest days, even with bottle-fed babies, fathers spent less time than mothers in feeding and related caretaking activities, which suggests that parental role allocation operates from the beginning of a child's life (see also Chapter 9, pp. 177–182).

Beyond the newborn period, fathers spend less time feeding and caretaking than mothers, and spend more time in play activities. Whereas mothers pick children up for caretaking activities such as nappy-changing, fathers pick them up to play with them. Not only do fathers play more with their children, but they also play differently to mothers. From as early as 8 months fathers engage in physical play, lifting, pushing and rough-and-tumble activities, whilst mothers engage in toy-stimulated play and reading to their children. These differences seem to be consistent throughout the early years, and lead to a preference for fathers as playmates, with more than two-thirds of children choosing to play with their father rather than their mother (Fig. 5.5). Research shows that the quality of the father's social, physical play is significantly related to the cognitive development of boys, whilst the quality of the father's verbal interactions with girls is important in female cognitive development.

The absence of a father is likely to be significant in a child's life. Apart from the poverty frequently found in families headed by a single mother, there is some evidence that IQ scores are lower, that achievement at school is poorer, and that 75 per cent of the children whose parents divorce feel rejected by their fathers, even when the fathers visit frequently (Wallerstein and Kelly, 1996). There is also some evidence that a father's absence is associated with psychiatric problems, lack of self-control and violent behaviour, particularly in boys. Girls seem to be less affected in this way.

Recent research in *father involvement* with young children in the UK has shown that there are some significant benefits for children later in their lives. Eirini Flouri, at the Oxford University Centre for Research Into Parenting and Children, has produced over 30 papers in the years between 1998 and 2003, based on the National Child Development Study of children born in 1958, and has shown that a strong father figure improves children's later mental health, makes antisocial behaviour (and for boys, trouble with the police) less likely, and makes young people more likely to gain 'A' level or higher qualifications, and to have more satisfactory partnerships in adult life. The four key criteria for gauging father involvement were reading to the

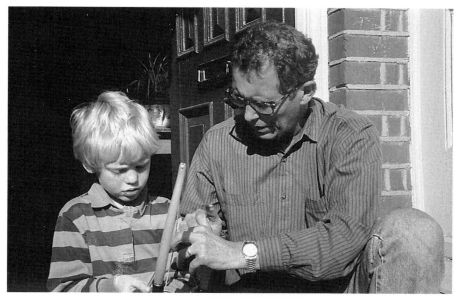

Figure 5.5   Children show a preference for playing with their fathers.

child, taking the child on outings, taking an interest in the child's education, and an equal role in managing the child. It is important to note that it is the continued presence of a father figure that matters. The family structure, whether he lives with the mother or not, and whether he is the biological father or not, did not make a difference. An older brother, an uncle, or even a friend, may suffice when the involvement is of good amount and quality (Flouri and Buchanan, 2003).

One of the areas thought to be very important in relation to fathers is that of sex-role development. First, fathers appear to prefer boys, and from birth onwards actually treat boys and girls differently. They encourage boys to be more 'masculine', and consistently pay more attention and give more stimulation to boys than to their daughters (although they cuddle their daughters more than their sons). They also appear to discriminate more than mothers in the treatment of male and female children, and seem to have somewhat rigid views about what constitutes appropriate sex-role behaviour, which they communicate to boys by providing masculine role models. Interestingly, boys who live in households without fathers generally show fewer sex-typed behaviours and attitudes than boys who live in intact families. The role of fathers is clearly important in a number of areas, yet there is also a pronounced discrepancy between popular cultural beliefs and actuality. To bring the two closer together, cultural support systems designed to encourage fathers' involvement, clearer role allocation and expectations, and better early socialization of males in nurturance and responsibility-taking, are all needed for the benefits to be realized.

SIBLING RELATIONSHIPS

The birth of a second child into a family is of significance not only to the parents but also to the first-born child. Until the early 1980s, there were few systematic studies of

sibling relationships (except for birth-order effects and
then there have been major developments in our underst
second child on the family, how sibling relationships deve
between parent–child relationships, and the effects of e
child's later friendships and adjustment. The leading in:
ments was Judy Dunn (Dunn and Kendrick, 1982), and
co-workers, to make important advances in this area (Dur

The commonly held view that a first-born child's rea
create behavioural problems, jealousy and rivalry seems t
disturbance of bodily functions, anxiety, withdrawal and
the immediate consequences to have been noted. Altho
first-born children show a range of reactions, ranging fro
empathy, through ambivalence to outright aggressiveness.
borns are keen to help to care for the new baby and to cud
her. One of the factors that influences the beginning of a :
way in which the mother talks to the first-born about the n
When mothers make reference to the expected baby, relationships between the siblings are subsequently much more friendly than when the newcomer has not been
introduced in discussion. Positive feelings between siblings are also more likely when
the parents have a positive relationship with each other.

The birth of a second child changes the existing relationships within a family.
Mothers may reduce the amount of time spent with the older child while they concentrate on the baby, and fathers often spend more time with the older sibling, whilst both
parents have less time for each other. Same-sex siblings seem to develop friendly
relationships with each other, particularly in families with first-born boys. Older
children seem to become particularly vigilant about the mother's interactions with a
new baby, and often demand absolute equality of maternal attention. The second-
born child is also very vigilant in monitoring the mother's relationships with her
older children, and it is out of this interest that a child's social understanding develops.

In the early years siblings serve a number of functions for each other. They provide affection and security, companionship and intimacy. They give support and
help to each other, provide models for imitation and the learning of both skills and
language, and through conflict and co-operation develop their own internal working
model of relationships, and an understanding of the feelings of others (Fig. 5.6).

There is some evidence that the quality of sibling relationships is associated with
the *security of attachment* each child has to its mother. That is, securely attached
older and younger siblings are likely to have friendly relationships with each other,
whereas insecurely attached children are more likely to have antagonistic relationships with one another. Although it is plausible that maternal attachment provides
a template for subsequent relationships, we must note that the evidence is correlational and as yet does not indicate a causal effect between attachment and the quality of sibling relationships.

One of the areas of sibling research that has received considerable attention in
recent years is concerned with differential parental treatment of children, especially
the notion of favouritism towards one of the siblings. Many adults who report a poor
sibling relationship in childhood often attribute this to their parents either positively
favouring one of the children, or scapegoating one of them. An early study found
that mothers were less affectionate and had less social interaction with second children than with first-born children (Jacobs and Moss, 1976), but in an even earlier
study Lasko (1954) found that parents were less warm and more coercive towards

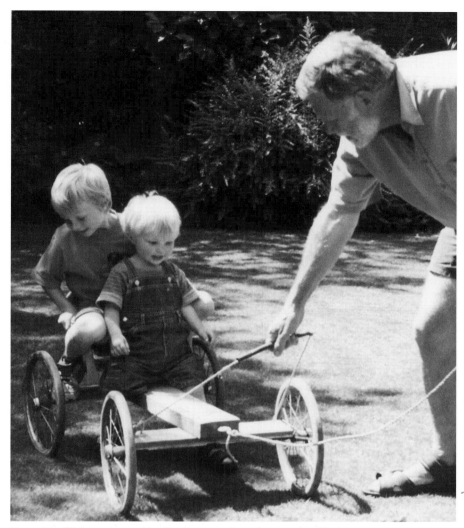

Figure 5.6   Siblings can provide affection, security and companionship.

their first-born children. Recent studies show a high level of consistency of treatment by mothers at 12 and 24 months, although in one study there was a sizeable group of mothers (34.5% of the sample) who appeared to treat their children differently (Ward *et al.*, 1988). This, of course, may be because their children's temperaments need differential treatment. At a given point in time with, say, a 12-month-old boy and a 24-month-old girl, maternal treatment may be quite different because of the age-determined or temperamental needs of the children.

What seems to be important in the different treatment of children by their parents is the *discrepancy* between one child and another. Bryant and Crockenberg (1980) found that, even when a child's own needs were being well met, if there was a discrepancy of treatment by the mother, that child would show more hostility and negative behaviour towards his or her sibling. Hetherington's study (1988) showed that it is the *relative* treatment of children that is significant, rather than the absolute parental behaviour that affects children most deeply. A sibling treated less warmly, less affectionately, more irritably or more punitively is likely to behave more aggressively and with less affection towards the other sibling. The favoured child is also more aggressive and unaffectionate towards the sibling. The *favouritism–hostility* hypothesis would seem to be supported. Recent research suggests that some children are particularly susceptible to differential treatment by parents. This seems to be related to the child's perception of having less responsive or unfair parents. The child attributes a negative meaning to parental actions, and may create a situation in which it is almost impossible for the parents to be perceived as fair. There is a growing research interest in this aspect of a child's interpretations of reality, and there are many questions yet to be answered about the effects of perceptions upon the child's future development. Conley (2004) argues that every family has a pecking order and that, in a complex, multilayered way, families select the most potentially successful sibling and invest considerably in their development.

One final point is that in many cultures around the world siblings provide and receive a great deal of caregiving – and therefore their socialization – from their siblings and not from adults, which is the usual pattern in Western societies. The implications of this will undoubtedly be explored as our knowledge of other cultures expands.

FRIENDS

In adults, friendships are based on the reciprocal exchange of benefits between equals, in which there is a sense of commitment and affection. Friendships are special in a way that simple peer interactions are not. Young children are clearly primarily attached to their parents in the first year or so of their lives, but they show increasing interest in other children, and by the age of 4 or 5 years most children have formed a special relationship with at least one other child. At school they develop relationships with about five children, a figure which continues into adolescence.

Children's conceptions of friendship begin somewhat simply, and become more elaborate and differentiated as the child grows older. Infants' conceptions are likely to focus on concrete aspects ('he lets me play with his toys'), whereas older children will use more complex and abstract ideas. Many psychologists argue that these differences are related to the general cognitive and language development of the child (Dunn, 2004).

Identification of a child's friendships has been attempted by several different methods:

- asking children to indicate their best friends;
- asking children who they 'like especially';
- observing the proximity between children.

In general, the level of agreement between these methods, although not perfect, has been very high. In general, a friend identified by a child will also be identified by a parent or a teacher, and the two children will clearly prefer to play together.

Children's friendships, like those of adults, move through a series of 'stages' (Levinger, 1983). A necessary condition for a child to begin a friendship is *proximity* – that is, being in the same place at the same time. However, this is not sufficient for the establishment of a friendship, because if the initial encounter is not rewarding at a superficial level, the relationship is unlikely to develop. At the second stage, the *build-up* of the relationship is characterized by repeated encounters which are mutually rewarding, in which the children communicate with each other and establish common interests by exchanging information and beginning the process of reciprocal self-disclosure. The *consolidation* of a friendship is marked by the development of a 'we feeling', where the two children develop a commitment to one another, and stable patterns of conflict resolution and successful management of the relationship occur. Sometimes the *deterioration* of a friendship happens when clear disagreements or conflicts are not successfully resolved. However, children's friendships often end without any clear argument and seem simply to fade away because the children stop interacting with one another, presumably because the interaction is no longer mutually satisfying. The *ending* of a child's friendship usually results in the children avoiding one another, reduced interaction and dependence, and usually little recrimination or conflict.

According to Hill (1987), the need for affiliation and relationships with friends serves four main functions. *Social comparison* allows children to establish their own position in relation to others ('My friend Tommy's got lots of guns, why can't I have some?'). *Emotional support* is provided by friends when a child is distressed ('Emily helped me when I fell over at nursery today'). *Positive stimulation* is provided by conversation, ideas and suggestions for play activities. *Attention* is paid by friends to a child's own being, and praise is offered for successes, raising the level of a child's self-esteem.

The functions of friendship in children probably vary with the age of the child, but a number of areas have been identified as important in child development. First, friendships are significant in the development of social competence. Howes (1983) found that in children aged 44–49 months, social behaviour with friends (as opposed to non-friends) was more elaborate, play was more co-operative, emotional exchanges were more positive, and vocalizing was increased. Friends are both cognitive and emotional resources for each other. They provide information about the world (not always accurately, e.g. 'My dad's a millionaire') and the opportunity for co-operative learning where, because of the nature of the relationship, the quality of the learning is likely to be better and problem-solving capacities are maximized. There is some evidence that friends increase the amount of laughing, talking, smiling and looking – that is, positive emotional feelings – and that they also increase a child's sense of security in a strange situation. Studies of adult relationships strongly suggest that friendships provide a buffer against the adverse effects of stressful life events such as divorce or a death in the family. Those with good-quality close relationships seem to suffer fewer physical illnesses or psychological disturbances than more isolated individuals. It would seem likely that this is true for children as well. Friends are judged second only to parents as sources of emotional support and their value increases as children get older.

Studies of adult friendship indicate that one of the major factors in the formation and continuation of relationships is *similarity*. Not only do we develop relationships with and eventually marry people similar to ourselves, but children, too, base their choices of friends upon similarity. Although choices are sometimes made on the basis of dissimilarity, for example higher status or more attractive or more popular children may be sought as friends, there is strong evidence of similarity between friends on a number of dimensions. From early childhood to adolescence children have friends of similar *age*. To some extent this is determined by the age structure of nurseries and schools and imposed by adults, but when given a free choice, most children usually form friendships with those of the same age. This is probably because of the egalitarian, horizontal power distribution between friends.

From pre-school years onwards, *same-sex* friendships predominate, and opposite-sex friendships are rare until adolescence, although even then only 5 per cent of friendships are with the opposite sex. Studies indicate that race, educational aspirations, attitudes towards achievement, and children's culture (e.g. music and sport) are all found to be similar between friends. Not only do children choose friends similar to themselves, but they actually become more similar to one another over time. Finding someone who is very like oneself is obviously highly rewarding, and the potential risks of conflict created by dissimilarity are significantly reduced.

The overall outcome of children's friendships is that they are important, if not absolutely necessary, for optimal development in a number of areas. Hartup and Rubin (1986) argue that most of the benefits of friendship may be achieved by other relationships – with parents, siblings or other family members. However, there is a developmental advantage for a child with friends. Perspective-taking, co-operation, altruism, social competence and adjustment and conflict management are all best learned within friendships.

Research into *popularity* shows that intellectual ability and physical attractiveness are important in a child being liked by other children. The 'beautiful is good' stereotype seems to operate from an early age, and it appears that the positive responses that bright, attractive children get from birth onwards help them to develop friendly, cheerful behaviours and skills which enable them to initiate interaction with other children, to maintain that interaction with sensitive communication, and to resolve conflict with agreeable and fair strategies. Popular children have more friends, and generally have high global self-worth scores (Berndt, 2002).

ABUSIVE RELATIONSHIPS

Child protection issues are fully discussed in Chapter 11, and full definitions of the different types of abuse are provided. This chapter, however, would not be complete without at least a brief mention of the implications of abusive relationships.

An ever-increasing body of evidence shows that, although a child's relationships with mother, father, siblings, grandparents and friends provide care and nurturance, they may also be the main sources of profound damage. It is usually someone to whom the child is closely connected by family or emotional ties who carries out acts of emotional, physical or sexual abuse or who neglects a child.

The results of the mistreatment associated with emotional abuse are thought to be severely injurious to the child's development of self-esteem, his or her perception of other people, and his or her future social relationships (Briere, 1995). Emotional neglect can also have serious cognitive and social consequences for the young child, with disturbances continuing into adolescence and adulthood.

The long-term effects of physical abuse – especially when combined with neglect or emotional abuse, as is often the case – can include post-traumatic stress reactions, cognitive distortions, altered emotionality and depression, identity confusion, poor self-image and difficulties in relating to important others (see for example Corby, 1993).

The effects of sexual abuse have been recently researched more fully than other forms of abuse. Survivors show a wide range of psychosocial symptoms, in both the short and long term. Sexual abuse occurring within a relationship of warmth and affection, with bribery and special privileges as well as secrecy and threats, is as likely to produce traumatic results as abuse that is based on violence and coercion. Anxiety, difficulty in giving and receiving affection, sexualizing of all relationships, depression, confusion, anger, aggression, psychosomatic illnesses, suicide attempts, self-mutilation, learned helplessness, sleep disturbance, moodiness and social isolation from peers have all been noted in children who have been victims of sexual abuse.

In adult survivors of sexual abuse, post-traumatic stress disorders sometimes occur, but major depression is the symptom most frequently recorded in child-abused adults. Anxiety is also common, with hypervigilance with regard to danger in the social environment, and a preoccupation with controlling threats or perceived dangers often present. Major difficulties are encountered in relationships with significant others, and problems with intimacy and trust, as well as sexual dysfunction (either promiscuity or sexual coldness), aggression, alcohol and drug abuse and also frequent suicide attempts by sexually abused survivors range from 51 per cent to 79 per cent (Briere, 1995). These are *failed* attempts, and the extent of successful suicides in sexually abused victims is not known.

Adults who have been sexually abused often become abusers of their own or other children. In the highly publicized case of Fred and Rosemary West, who physically and sexually abused – and indeed murdered – at least 12 young females, both of the abusers had been physically and sexually abused themselves as children, and appear to have continued and elaborated the abuses perpetrated upon them. However, not all abused children are destined to become child-abusing adults. Therapeutic help, support from family and friends, and sympathetic and understanding partners in adulthood may all diminish the adverse effects of sexual abuse and prevent the repeated pattern of abusive behaviour.

Conclusion

In reviewing the ideas, theories and evidence discussed in this chapter, the importance of a child's relationships becomes apparent. Relationships of high quality – whether they are with mother, father, siblings or friends – have a profound and long-lasting effect on the emotional, cognitive and social development of children. Although all children have their own unique characteristics, they are very responsive to the influences of their culture, their family and all of those with whom they interact. Widening our understanding of the reciprocal nature of these interactions and revealing the complex subtleties of a child's relationships are tasks which are now well established, although incomplete. Enriching our understanding through the growth of new knowledge from the fascinating and diverse cultures of the world is the next major task.

Student activity

For at least 30 minutes, observe the interaction between two (or more) siblings under 8 years of age. Identify instances of: affection; empathy; concern; jealousy/rivalry; aggression. Consider your observations in the light of theory from this chapter and discuss with a tutor, colleague or fellow student.

REFERENCES

Ainsworth, MD (1978): *Patterns of Attachment: a Psychological Study of the Strange Situation*. Hillsdale, NJ: Erlbaum.

Anderson, SA and Sabatelli, RM (2003): *Family Interaction*, 3rd edn. Boston, MA: Allyn & Bacon.

Barbarin, O and McCandies, T (2002): African-American families. In Ponzetti, J, Hamon, R, Kellar-Guenther, Y, Kerig, PK, Laine Scales, T and White, JM (eds), *International Encyclopaedia of Marriage and Family*, 2nd edn. New York: MacMillan Reference, USA.

Baumrind, D (1971): Current patterns of parental authority. *Developmental Psychology Monographs*, **4**, 1–103.

Baumrind, D (1991): The influence of parenting style on adolescent competence and substance use. *Journal of Early Adolescence*, **11**(1), 56–95.

Berndt, TJ (2002): Friendship quality and social development. *Current Directions in Psychological Science*, **11**, 2–10.

Bowlby, J (1953): *Child Care and the Growth of Love*. Harmondsworth: Penguin.

Briere, JN (1995): *Child Abuse Trauma*. London: Sage.

Bryant, B and Crockenberg, S (1980): Correlates and dimensions of prosocial behaviour. *Child Development*, **51**, 529–544.

Buss, DM (1999): *Evolutionary Psychology*. Boston: Allyn & Bacon.

Cassidy, J and Shaver, P (1999): *Handbook of Attachment Theory, Research and Clinical Applications*. New York: Guilford Press.

Conley, D (2004): *The Pecking Order: Which Siblings Succeed and Why*. New York: Pantheon Books.

Corby, B (1993): *Child Abuse – Towards a Knowledge Base*. Buckingham: Open University Press.

Dinkmeyer, D and McKay, G (1996): *Raising a Responsible Child*. New York: Fireside.

Dunn, J (2002): Sibling relationships. In Smith, PK and Hart, CH (eds), *Blackwell Handbook of Childhood Social Development*. Madden, MA: Blackwell Publishers.

Dunn, J (2004): *Children's Friendships: The Beginnings of Intimacy*. Malden, MA: Blackwell Publishers.

Dunn, J and Kendrick, C (1982): *Siblings: Love, Envy and Understanding*. London: Grant McIntyre.

Evans, GW (2004): The environment of childhood poverty. *American Psychologist*, **59**(2), 77–92.

Flouri, E and Buchanan, A (2003): The role of father involvement in adolescents. *British Journal of Social Work*, **33**, 399–406.

Hartup, WW and Rubin, Z (eds) (1986): *Relationships and Development*. Hillsdale, NJ: Erlbaum.

Hetherington, EM (1988): Parents, children and siblings. In Hinde, RA and Stevenson-Hinde, J (eds), *Relationships within Families*. Oxford, Open University Press.

Hill, AC (1987): Affiliation: people who need people. *Journal of Personality and Social Psychology*, **52**, 1008–1018.

Holmes, TH and Rahe, RH (1967): The social readjustment rating scale. *Journal of Psychosomatic Research*, **11**, 213–218.

Howes, C (1983): Pattern of friendship. *Child Development*, **54**, 1041–1053.

Jacobs, BS and Moss, HA (1976): Birth order and sex of siblings. *Child Development*, **47**, 315–322.

La Freniere, P and Sroufe, LA (1985): Profiles of peer competence in the pre-school: interrelations between measures, influence of social ecology, and relation to attachment history. *Developmental Psychology*, **21**, 56–59.

Lamb, ME (1987): *The Father's Role: Cross-cultural Perspectives*. Hillsdale, NJ: Erlbaum.

Lamb, ME (ed.) (1997): *The Role of the Father in Child Development*. New York: John Wiley & Sons Ltd.

Lasko, JK (1954): Parent behaviour toward first and second born children. *Genetic Psychology Monographs*, **49**, 97–137.

Levinger, G (1983): Development and change. In Kelley, H *et al.* (eds), *Close Relationships*. New York: Freemans.

Maccoby, EE and Martin, JA (1983): Socialisation in the context of the family. In Mussen, PH and Hetherington, EM (eds), *Handbook of Child Psychology*, Vol. 4, 4th edn. New York: John Wiley & Sons Ltd.

Main, M and Solomon, J (1986): Discovery of a disorganized/disorientated attachment pattern. In Brazelton, TB and Yogman, MW (eds), *Affective Development in Infancy*. Norwood, NJ: Ablex.

McCubbin, HI, Thompson, AI and McCubbin, MA (1996): *Family Assessment: Resiliency, Coping and Adaptation*. Madison: University of Wisconsin Publishers.

Olson, DH and DeFrain, J (2000): *Marriage and Family: Diversity and Strengths*, 3rd edn. Mountain View, CA: Mayfield Publishing.

Olson, DH, McCubbin, HI, Barnes, H, Larsen, A, Muxen, M and Wilson, M (1989): *Families: What makes them Work*, 2nd edn. Beverley Hills, CA: Sage.

Parke, RD (1981): *Fatherhood*. Cambridge, MA: Harvard University Press.

Richards, M (1995): Family relations. *The Psychologist*, **8**, 70–72.

Rode, S, Chang, P, Fisch, R and Sroufe, LA (1981): Attachment patterns of children separated at birth. *Developmental Psychology*, **17**, 188–191.

Wallerstein, JS and Kelly, JB (1996): *Surviving the Breakup*. New York: Basic Books.

Ward, MJ, Vaugh, BE and Robb, MD (1988): Social-emotional adaptation and infant–mother interaction in siblings. *Child Development*, **59**, 643–651.

Whiting, BB and Edwards, CP (1988): *Children of Different Worlds*. Cambridge, MA: Harvard University Press.

FURTHER READING

Barnes, P (1995): *Personal, Social and Emotional Development in Children*. Oxford, Blackwell.

Boer, F and Dunn, J (1992): *Children's Sibling Relationships*. Hillsdale, NJ: Erlbaum.

Bornstein, MH (ed.) (2002): *Handbook of Parenting*, 2nd edn, Vol. 3. Hove: Erlbaum.

Buss, DM (1999): *Evolutionary Psychology*. Boston: Allyn & Bacon.

Conley, D (2004): *The Pecking Order: Which Siblings Succeed, and Why*. New York: Pantheon Books.

Corby, B (2000): *Child Abuse*. Buckingham: Open University Press.

Dunn, J (2002): Sibling relationships. In Smith, PK and Hart, CH (eds), *Blackwell Handbook of Childhood Social Development*. Madden, MA: Blackwell Publishers.

Dunn, J (2004): *Children's Friendships: The Beginnings of Intimacy*: Madden, MA: Blackwell Publishers.

Erwin, P (1993): *Friendships and Peer Relations in Children*. Chichester: John Wiley & Sons Ltd.

Erwin, P (1998): *Friendship in Childhood and Adolescence*. London: Routledge.

Frude, N (1990): *Understanding Family Problems*. Chichester, John Wiley & Sons Ltd.

Lamb, ME (ed.) (1997): *The Role of the Father in Child Development*. New York: John Wiley & Sons Ltd.

PLAY, LANGUAGE AND LEARNING

6

Anne Greig

This chapter aims to:

■ explore the nature of, and interrelationship between, play, language and learning.

INTRODUCTION

Consider the following scene from a Wendy house, involving Simon and Rebecca, both aged 4 years, who are not friends:

S: Oh, it's half-past one! Cor, I think it's time we've to go to bed!
R: (Ignores him)
S: Goodnight! I'm going to bed.
R: (Ignores him)
S: I'm going to bed!
R: But mummies and daddies stay up for late … take a book to bed … let's take our babies to bed!
S: I'm going to sleep, I won't bother (mutters).
R: (Follows him). It's time to go to sleep now.
S: Come on, shut the curtains shall we? I'm going to have some water and then I put some aspirin in a cup. I got a poorly head.

(extract from Greig, 1993)

According to Garvey (1991), we may regard this play-scene as charming, silly or disturbingly perceptive in its portrayal of adult behaviour. However, for the serious student of the child, there is much more to discern and discover. It can tell us, for instance, about relationships on many levels – between the children themselves, with adults at home, and in the little cultural rituals of going to bed. It tells us about their communicative and social competencies, and also how they think, learn and feel. Researchers from a variety of disciplines that include child development, anthropology and psychotherapy, examine hundreds of such encounters between children in order to detect the patterns and rules which govern their interaction and communication (for recent accounts, see James, 1998; Blatchford, 1998; Goodwin, 1997; Howe *et al.*, 2002).

In this chapter we shall explore the nature of this play with its associated language and learning, and examine their role in early childhood. We shall also focus on the complex and special relationship between these three aspects of early childhood. Our approach to early childhood has been expressed as an holistic one, and the nature of the relationship between play, language and learning is an example, par excellence, of the holistic nature of the child. Children play, learn, talk, build relationships – and more besides – all at once, making the child observer's task a difficult one. In addition, specifying the exact nature of interacting elements is often contentious. For instance, does the child develop language after, before or in parallel to the development of cognition? The relationship between play, language and learning is of this highly complex and contentious nature. An apt analogy to introduce the nature of the relationship comes from Bjørkvold (1987), who describes the Swahili concept of ngoma. This is a special word meaning 'dance-ritual-song', activities which in the Swahili culture are inseparably moulded together – no song without dance, no dance without words and song. It is a nice idea, and in considering the play of Simon and Rebecca, it is apparent that their play, language and learning are inextricably linked, but would we go so far as to say 'no play, no language, no learning' or 'no language, no play, no learning'? Clearly there are links, but to what extent and in what way? Finding the answers to these questions is the ongoing and daunting task of both theoreticians and practitioners.

The study of language is a very large, well-defined research area in itself, including specialized research on acquisition, including literacy, oracy, reading, bilingualism, linguistics, psycholinguistics, sociolinguistics, applied linguistics, grammars, phonology, syntax and semantics, language and mind, semiotics and signs, non-verbal communication and paralinguistics (see Whitehead, 1990; Chapman, 2000, for a contemporary analysis). Learning theory has a variety of perspectives, and it has been claimed that, although research on play has produced some valuable results, the overall pattern is disconnected, much of it not following a clearly thought-out or promising agenda (Nicolopoulou, 1993; Hunter, 1998). Our agenda is to introduce the available theoretical approaches to play, language and learning. The field will also be delimited in that we are focussing on early childhood, and the relevant theorists (mainly Piaget and Vygotsky) who, in addition to being learning theorists, subscribe to theories on play and the role played by language. Consequently, the chapter will have a theoretical flavour, with less attention being given to more applied, practical specialisms.

SPECIAL ISSUES AND INFLUENTIAL THEORIES ON PLAY, LANGUAGE AND LEARNING

As we do not have to whip children into playing and learning how to say 'mama', most people would be happy to agree that play, language and learning are all spontaneous activities. None the less, they need examination with regard to the influences of genes, environment, or both. For example, are cognition and language both natural and equally spontaneous activities? That is, to what extent is each innate or acquired? Consequently, the nature-nurture controversy will be a recurring theme in this chapter (see also Chapter 1, p. 4). In addition, the special relationship between language and learning promotes a debate as to which one has supremacy. Does language determine thought, or is it a by-product of the learning process? Both language and learning are relatively easy to define, and research on language usually refers either directly or indirectly to research on learning, and vice versa. They need not, however, refer to play. 'Play' seems to be one of those words, like 'beautiful' or 'pornographic', that you know when you see it, but that is difficult to define (Goodman, 1994). There is an emerging consensus that, given the width of the concept of play within and across cultures, it is important not to be bound by limited definitions of play (Hunter, 1998; James, 1998) and, despite passionate writings on the subject, there remains a need for more systematic research into the functional aspects of play (Scott, 1998).

In this section we shall focus on play, language and learning, together with their special issues. Furthermore, because play is usually viewed as the context for the display or improvement of learning and language, the sequence of discussion will be learning, followed by language, and finally play. Towards the end of the chapter consideration will be given to the relationship between play, language and learning.

SPECIAL ISSUES IN LEARNING

The question of how children learn has been much studied. The first few years of a child's life are a period during which the child will learn more than in the rest of his or her lifetime. The early years, including the time in the womb, are regarded as critical in terms of vulnerability to infection, damage and environmental modification. Consequently, it is important to understand this early learning process so that we are in a position to enhance it, intervene and develop new theories. In essence, learning theories occupy various positions in the nature–nurture controversy. As you will already be aware, these positions are known as nativist, empiricist, and constructivist views.

You will recall from Chapter 1 that nativists argue that we are born with the knowledge we have. As such, they are biologists who argue that the child is genetically pre-programmed to unfold in certain ways, and that attainment of knowledge takes place only gradually and via inherent maturational mechanisms. (For a contemporary, nativist approach to the genetic pre-wiring of cognitive processes, see Karmiloff-Smith, 1995.) Empiricists argue that the child is not born with genetic blueprints, but is instead a tabula rasa or blank slate which is filled only as a consequence of environmental experience. This is the approach of behaviourists such as Pavlov and Skinner, who believed that learning is the process of forming associations between external stimuli and internal responses. This type of learning is mainly passive, with the child responding to the environment, although operant conditioning sees the child or organism as operating on the environment. Constructivists represent a combination of both genetic pre-programming and environmental adaptation or experience. The child actively constructs a version of reality from his or her unique experiences. It is this approach which has been most influential in educational research, and has greater holistic relevance.

Influential learning theories

The constructivists Piaget, Vygotsky and Bruner all share an interest in the relationship between the inner, biological, individual child and the outer, environmental, social child – that is, the extent to which a child's knowledge is determined biologically and culturally, compared with the child's freedom to act independently and creatively. All three theorists agree that the child is both determined and a determiner of knowledge and understanding. Where they differ is in the emphasis that they each place on the direction of the relationship.

In the process of learning, Piaget's child is an isolated individual who attempts to adapt to the world around him or her. This process of adaptation takes place via four important processes: schemas; assimilation; accommodation; and equilibration. Schemas are present from the start, and are initially purely physical or sensory actions. The infant does not plan, intend or internally represent objects by means of mental pictures, but instead responds only to stimuli that are immediately available.

For instance, the infant will have a looking schema, a holding schema and a grasping schema. As the child develops, he or she acquires more obviously mental schemas, such as categorization and comparison of objects. After further maturation, more complex schemas are added, such as deductive analysis. It is, however, the three basic processes of assimilation, accommodation and equilibration which enable development from the simple action schemas of infancy to the increasingly complex mental schemas of later childhood. Assimilation involves taking in and absorbing experiences into existing schemas. Thus, when a child already knows how to pick up one object, new objects and situations can be acted out and understood within the existing schema. There is also room for subjectivity in the process, because a child may assimilate a roundish object into a round schema and remember it as being more round than it actually is.

Accommodation occurs when the child changes an existing schema as a result of new information taken in by assimilation. For instance, a child will have a sucking schema for the breast which will have to be adapted to a new form of action in order to cope with a bottle, and subsequently to drink from a cup. Subtle sensorimotor changes will be necessary in order to cope with the less familiar objects. In this way, accommodation is crucial for the developmental progress. As the child adapts existing schemas to new ones presented in the environment, Piaget believed the child to be seeking a balance in his or her understanding of the world, and this he termed 'equilibration'. The child strives to create a coherent and internally consistent understanding and knowledge. According to Piaget, there are four crucial stages when the child is faced with challenges resulting in disequilibrium, after which, through adaptation, the balance is restored and the child achieves a significant shift on to a higher level of understanding. In essence, then, the child is inner, biological and individual – many adults and educators have believed that they must wait for the child to reach the appropriate level of development before they can enhance his or her emerging capabilities. While such a strict interpretation of the theory has not been advocated recently in practice, the Piagetian approach does, to a considerable extent, place the responsibility for learning on the child who develops in isolation, making and testing theories as he or she constructs understanding by operating or acting on his or her environment. Piaget's child therefore becomes social only gradually as his or her cognitive capacity to do so matures.

Vygotsky's child, by contrast, is the child in society. The social nature of the child is present right from the beginning when the infant arrives into a complex world of social relationships and culture – a culture which itself has an historical development. Vygotsky proposed two lines of development for the child: the natural line of organic growth and maturation; and the line of cultural improvement of the psychological functions. At a certain point, they meet up, mediated by speech (Vygotsky writes about speech rather than language) and external, cultural knowledge becomes internal. Whilst Vygotsky viewed individual forces and cultural forces of development as being equally important, his general emphasis is often regarded as being on the impact of culture on the child. Vygotsky does not accept that a child is in the position of creating a conceptual world 'from scratch', but believes that they need instead to appropriate the conceptual resources of the pre-existing cultural world which are transmitted to them by parents, adults and peers. He argued that psychological functions originate in interaction with other people and therefore such knowledge appears initially in interaction with others or interpersonally, and only later becomes intrapersonal (within the child). The example of this cited in *Mind in Society* (Vygotsky, 1978) is the development of pointing, highlighting the importance of gesture and communication in cognitive development.

'*Initially, this gesture is nothing more than an unsuccessful attempt to grasp something… At this initial stage, pointing is represented by the child's movement… that and nothing more… When the mother comes to the child's aid and realises his movement indicates something, the situation changes fundamentally… Pointing becomes a gesture for others… consequently, the primary meaning of that unsuccessful grasping movement is established by others.*'

(Vygotsky, 1978, p. 56)

The facilitative role for the more competent other is further developed by Vygotsky in his theory of the zone of proximal (next) development. He complained about the generally accepted method of assessing a child's level of development using standardized tests, because these do not differentiate between the child's actual developmental level and what he or she might reasonably achieve with some assistance (see also Chapters 3 and 7). In this situation, individual children will demonstrate greater interpersonal variation in terms of potential development. According to Vygotsky, then, the zone of proximal development (ZPD) is '… the distance between the actual developmental level as determined by independent problem solving and the level of potential development as determined through problem solving under adult guidance or in collaboration with more capable peers' (Vygotsky, 1978, p. 86).

Vygotsky's child is therefore a social, outer, culturally determined child. None the less, through the ZPD any child is capable of making a unique contribution to his or her learning, knowledge and understanding.

Bruner's approach to learning was influenced by both Piaget and Vygotsky, but ultimately owes more to Vygotsky. Bruner's child assimilates and accommodates, but the nature of mental representation is crucially influenced by the child's social interactions and environment. Children learn to think in actions (enactively), in pictures (iconically) and in words (symbolically), because actions, pictures and words are used by people around them. That is, learning and knowledge are social in origin and, although the developmental sequence is enactive, then iconic and finally symbolic, Bruner believes that all three remain available to adults. Although he has not presented a unified theory of learning, his work has formalized many of Vygotsky's ideas into educational strategies such as 'scaffolding' (a culturally imposed framework for learning) and the 'spiral curriculum' (the notion that any subject can be taught effectively in some intellectually honest form to any child at any stage of development) (Bruner, 1972, 1990; for a critical review, see Newman and Holzman, 1993).

SPECIAL ISSUES IN LANGUAGE

In defining language, in order to be consistent with our holistic views elsewhere, it is necessary to make our definition in the broadest sense of both verbal and non-verbal communication. Smith *et al.* (2003) discuss how communication systems exist within almost all species, yet what sets humans apart is the creative flexibility of generating new meaningful utterances, communication of ideas, shared thoughts and consideration of themes that are remote in time and place. As such, communication is an excellent example of complex human behaviour, recruiting information processing to the full. The fact that children have already quickly mastered the complexities of communication by the pre-school years is an ongoing research interest. Are children born pre-programmed to learn language? What is the effect of the environment?

How does language develop? These questions are directly relevant to learning and the nature versus nurture issue already mentioned.

The recognition that there is a fundamental connection between language and thinking has existed since the time of Aristotle. However, the general claim that thought and language are intrinsically related raises a number of questions. Can there be thought without language? Do different languages reflect different ways of thinking? Do different languages cause differences in the ways in which people think? The view that language determines thought and mentality is traditionally known as linguistic determinism, and consistent with this is linguistic relativity, which means that differences in languages cause differences in thinking. From a developmental point of view, there has always been some debate about which develops first – thought or language – and the exact nature of the interdependence between them. The contention that it is language which dictates thought has serious implications for children and their free will – children will be socialized into a restricted world view, habitual patterns of language use in some subcultures will disadvantage children educationally, thought will not exist without language, thought will not develop before language, and communication across cultures will at best be limited. Such views have been attacked as being narrow and pessimistic, and a number of alternatives have been in circulation for some time (Mead, 1934; Piaget, 1959; Vygotsky, 1962; Chapman, 2000). Other theorists have examined cognitive development empirically and have differing notions of the role played by language, culture and social relationships. The two main approaches could be described as Western (Piaget, 1959) and Eastern (Vygotsky, 1962). Piaget and Vygotsky agree that thought does not originate in language. However, Piaget virtually ignored language except in relation to the unsocial nature of egocentric speech – a view he later revised – and how the child's stage of cognitive development is manifested in the language of the child. This egocentric speech reflects the child's cognitive developmental level as being unable to take the 'social' point of view of others. Whilst acknowledging the importance of peers over parents for cognitive development, because of the opportunity they present for interaction on an equal footing,

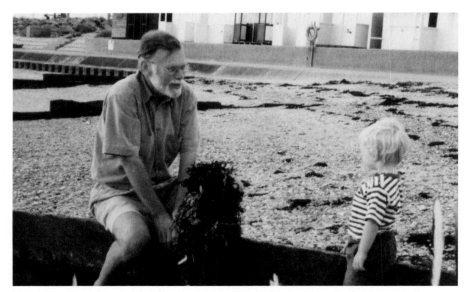

Figure 6.1 Vygotsky considered language and adults to be crucial for the development of cognitive processes.

Piaget none the less gave the child's inherent creativity and individuality precedence over social factors in cognitive development. Vygotsky, on the other hand, considered both language and adults to be crucial for the development of cognitive processes.

Language and thought, which are initially separate functions, join forces at about 2 years of age to transform the inner mental life of the child. A child initially uses overt speech (egocentric) to organize the inner mind, and the overt speech then becomes covert or inner thought. Speech is a powerful source of signs, and empowers the child to restructure his or her environment. In addition, language is an important feature for internal cognitive restructuring – as the child plays, he or she will often maintain a monologue on what he or she is doing. The outer speech is not unlike the commentary that adults provide for very young children, for example counting out loud as the child climbs the stairs '... one ... two ... oops ... two ... three'. Such monologues represent over-socialized speech, which eventually becomes internal or silent inner speech, thus enabling verbal thought (for a modern account of egocentric speech see Bråten, 1991; Diaz and Berk, 1992).

The ideas from the seminal works of interactionists such as Donaldson (1978), Youniss (1980) and Trevarthen (1987), taking account of both individual and social influences on language and thought, continue to be well represented in modern developmental research (e.g. Trevarthen and Aitken, 2001).

Influential language theories

The main theoretical approaches to language acquisition are:

- learning;
- nativist;
- cognitive;
- social interactionist.

The learning theory or behaviourist approach to language explains acquisition as a matter of imitation and reinforcement. As an infant says 'goo goo', babbles, etc., the sounds are shaped by adults until they become words. It is also argued that when a child imitates an adult, the adult rewards the child, and these words will then be learned and used again under similar stimulus conditions. Whilst one can readily find examples of imitation, reinforcement and shaping in language, they do not necessarily occur in all utterances. It is too simplistic to account for the child's spontaneous, original speech efforts and their sensitivity to the regularities of speech evident from their systematic errors as they try to generate meaningful utterances.

The nativist view of Chomsky is one in which infants are pre-programmed to learn a language and are highly sensitive to the linguistic features of their environment. As Chomsky was concerned with the mental structures within the mind, he spoke of an internal Language Acquisition Device (LAD), namely the mental apparatus that supposedly innately programmes human beings to a universal grammar, thus making it possible for them to speak and comprehend language. Examples of the evidence which suggests that children do generate their own language around rules might include their tendency to over-generalize a rule such as plurals (e.g. 'mans') and tenses (e.g. 'goed'). The traditional cognitive (Piagetian) view of language acquisition is that it is seen as part of general cognitive development. In effect, language acquisition must wait for sensorimotor thinking to develop first.

The importance of the role played by adult and child relationships in learning has, however, been applied to the study of language acquisition. As a social interactionist, Bruner proposed, in addition to the LAD, a 'sister' known as a Language Acquisition Support System (LASS). 'If there is a Language Acquisition Device, the input to it is not a shower of spoken language but a highly interactive affair shaped ... by some sort of an adult Language Acquisition Support System' (Bruner, 1983, p. 39). This approach is pragmatic in that it emphasizes language use and its social functions. According to Bruner, the LASS is not exclusively linguistic, but forms part of an overall system for passing on the culture of which language is both instrument- and creator-passed on through a complex system of rules (for a critical analysis, see Newman and Holzman, 1993).

Aitchison (1983) proposed that something specific to language is innate, even though we are not entirely sure what that 'something' consists of. Neither can language be explained as a general offshoot of general intelligence, although we undoubtedly use it when we speak in an as yet undefined way. Aitchison considers learning theories such as those of Skinner to have failed dismally as an explanation of how children acquire language. Chapman (2000) gives an interesting account of language learning which is 'interactionist'. He argues that, in light of improved methodologies and shifts in our understanding of children's general cognitive development (e.g. integration of infancy research with later childhood, thinking as a collaborative process and theory of mind to name a few), language learning needs to be reconceptualized as an integration of learning in multiple domains:

> *'Much of what appears given or innate in young children's developing cognition and language, may on closer inspection, be shown to arise from the statistical structure of the encountered world and the correlations arising in action upon it, in a manner shared with other species. ... Such an enterprise is initially discomfiting, in a world of narrow and traditional disciplines of study and discourse; it suggests a reality so multi-layered and complex that it is dizzying to think about'*
>
> (Chapman, 2000, p. 45)

There have been many studies of the relationship between language and learning (see, for example Wells, 1987, and Roskos and Christie, 2000).

SPECIAL ISSUES IN PLAY

Play and childhood usually go together. Indeed, much of what children do is regarded as play. However, much of what children do is also clearly not play (Garvey, 1991). Different cultures may view play and childhood differently (see Introduction and Chapter 9 for further discussions around this topic; also see James, 1998). In the Greek language, for example, the word for play comes from the word for child, and a separate word is used for organized games or contests, mostly associated with adult life. The English 'play' comes from the Anglo-Saxon 'plega', which referred to play or rapid bodily movement, and was also used to mean performing with musical instruments. However, Roman languages (e.g. French and Italian) do not distinguish between play and games, and use one word for both.

Although play has been passionately and widely studied, authors have repeatedly noted that the most troublesome aspect of studying play arises from the fuzziness of the concept and the lack of a precise behavioural definition (e.g. Fein, 1981; Pelligrini and Smith, 1998; Scott, 1998). There are many ways of approaching play, and there are also many different kinds of play (see Pelligrini and Smith, 1998; Smith *et al.*, 2003), so it is perhaps unsurprising that a firm working definition eludes us. Consider a baby babbling in his or her cot or shaking a rattle, or two boys chasing each other and wrestling on the floor, or the elaborate role play of 4-year-old doctors and nurses. Play may be viewed differently depending on personal characteristics such as age, gender, culture, social class, features of the environment (e.g. space, weather and equipment) and cultural factors (e.g. behavioural conventions and fashions). These are some of the factors which are known to influence play and the difficulty in defining it. Consequently, whilst authors agree that it is best not to define play, most of them have attempted to identify the general characteristics of/criteria for play (Hunter, 1998; Lillemyr *et al.*, 2001). It is generally agreed that play is non-literal, that is, a non-serious attitude to reality (Garvey, 1974), and that play is pleasurable, enjoyable and indexed by laughter. Other more contentious characteristics include freedom from extrinsic motivation; that is, play is unconstrained by external rules or social demands, but is engaged in for its own sake (Bruner, 1976); the flexibility of play in utilizing alternatives for action, which means variation in the form and content of the play, and play as having a means rather than ends orientation (e.g. Hutt, 1979; Smith *et al.*, 2003). Sutton-Smith and Kelly-Byrne (1984) accuse researchers and practitioners alike of over-emphasizing the importance and positive aspects of play. Instead, they remind us that play can be non-egalitarian (e.g. dominance and conflict), may not be voluntary, spontaneous or intrinsically motivated (obligation to and the power of friends and restricted environments), often manifests negative affect (fighting, brutal teasing), and finally, can be dysfunctional. Smith (1993) urges theoreticians, practitioners and students of play to proceed with caution and to take a balanced view of play and its value and relationship to children. It is both ambiguous and paradoxical, and the preferred definitional common ground noted above remains unsteady. None the less, most practitioners are convinced of the empowering potential of play for developing language and learning, and this view has been reflected in the burgeoning interest in play in the fields of psychology, education, anthropology and sociology, and also in the recommendations of policy-makers and practitioners (e.g. Lillemyr *et al.*, 2001).

Mellou (1994), in a review of play theories, prefers to view them as either classical (early) theories (e.g. surplus energy theory, recreation/relaxation theory, practice theory, recapitulation theory) or modern theories (e.g. psychoanalytical theory, metacommunicative theory, cognitive theory). More will be said about these theories later, but Mellou is keen to point out that the much-criticized early theories actually provide a basis for the modern theories. In all theories, she claims, there is a duality in the process of play in terms of personal expression versus social adaptation.

Influential play theories

The forum for the discussion of the nature and purpose of play was opened by the German poet and philosopher, Schiller, in the eighteenth century with his letters on the Aesthetic of Man. He was responsible for formulating the evolutionary-type theory, notably what became known as the surplus energy theory of play, according to which the young of both animals and humans have large quantities of superfluous energy that are invested in the aimless activity of play. Smith *et al.* (2003) cite the classic theorists on play (Spencer, Lazarus, Patrick, Hall and Groos). Spencer's (1873) elaboration of this notion included classification of types (e.g. sensorimotor, artistic-aesthetic, memetic, games) of play. Other evolutionary/biological theories include those of recreation and relaxation (Lazarus, 1883) and Patrick (1916), who argued that play was needed by adults and children as a natural consequence of experiencing fatigue. Thus, the function of play was to renew the organism by way of its alternative and more primitive source of energy. An extreme evolutionary theory is Hall's recapitulation theory, in which the development of the individual mimics the development of the species. In this way, children's play was seen to represent the evolutionary history of our species. For example, climbing was related to the early animal stage of mankind, whilst playing with dolls was linked to a later agricultural/patriarchal stage. One particularly influential evolutionary theory was that of Groos (1901). Under a Darwinian influence, he proposed practice theory, according to which the young of various species went through more or less extensive periods of immaturity during which they had the chance to practise skills that would prove indispensable to them in adult life. These included the practice of physical, mental and social skills. The results of such playful activities were regarded as being of secondary importance, as what mattered most was the behaviours involved in the process. For a critical appraisal on the types and functions of play, see Pelligrini and Smith (1998) and Smith *et al.* (2003).

Many widely accepted theories of play are of a more psychological nature, dealing with the emotional, social and cognitive functions. First, play is presented as being important in the emotional life of individuals – it helps to overcome problems of reality and it satisfies basic emotional needs. Second, the social functions of play, normally studied by sociologists or social anthropologists, are what could be described as affiliative in that play is akin to ritual in social groups and contributes to a temporary inversion of reality and of given social structures, offering a sense of 'togetherness'. This approach is still only represented by a few studies in developmental research (e.g. Corsaro, 1979). The social function of play is perhaps more commonly studied in conjunction with cognition (socio-cognitive) as, for example, in the work of Leslie (1987), Bateson (1955), Bruner (1976) and Vygotsky (1967), or in conjunction with emotion (socio-emotional), as in the work of Freud (1920). Third, the purely cognitive function of play is the domain of Piaget, who differs from the socio-cognitivists noted above, not only with regard to their interest in the social context, but also in the role that language plays in the development of the cognitive function. We shall now consider each of these approaches to play in slightly more detail.

For the *psychoanalysts*, play has an important role in resolving the emotional conflicts that arise as a consequence of the child's relationships with others. Children and adults alike are subject to anxiety and neuroses, the foundations of which begin in childhood and persist into later life. Psychoanalysts therefore view childhood as critical and the role of play as therapy as particularly important (Alvarez and Phillips, 1998; Woolgar, 1999). For *psychotherapists*, play is a serious business (Winnicot, 1971). For children who have been deprived of a normal access to play there can be serious consequences (e.g. Levin, 2002). Play that is therapeutically facilitated by adults can give these troubled children a sense of emotional 'containment' (Bion, 1962). This refers to an emotional 'gathering together' of the child who is distressed, so that emotions can be managed, the child has the security of being heard and learns a model of how to deal with distress and think about feelings. The need to feel secure in order to play productively is a crucial concept in attachment theory (see also Chapters 4 and 5). It is this psychoanalytical approach to play which has established the play therapy system currently used for highly disturbed children, although there are many different therapeutic approaches (e.g. Erikson, 1963). Erikson argued that children are partners with their futures in play because their 'as-if' play seemed to serve as a metaphor for their lives. When children grow up, their adult life-style will have been implicit in their

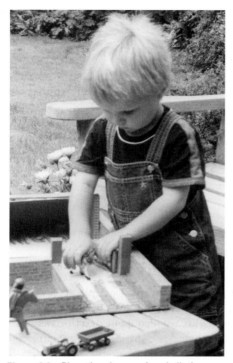

Figure 6.2 Piaget's primacy of assimilation – the child incorporating events and objects into existing mental structures.

childhood free-play. It is through play that they learn to deal with disappointment and failure, and learn to approach life with a sense of increasingly focused purpose.

Piaget considered play to be characterized by the primacy of assimilation over accommodation – the child incorporates events and objects into existing mental structures. As the child evolves through cognitive developmental stages, there is an equivalent manifestation in play behaviours. First, sensorimotor play is practice play involving repetitious actions which gradually become purposive. When language and representation emerge, the child is able to play symbolically. However, this is a solitary affair, directed initially towards self, and is a simple ability, for instance, to pretend to go to sleep out of the context of reality. Soon, the child will move from this self-reference to other-reference – for example, he or she will put teddy to sleep (Fig. 6.3). This is followed by the ability to use objects symbolically; for example, a peg serves as a substitute for a doll. Finally, the child is able to make sequential combinations – that is, a whole play-scene. Socio-dramatic play is evident between 4 and 7 years, when

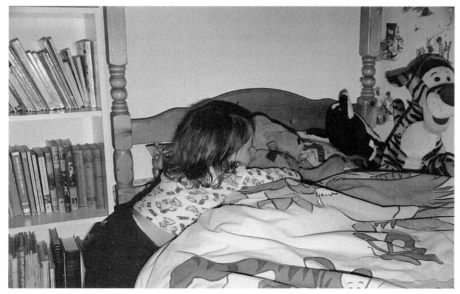

Figure 6.3 Putting teddy to sleep: children move from self-reference to other-reference.

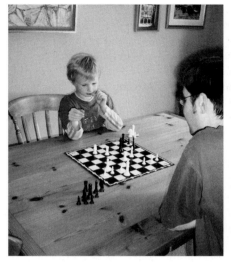

Figure 6.4 Chess: children later play games with explicit rules but an imaginary situation.

the child engages in pretend-play with others. Between 7 and 11 years the child moves into the realm of collective symbols, rules and games with rules, and it is this play which marks the transition to a socialized individual. Play thus moves from purely individual, idiosyncratic, private processes and symbols to social play and collective symbols. As play is about assimilation, pretend play serves to enable the child to relive past experiences, rather than to create possible future ones.

The other play theorists who have been concerned with cognition have, without exception, also addressed how language and the social environment interact with the child's learning or developing cognitive abilities. Vygotsky discussed play as arising from social pressures, that is, for social and emotional needs. For Vygotsky (1967), play is always a social symbolic activity. Even when a child plays alone, there will be implicit socio-cultural themes; for example, toys are cultural inventions, and role-play entails socially constructed rules for behaviour and interaction. Vygotsky believed that solitary play was a later development than social play, and that genuine play emerged at about 3 years of age. Genuine play has two main characteristics, namely the imaginary situation and the rules implicit in that imaginary situation. For example, a child playing as a 'mother' can freely select her behaviour, but must also follow the rules of maternal behaviour as she understands them, and this entails cognitive effort. Later on, pretend-play with games and rules, such as chess, involves explicit rules but an imaginary situation (Fig. 6.4). The function of play is socio-emotional – the child desires to act in the ways of an adult, but is not yet able to do so. This need can be satisfied through fantasy. Furthermore, in submission to implicit and explicit rules, children are empowered with self-control over their impulsive desires. Importantly, play also contributes to cognitive development rather than simply reflecting it. It is through early play that the child first creates the zone of proximal development:

> 'In play a child is always above his average age, above his daily behaviour; in play it is as though he were a head taller than himself'.

(Vygotsky, 1967, p. 6)

Consider also a pretend world in which a piece of wood can be used as a substitute for a doll or a horse or a car. This is the creation of a world dominated by meanings – one in which action arises from ideas rather than from objects – and this paves the way for abstract internalized thought (for a critical review of Piaget and Vygotsky, see Nicolopoulou, 1993).

Bruner (1976), clearly influenced by Groos and Vygotsky, noted that the increased dominance of play during immaturity among higher primates serves as practice for the technical social life that constitutes human culture. He also realized the practical educational implications of his theory and the role played by others (especially adults), in particular, referring to interactional routines such as 'peek-a-boo' as 'scaffolding'. It is such conventional routines and formats of games which prepare children to take their place in society and culture.

The remaining socio-cognitive theorists have developed further the importance of communication and language in play or, more precisely, pretend-play, for the development of knowledge and understanding. There is more consideration given to the nature of mental representation and the child's ability to comprehend his or her own understanding and that of other people. Bateson (1955) was interested in the 'not really serious' aspect of play which pre-supposes that children are well able to distinguish between what is play and what is not. This ability to stand back from their activities and represent it as 'not serious' is a particular type of higher understanding between players which Bateson termed 'metacommunication'. Play behaviour signals convey the message 'what I am about to say is not to be taken exactly as I say it'. Thus, it is in play that a child learns about the different ways in which social rules can be 'framed' and 'reframed'. According to Bateson, then, what a child actually learns in play is about learning itself.

In a similar vein, Leslie (1987) focused on pretend-play as a means whereby a child develops knowledge about his or her own and other peoples' thinking or metacognition. When children engage in imaginary role-play, some statements may be true (e.g. 'this cup is empty') and others false (e.g. the imaginary tea 'is cold') (where both statements are used with reference to a child's empty play cup). Children know that, whilst it is true that the cup is empty, any tea in the cup will be imaginary. Thus, pretend-play is about the overall understanding of the situation, and not the truth value of statements within the situation. Consequently, the emergence of pretend-play between 18 and 24 months can be seen as the development of the faculty of metarepresentation.

The most influential of these theorists for educational policy and reform have been Piaget, Vygotsky and Bruner (1972). However, these theorists are essentially psychologists. There is another species of theorist for whom the philosophy of education is the direct and principal concern, including Froebel (1782–1852), McMillan (1860–1931), Dewey (1859–1952) and Isaacs (1885–1948). Another way in which these theorists differ from those already mentioned is in their eclectic approach to the holistic well-being of the whole child – physical, mental, emotional, social and spiritual (for a detailed overview, see Bruce, 1991). Froebel believed play to be a unifying mechanism which integrated the child's learning, and as the highest phase in the child's functioning, viewed play as a spiritual activity. McMillan developed the free-play side of the curriculum, seeing greater cohesion between Froebelian ideas and practical application. In the twentieth century, Dewey helped teachers to take play seriously in the classroom, whilst Isaacs was more specific about the emotional nature of the child and how play helps to meet his/her emotional needs. Despite the views of these leading educational minds, the emotional, spiritual and playful dimension to learning is still a much neglected area of early childhood provision.

SUMMARY AND INTERPLAY OF THE THEORIES

A discussion of the interplay between play, language and learning presents a considerable challenge. The task is a thesis in itself, and specific research on this complex three-way relationship is scant. However, if we turn to developmental psychology, we find many exciting and relevant developments. In her 1996 review of theory and research,

Dunn describes the links between emotion, cognition and interpersonal relationships. This work illustrates what is currently missing from many traditional, early education-based programmes which feature play, language and learning as a single unit. Leading researchers are now integrating the play, language and learning notion in a 'Play and Literacy in Early Childhood' approach (Roskos and Christie, 2000). We now also know much more about the social and emotional lives and abilities of young children, and so cannot ignore their obvious impact on children's play, language and learning (see Chapter 4 for a detailed discussion). Indeed, an holistic approach to child development and behaviour demands that we paint on a much broader canvas.

In summarizing this chapter, some of the common ground shared by classical and modern theories of play includes the following:

- The categorization of types of play (e.g. functional, sensorimotor, artistic-aesthetic, memetic, games), all of which appear in the work of Spencer and Piaget in various forms.
- The non-literal ('as-if') nature of play. This is crucially important for all modern cognitive theorists, such as Bateson and Leslie, as well as for the classical theorists.
- The importance of the lengthy period of childhood for the purpose of practising skills through play features in the work of Groos, Piaget and Bruner.
- The emotional functions of play. Interestingly, a diversity of authors agree on this. Piaget (1962) describes play as 'pleasure in mastery … illusion of omnipotence', while Vygotsky (1962) describes play as 'wish-fulfilment' after having experienced early disappointment, and for psychoanalysts play is described as the only remedy that children (and sometimes adults) have at their disposal after confronting the real side of living with others. The views of Piaget, Vygotsky and Freud have been seized upon by the holistic education theorists.

Those features of play which relate closely to learning include play as pressure-free – in that the consequences of success or failure are very different in play and in reality, play as symbolic and play as interactive. Such theories include ideas from cognitive science, such as script theory – knowledge acquisition through social interaction (Nelson, 1981) – and schema theory (Athey, cited in Nutbrown, 1993), which is based on Piagetian concepts. From sociology comes the frame analysis of Goffman, which has a dramaturgical approach, sharing much with script theories. There is a body of literacy-play research (e.g. Butterworth, 1993) in which the social constructivist theory helps to show that play and literacy share certain mental processes such as representational and narrative abilities (Meek, 2000). Narrative approaches to early literacy learning (Roopnarine *et al.*, 2000; Fein *et al.*, 2000) argue that children have an abundant store of narrative tools for narrative organization that pave the way for language acquisition (Pellegrini and Galda, 2000; Bruner, 1990). For young children, literacy certainly involves the ability to talk about and reflect on oral and written language, and this is often represented in the narrative genre (Fein *et al.*, 2000). Higher-order abilities of metacommunication and metarepresentation, such as thinking about thinking, thinking about talking and thinking about reading, playing and learning are also noted as important for positive outcomes (Howe *et al.*, 2002).

Additionally Meek (2000, p. viii) reminds us that:

'literacy is neither a single entity nor a cloistered individual virtue. Its labyrinthine past locates it in recurrent social practices and conventions related to textual transmission

before printing … it is helpful to remember that cognitive aspects of literacy are always deeply entwined with cultural ones.'

Since play is evident before speech and language, it is apparent that children enjoy the ludic nature of words from the start. Meek refers to classic studies on children's delight at word play and the strange, incongruous worlds of stories and nursery rhymes (see also Smith *et al.*, 2003), humour and teasing.

Most developmentalists stress the importance of relationships and the interpersonal context in which language, imagination and cognition flower (Hobson, 1989). In addition to relationships with parents, children form friendships, have siblings and spend a lot of time with peers at school. If this context is not there or is maladaptive, there will be consequences for the child and for society, because it is in these early social interactions that children first learn to partake in their culture (Stern, 1985; Trevarthen and Hubley, 1978). More recent studies express concern at growing negativity towards play at school and the impact of playtime on children's learning (Blatchford, 1998; James, 1998). The importance of adult mediation in the playground and at home in order to scaffold social problem-solving with peers and siblings has also been noted (Levin, 2002; Howe *et al.*, 2002). It is interesting that, despite clear indications by leading educational thinkers and practitioners of the importance of emotional and spiritual development in children's play, language and learning, there has been a glaring gap in relevant research and practice for quite some time. This topic, however, is pursued in detail in Chapter 4.

Conclusion

Simon and Rebecca could be anywhere one might expect to find children playing – in their own home, at pre-school, in a hospital, in a care facility, or with a child-minder. What do all of these theories and special issues on play, language and learning mean for them and the adults who are caring for or studying them? At once it is clear that children are both fascinating and complex individuals and, given the holistic nature of the child, it is important to concede that no single special issue or theory is absolutely correct and able to account for the total complexity of behaviour involved in play, language and learning.

Student activity

Observe a group of young children at play. Use the narrative report technique (see Chapter 1) to record their actions and utterances. Afterwards, analyse the children's language and play, identifying ways in which the two are linked, and noting any learning that occurred as a result of the language and play.

REFERENCES

Aitchison, J (1983): *The Articulate Mammal: an Introduction to Psycholinguistics*, 2nd edn. London: Hutchison.

Alvarez, A and Phillips, A (1998): The importance of play: a child psychotherapist's view. *Child Psychology and Psychiatry Review*, **3**(3), 99–103.

Bateson, GA (1955): A theory of play and fantasy. *Psychiatric Research Reports*, **2**, 39–51.

Bion, WR (1962): *Learning from Experience*. London: Heinemann.

Bjørkvold, JR (1987): Our musical mother tongue – world-wide. In Soderbergh, R (ed.), *Children's Creative Communication*. Lund: Lund University Press.

Blatchford, P (1998): The state of play in schools. *Child Psychology and Psychiatry Review*, **3**(2), 58–67.

Bråten, I (1991): Vygotsky as precursor to metacognitive theory. II. Vygotsky as metacognitivitist. *Scandinavian Journal of Educational Research*, **35**, 305–320.

Bruce, T (1991): *Time to Play*. London: Hodder & Stoughton.

Bruner, JS (1972): *The Relevance of Education*. London: Allen & Unwin.

Bruner, JS (1976): Functions of play in immaturity. In Bruner, JS, Jolly, A and Sylva, K (eds), *Play: its Role in Evolution and Development*. New York: Basic Books, pp. 28–64.

Bruner, JS (1983): *Child's Talk: Learning to use Language*. New York: W.W. Norton & Co.

Bruner, JS (1990): *Acts of Meaning*. Boston, MA: Harvard University Press.

Butterworth, G (1993): Context and cognition in models of cognitive growth. In Light, P and Butterworth, G (eds), *Ways of Learning and Knowing*. Hillsdale, NJ: Lawrence Erlbaum Associates.

Chapman, RS (2000): Children's language learning: an interactionist perspective. *Journal of Child Psychology and Psychiatry*, **41**(1), 33–54.

Corsaro, WA (1979): We're friends, right? Children's use of access rituals in a nursery school. *Language in Society*, **8**, 315–336.

Diaz, RM and Berk, LE (1992): *Private Speech: from Social Interaction to Self-regulation*. Hillsdale, NJ: Lawrence Erlbaum Associates.

Donaldson, M (1978): *Children's Minds*. London: Fontana.

Dunn, J (1996): The Emmanuel Miller Memorial Lecture 1995. Children's relationships: bridging the divide between cognitive and social development. *Journal of Child Psychology and Psychiatry*, **37**, 507–518.

Erikson, E (1963): *Childhood and Society*. London: Routledge and Kegan Paul.

Fein, G (1981): Pretend play in childhood: an integrative review. *Child Development*, **52**, 1095–1118.

Fein, G, Ardila-Rey, AE and Groth, LA (2000): The narrative connection: stories and literacy. In Roskos, KA and Christie, JF (eds), *Play and Literacy in Early Childhood: Research from Multiple Perspectives*, pp. 27–43.

Freud, S (1920): *Three Contributions to the Theory of Sex. Nervous and Mental Disease Monographs No. 7*. New York: Nervous and Mental Disease Publishers.

Garvey, C (1974): Some properties of social play. *Merrill-Palmer Quarterly*, **20**, 163–180.

Garvey, C (1991): *Play*, 2nd edn. London: Fontana.

Goodman, JF (1994): 'Work' versus 'play' and early childhood care. *Child and Youth Care Forum*, **23**, 177–196.

Goodwin, M (1997): Children's linguistic and social worlds. *Anthropology Newsletter*, **38**, 1–4.

Greig, A (1993): *Communication at Playgroup: A Relationships Approach*. Unpublished doctoral dissertation, Cambridge University.

Hobson, P (1989): Beyond cognition: a theory of autism. In Dawson, G (ed.), *Autism: Nature, Diagnosis and Treatment*. New York: Guilford Press.

Howe, N, Rinaldi, CR, Jennings, M and Petrakos, H (2002): 'No! The lambs can stay out because they got cozies': constructive and destructive sibling conflict, pretend play, and social understanding. *Child Development*, **73**(5), 1460–1473.

Hunter, M (1998): Play across the spectrum. *Child Psychology and Psychiatry Review*, **3**(3), 115.

Hutt, C (1979): Play in the under-fives: form, development and function. In Howells, JG (ed.), *Modern Perspectives on the Psychiatry of Infancy*. New York: Brunner/Marcell.

James, A (1998): Play in childhood: an anthropological perspective. *Child Psychology and Psychiatry Review*, **3**(3), 104–109.

Karmiloff-Smith, A (1995): *Beyond Modularity: a Developmental Perspective on Cognitive Science*. Cambridge, MA: MIT Press.

Leslie, A (1987): Pretence and representation: the origins of 'theory of mind'. *Psychological Review*, **94**, 412–426.

Levin, DA (2002): Aggression in the playroom. In Render-Brown, C and Marchant, C (eds), *Play in Practice: Case Studies in Young Children's Play*. Early Childhood Consortium, St Paul, MN: Redleaf Press.

Lillemyr, OF, Fagerli, O and Søbsted, E (2001): *A Global Perspective on Early Childhood Care and Education: A Proposed Model*. Paris: UNESCO.

Mead, GH (1934): *Mind, Self and Society*. Chicago: University of Chicago Press.

Meek, M (2000): Foreword. In Roskos, KA and Christie, JF (eds), *Play and Literacy in Early Childhood: Research from Multiple Perspectives*, p. viii.

Mellou, E (1994): Play theories: a contemporary review. *Early Child Development and Care*, **102**, 91–100.

Nelson, K (1981): Social cognition in a script framework. In Flavell, J and Ross, L (eds), *Social Cognitive Development*. New York: Cambridge University Press, pp. 97–118.

Newman, F and Holzman, L (1993): *Lev Vygotsky: Revolutionary Scientist*. London: Routledge.

Nicolopoulou, A (1993): Play, cognitive development and the social world: Piaget, Vygotsky and beyond. *Human Development*, **36**, 1–23.

Nutbrown, C (1993): *Threads of Thinking*. London: Paul Chapman Publishing.

Pelligrini, AD and Galda, L (2000): Cognitive development, play and literacy: issues of definition and developmental function. In Roskos, KA and Christie, JF (eds), *Play and Literacy in Early Childhood: Research from Multiple Perspectives*, pp. 63–74.

Pelligrini, AD and Smith, PK (1998): The development of play during childhood: forms and possible functions. *Child Psychology and Psychiatry Review*, **3**(2), 51–57.

Piaget, J (1959): *The Language and Thought of the Child*. London: Routledge and Kegan Paul.

Roopnarine, JL, Shin, M, Donovan, B and Suppal, P (2000): Sociocultural contexts of dramatic play: implications for early education. In Roskos, KA and Christie, JF (eds), *Play and Literacy in Early Childhood: Research from Multiple Perspectives*, pp. 205–220.

Roskos, KA and Christie, JF (2000): *Play and Literacy in Early Childhood: Research from Multiple Perspectives*. Mawah, NJ: Lawrence Erlbaum Associates.

Scott, S (1998): Forum on play: introduction. *Child Psychology and Psychiatry Review*, **3**(2), 50–51.

Smith, PK (1993): Play and the uses of play. In Moyles, JR (ed.), *The Excellence of Play*. Buckingham: Open University Press, pp. 15–26.

Smith, PK, Cowie, H and Blades, M (2003): *Understanding Children's Development*, 3rd edn. London: Basil Blackwell.

Stern, D (1985): *The Interpersonal World of the Infant*. New York: Basic Books.

Sutton-Smith, B and Kelly-Byrne, D (1984): The idealisation of play. In Smith, PK (ed.), *Play in Animals and Humans*. Oxford: Basil Blackwell, pp. 305–321.

Trevarthen, C (1987): Infants trying to talk: how a child invites communication from the human world. In Soderbergh, R (ed.), *Children's Creative Communication*. Fourth International Congress for the Study of Child Language. Lund: Lund University Press, pp. 9–31.

Trevarthen, C and Aitken, KJ (2001): Infant intersubjectivity: research, theory, and clinical applications. *Journal of Child Psychology and Psychiatry*, 42(1), 3–48.

Trevarthen, C and Hubley, P (1978): Secondary intersubjectivity: confidence, confiding and acts of meaning in the first year. In Lock, A (ed.), *Action, Gesture and Symbol: The Emergence of Language*. London: Academic Press.

Vygotsky, LS (1962): *Thought and Language*. Cambridge, MA: MIT Press.

Vygotsky, LS (1967): *Play and its Role in the Mental Development of the Child*. Soviet Psychology 3.

Vygotsky, LS (1978): *Mind and Society*. Cambridge, MA: Harvard University Press.

Wells, G (1987): *The Meaning-makers: Children's Learning, Language and Using Language to Learn*. London: Hodder & Stoughton.

Whitehead, M (1990): *Language and Literacy in the Early Years*. London: Paul Chapman Publishing.

Winnicot, D (1971): *Playing and Reality*. London: Tavistock.

Woolgar, M (1999): Projective doll play methodologies for preschool children. *Child Psychology and Psychiatry Review*, 4(3), 126–134.

Youniss, J (1980): *Parents and Peers in Social Development. A Sullivan–Piaget Perspective*. Chicago: Chicago University Press.

FURTHER READING

Kane, SR and Furth, HG (1993): Children constructing social reality: a frame analysis of social pretend play. *Human Development*, 36, 199–214.

Lee, V and Das Gupta, P (1995): *Children's Cognitive and Language Development*. Oxford: Basil Blackwell in association with the Open University.

Mead, GH (1932): *The Philosophy of the Present*. La Salle, IL: Open Court Publishing Company.

Meadows, S (1993): *The Child as Thinker: The Development and Acquisition of Cognition in Childhood*. London: Routledge.

Moll, LC (ed.) (1992): *Vygotsky and Education: Instructional Implications and Applications of Socio-historical Psychology*. Cambridge: Cambridge University Press.

Moyles, JR (1989): *Just Playing*. Milton Keynes: Open University Press.

Nelson, K (ed.) (1989): Monologues in the crib. In Nelson, K (ed.), *Narratives from the Crib*. Cambridge, MA: Harvard University Press.

Nelson, K and Seidman, S (1984): Playing with scripts. In Bretherton, I (ed.), *Symbolic Play*. London: Academic Press Inc., pp. 45–71.

EARLY CHILDHOOD EDUCATION AND CARE

7

Margaret Woods

This chapter aims to:

- explore why we should have high quality early childhood education and care;

- examine the nature of that quality.

The focus is primarily on children aged 3–5 years.

INTRODUCTION

The United Nations (UN) Convention on the Rights of the Child affirms children's fundamental right to education and care (Articles 28 and 3).

Care is described by the United Nations Children's Fund (UNICEF) as ensuring and promoting children's 'survival, protection, growth and development in good health with proper nutrition … in a safe environment that enables them to be physically healthy, mentally alert, emotionally secure, socially competent and able to learn' (UNICEF, 2003, p. 15/16). The philosophy of holism and the link with education are obvious.

Education seems a little more complex to define (and UNICEF doesn't try). Vygotsky, currently one of our most favoured educational theorists, viewed education as a 'quintessential socio-cultural activity … central to cognitive development' (Moll, 1990, p. 1). It was the means of developing every child's potential and transmitting the culture within a particular society. With this dual notion of constructivism, the individual develops cognitively by building on his/her previous learning and experience, and society develops as new understanding extends the frontiers of human knowledge.

The recommendation that education should prepare children to cope effectively with the changing demands of society is expounded by Dahlberg and Asen (1994); this accords with the current emphasis on learning how to learn and is endorsed by the Organisation for Economic and Cultural Development (see OECD website).

Dahlberg and Asen view education as a 'pedagogical challenge' with the primary intent to achieve 'the integration of the next generation into society' (p. 164–5); for them, this integration is essential if society and its inhabitants are to thrive.

UNESCO (United Nations Educational, Scientific and Cultural Organisation), in one of its early childhood initiatives, depicts early childhood education (including family education) as a means 'to improve children's development and well-being, increase their health, self-esteem and learning capacities and improve the skills of families and communities' (UNESCO website). Once more, we have the clear merging of education and care underpinned by the holistic philosophy and with clear benefits for children and society. UNICEF (2000) does, however, caution against too narrow a focus on children's experiences in early years settings, since all their environments – 'families, communities, with peers' – interlink and are 'essentially learning opportunities' (p. 14).

In this chapter, in order to reflect the international philosophical and organizational shifts towards greater co-ordination of early childhood provision and the philosophy of holism, we combine education and care and adopt the increasingly used term 'Early Childhood Education and Care' (ECEC) (Bertram and Pascal, 2002). The search for the perfect (but elusive) term to portray integrated education and care does, however, continue (Martin, 2004). We define ECEC for 3- to 5-year-olds as a socio-cultural activity, contributing to the enrichment and advancement of society and indicative of society's responsibility to young children. This should be an enjoyable time for children, and have the potential to promote their all-round development and overall well-being; it should also support them in becoming competent learners and in functioning healthily and effectively within their daily lives. The interworking of all of a child's pre-school environments and experiences should be utilized to make ECEC wholly meaningful for each child.

WHY WE SHOULD HAVE GOOD QUALITY EARLY CHILDHOOD EDUCATION AND CARE

Froebel (1782–1852), one of the most famous early childhood pioneers, was in no doubt about the reason: 'The earliest age is the most important ... because the beginning decides the manner of progress' (Froebel, 1877, p. 143). In the Introduction of this book there is a similar sentiment taken from Plato. Professor Lilian Katz summarizes the situation in the early twenty-first century: '... no one today with serious educational and social policy-making responsibility for a community or a country all round the world would now argue against the proposition that the experiences of the early years of life have a powerful influence later on' (Katz, 2003, p. 14). Also, going to pre-school has a positive impact '... compared to not going at all' (Siraj-Blatchford, 2003, p. 11) and '... over and above important family influences' (Sylva *et al.*, 2003, p. 5).

Let us now summarize the established benefits to children, their families and society of children experiencing good quality ECEC. We should note that these emanate from valid research and experience, although it must be acknowledged that several studies relate to disadvantaged children and some gains were short term, while others were long term.

(i) Recognized human rights

Children have a right to experiences that enable them to develop to their full potential and improve the quality of their lives. ECEC can help realize this right [Bernard van Leer Foundation (BVLF), 2004; Levin-Rozalis and Shafran, 2003; UNICEF, 2003].

(ii) Developmental benefits

Positive developmental effects – social, emotional, cognitive, communication and cultural – have been noted by many (e.g. BVLF, 2004; Papps and Dyson, 2004; Burchinall and Cryer, 2003; Heymann, 2003; Hicks, 2003; Katz, 2003; Fleer, 2002a;

Ramey and Ramey, 2002; Sylva *et al.*, 2003; Pascal and Bertram, 2001; Prince *et al.*, 2001; UNESCO, 2001; UNICEF, 2000).

(iii) Improved academic achievement

There is evidence of:

- Children who attended ECEC having higher scores on a variety of achievement tests; for example, mathematics, literacy, communication, logical problem solving and reading (Papps and Dyson, 2004; Bracey and Stellar, 2003; Heymann, 2003; Hicks, 2003; Wylie and Thompson, 2003; Fleer, 2002b; Reynolds and Stevens, 2002).
- Children who attended ECEC staying longer in education with fewer special educational placements (Fleer, 2002b; Landry, 2002; Prince *et al.*, 2001).
- ECEC establishing or encouraging attitudes and behaviour patterns which impact positively on educational motivation and competence (Wylie and Thompson, 2003; Fleer, 2002b; Lillemyr *et al.*, 2001).
- ECEC being linked to a reduction in the gap between the academic performances of advantaged and disadvantaged youngsters (Bracey and Stellar, 2003; Sylva *et al.*, 2003; Espinosa, 2002; Fleer, 2002b; DfES, 2001; Prince *et al.*, 2001).

(iv) Societal benefits

Several long-term societal benefits have been identified in addition to the educational and social equity benefits mentioned above. Examples include ECEC graduates claiming fewer state benefits and having:

- higher levels of employment;
- greater earning power;
- reduced instances of delinquency;
- fewer arrests and social exclusions;
- more settled behaviour;
- stronger involvement in community developments (BvL, 2004; Papps and Dyson, 2004; Bracey and Stellar, 2003; Raban *et al.*, 2003; Fleer, 2002b; Reynolds and Stevens, 2002; Pascal and Bertram, 2001; Prince *et al.*, 2001).

Also, though Myers (2001, p. 16) claims that the research requires '… leaps of faith when interpreting results', the cost effectiveness of providing quality ECEC seems to have been well proven (Bracey and Stellar, 2003; Hicks, 2003; Espinosa, 2002; Fleer, 2002a,b; Reynolds and Stevens, 2002; Zietlow, 2002; Pascal and Bertram, 2001).

Moreover, Schweinhart (2003) emphasizes 'the strong robust evidence' of the beneficial effects of high quality pre-school experiences on 'young children living in poverty' (p. 1), while Sylva *et al.* (2003) reach a similar conclusion. Additionally, the Department for Education and Science (now Skills) (DfES, 2001) sees effective ECEC helping local authorities deliver targets for employment and education by enabling parents to work or train, alleviating disadvantage and child poverty and altogether providing 'significant benefits for children, parents and communities' (p. 3). These are sentiments echoed by the Bernard van Leer Foundation (BVLF), the outcomes from their numerous international projects indicating that ECEC can bring about 'an improvement in the social fabric of the community itself', providing 'a springboard for wider social change and community development' (BVLF, 2004, p. 4).

With such strong evidence, one is compelled to agree with Gammage (1994, p. 4) that 'we neglect early childhood education at our peril'. If, however, we wish to ensure the most advantageous outcomes for children, their families and society, then ECEC must not merely exist, but be of the highest quality attainable (Mitchell, 2004; Bracey and Stellar, 2003; Burchinal and Cryer, 2003; Katz, 2003; Wylie and Thompson, 2003; Fleer, 2002a,b).

QUALITY IN EARLY CHILDHOOD EDUCATION AND CARE

Quality certainly seems to have become a national buzz-word, and a universal business and educational aim. Indeed, Moss *et al.* (2000) claim that 'we live in what might be called the "age of quality" … quality is measured, managed, assured and improved' (p. 103). Yet a concise, straightforward definition remains elusive. Policy documents often present quality as 'objective, real, universal and knowable' (Moss *et al.*, 2000, p. 100), but actually there is broad agreement that quality is a socially-constructed, culturally bound, context-specific and dynamic concept (Mooney *et al.*, 2003; Raban *et al.*, 2003; Ceglowski and Bagalup, 2002; Edwards *et al.*, 2002; Goodfellow, 2001; Ilfeld, 2001; Laevers, 2000; Moss *et al.*, 2000).

To help us begin to understand quality in relation to early years practice, we shall consider briefly a few interpretations/frameworks, selecting those that seem most able to accommodate diversity of circumstances and viewpoints and reflect the philosophy of holism.

Experiential education

First, let us outline the framework of Laevers (1994, 2000) and his Experiential Education, which purports to evaluate as well as improve quality. This has been applied successfully in England by Pascal and Bertram (Pascal, undated).

Laevers specifies three dimensions. The first consists of the *context/treatment variables*, for example the classroom environment, programme content, teacher style, level of training and educator/child ratios.

Laevers' second dimension is ascertained via measurement of the *effects or outcomes of ECEC programmes* and retrospective identification of their determinants. Whilst undoubtedly valuable, the long-term nature of outcome evaluation does not actually improve the quality of experience for children currently in the settings.

Laevers (1994, 2000) consequently focuses on the third category as the most interesting and fruitful, namely the *process variables*. These are considered to describe, as well as improve, quality by focussing on the extent of children's emotional well-being and their level of involvement in activities. Children's *involvement* is characterized by Laevers as concentration, persistence, motivation, fascination and intensity of experience leading to deep learning and development. The provision of appropriately challenging activities is deemed imperative, as are positive relationships and children being happy and secure in a stable, caring and stimulating environment.

SureStart

Similarities with Laever's concept of quality can be identified in that of SureStart (Mooney *et al.*, 2003). SureStart is a UK government programme encouraging integration of education, health and family support services for young children and families in disadvantaged areas. It is working towards providing the best possible start in life for these children, with particular emphasis on reducing poverty. From an examination of cross-national evidence from 15 countries, Mooney *et al.* developed a set of three inter-dependent indicators of quality to support SureStart ECEC programmes:

- *Structural features*, for example adequate funding, equity of access, affordability, staff qualifications and training, staff–child ratios, and group size.
- *Process features*, for example developmentally appropriate activities, sensitive interactions between children and adults.
- *Outcomes*, for example cognitive development, school readiness, academic skills, parents' satisfaction with provision.

Self-evaluation and partnership with parents were also deemed significant elements of quality and, together with the above features, seemed to be correlated with higher quality ECEC.

Espinosa (2002) offers a very similar model derived from what 'researchers have consistently found' (p. 3); this comprised structural and process quality.

Starting Strong: Early Childhood Education and Care (ECEC)

Improving the quality of ECEC is a major priority for the Organisation for Economic Cooperation and Development (see OECD website). Starting Strong (OECD, 2001) makes a broad holistic comparison of early years policy and practice in 12 countries. While much attention is given to acknowledging and reconciling diversity in the range of contexts, values and perspectives, a consensus quality framework emerges and similarities with the models of Laevers, SureStart and Espinosa can be detected. There are four elements:

- At systemic level: sufficient investment, efficiently co-ordinated management structures, adequate staff training and conditions, clear pedagogical frameworks; procedures for monitoring and evaluation.
- At programme level: duration and intensity of programmes, favourable group size and adult–child ratios, suitable environment and equipment.
- Process variables: sensitive adult–child interactions, active partnership with parents, effective learning and social opportunities.
- Outcome variables: short- and long-term measurement of, for example, children's development and achievements.

The Effective Provision of Pre-school Education (EPPE)

This rigorous English longitudinal study, which set out to assess the impact of ECEC experiences on children and to identify the characteristics of effective provision, claimed that their findings on early years quality were consistent with those of other large-scale studies (Sylva *et al.*, 2003). They employed a rich range of methodologies – observations, interviews, questionnaires, intensive case studies and the extended Early Childhood Environment Rating Scale (ECERS-E) to assess quality. Great pains were taken to ensure fair comparisons between different early years contexts and account for background influences on children's development. High quality was associated with:

- Integrated centres and nursery schools.
- Sensitive educator–child interactions, with adults showing warmth and being responsive to individual children. 'Sustained shared thinking' (p. 4) and open-ended questioning were significant.
- Highly qualified practitioners (especially graduate teachers), who were knowledgeable about the curriculum and children's learning.
- Promotion of positive social interaction amongst children.
- Effective pedagogy which included 'teaching' activities and 'freely chosen yet potentially instructive play activities' (p. 5). Sometimes the educator leads, sometimes the child does. Activities must be intellectually challenging and academically focussed.
- Small groups.
- Effective working with parents, especially by sharing information and involving parents in decisions.

Excellence in Early Childhood (EECL)

After reviewing much research data, Raban *et al*. (2003) developed a three-dimensional consensus framework to define quality:

1. An intellectually, aesthetically and physically stimulating, well-organized and resourced learning environment that accommodates children's emotional and social needs.
2. Pedagogy which comprises process elements such as:
   – promotion of independence and interdependence;
   – 'curriculum design and implementation' assuring a 'range and variety of teaching/learning experiences';
   – 'recognition of children's work';
   – 'sustained attention to activities';
   – 'review and reflection on teaching and learning'.
3. 'Partnerships with children, families, communities and staff' involving considered attention to children's emotional and social well-being, health and safety and continuity of care. Adult 'interactions with children through dialogue'; staff professional development and communication were also important elements.

(Adapted from Raban *et al*., 2003, p. 74)

Once again, parallels with previous descriptions of quality can be ascertained.

Reggio Emilia

Early childhood services in Reggio Emilia (a city in Northern Italy) are recognized worldwide as a source of inspiration for early years educators. Many have sought to capture the essence of their quality (e.g. McGavin, 2003; Edwards *et al*., 2002; Hewett, 2001; Dahlberg, 2000; Moss *et al*., 2000; New, 2000).

Reggio Emilia adopts a social-constructivist approach (see Chapter 1, p. 5), with children regarded as active co-constructors in their own development. Relationships with children, families, other educators, community members and amongst children are considered crucial to positive educational and developmental outcomes; consequently they are carefully nurtured. There is a strong emphasis on multiple forms of knowing, and on symbolic representation of ideas and feelings through the famous 'hundred languages' (see Edwards *et al.*, 1998). There is no predetermined curriculum; the understanding, experiences and interests that children bring to the setting constitute the starting points for learning. Sensitive interaction and responsiveness are much emphasized in the teaching and learning process with considerable use of projects, thoughtful observing of children and careful documenting of their progress and activities, well supported by the shared reflective practice of stakeholders. While the lack of a specified curriculum has led to criticism on grounds of accountability, advocates cite in defence the detailed recording undertaken by educators and the numerous early years visitors to the centres.

Children's views

Children's views on what constitutes quality are important. Mooney and Blackburn (2003) were commissioned by the Department for Education and Skills (DfES) to ascertain children's views to inform consultation for Investors in Children. They reviewed much literature, surveyed Early Years Development and Childcare Partnership consultations, and consulted with children from different ECEC settings. They summarize children's views on quality:

- friendships should be encouraged and supported;
- a wide range of activities, regularly changed to suit children's interests and needs with sufficient indoor and outdoor space;
- children and staff should have fun, with staff facilitating activities;
- staff show respect for children, are caring, take time to listen, avoid raising their voices, and interact sensitively with children;
- there is a choice of attractive, enjoyable food with ready access to drinks;
- children's views to be regarded seriously and children encouraged to participate in programme decisions.

(Adapted from Mooney and Blackburn, 2003)

Most of those indicators could be accommodated within the earlier quality frameworks described above, and of course they accord with the UN Convention on the Rights of the Child, Article 12 – acknowledging and responding to the voice of the child.

We have briefly explored ECEC quality from a range of international sources which incorporated the views of different stakeholders – children, educators, parents, policy-makers, community members, researchers. All of the models have applicability for diverse early years settings, and some degree of consensus has emerged.

A CONSENSUS FRAMEWORK FOR QUALITY EARLY CHILDHOOD EDUCATION AND CARE

Quality early childhood education and care probably would:

- adopt an holistic philosophy and an integrated/multiprofessional approach to the education and care of young children;

- create an atmosphere of respect that values each child, ensures children's social and emotional well-being and is anti-discriminatory;
- make certain that educators have the appropriate knowledge, understanding, skills and attitudes to interact and work effectively with young children, providing a range of appropriate and challenging learning activities;
- work in partnership with children's families;
- enhance quality through reflective practice and evaluation;
- maintain a rich, stimulating, child-focussed learning context with adequate indoor and outdoor space, equipment/materials and time for a wide range of activities;
- be adequately funded with a favourable ratio of educators to children;
- promote effective management of highly trained educators who are given regular opportunities for continuing professional development.

This consensus does not constitute a check-list, but rather a framework from which to develop a rich understanding of quality. By entering into a dialogic process with stakeholders and taking account of the range of perspectives, educators can work more democratically towards contextually appropriate quality within their particular setting. To aid such debate we shall now consider, in a little more detail, the process-oriented variables from this consensus viewpoint.

An holistic philosophy and integrated/multiprofessional approach to early childhood education and care

Readers should return to the Introduction of this book for a more detailed account of our holistic philosophy and integrated/multiprofessional approach which endeavour to view the child as a whole and avoid artificial segregation of care and education. Collaboration is required amongst stakeholders and relevant professionals.

Stakeholders in ECEC settings would be the early years professionals, parents/guardians, children, ancillary staff and community representatives, for example from the Local Education Authority (LEA), local schools, playgroups, Early Years Development and Care Partnerships, or SureStart.

The professionals with whom ECEC educators might liaise could include reception-class teachers, headteachers, practitioners from other early years settings, early years/special needs advisers, health visitors, social workers, family doctors, speech therapists, school nurses, educational psychologists, physiotherapists, college tutors, researchers and police.

Obviously the co-ordination of such a wide range of expertise, for example as intended in the Children Act 2004, could, with strong commitment and adequate resourcing, take settings closer to providing the ideal of integrated ECEC.

Creating an atmosphere of respect that values each child, ensures each child's social and emotional well-being and is anti-discriminatory

There is considerable consensus amongst educators of the benefits to young children of a climate of respect in their ECEC setting (Pianto and La Paro, 2003). Respect is related to educators being sensitive and responsive to children's needs, interests, motivation and circumstances and also 'attuned to each child's emotional well-being' (Goodfellow, 2001). It would be evident in interactions and in the way individuals are treated and treat others. The Early Childhood Education Forum (ECEF, 1998) expands the concept to comprise 'respect for children as individuals for their ability/disability, sex/gender, as members of families and as members of ethnic/racial, linguistic, social, cultural and religious groups' (p. 51); also included is respect for parents and their child-rearing practices and decisions.

National representatives at the UN Special Session on 10 May 2002 declared their determination '… to respect the dignity and to secure the well-being of all children' (Declaration 4, UNICEF, 2003). Respect features in many official policy and advisory documents and sets of principles (e.g. Ofsted, 2001; QCA/DfEE, 2000). Educators in Reggio Emilia are 'clearly respectful of children' (Edwards *et al.*, 2002). Espinosa (2002) emphasizes the criticality for children of being 'respected, nurtured and challenged', and of their home language and culture being 'respected, appreciated and incorporated into the curriculum and the classroom'; she also affirms the link with 'close warm relationships between educators and children' (p. 5). Rimm-Kaufman *et al.* (2003) cite several studies confirming this correlation between warm, positive relationships and children's enhanced social and emotional learning, as well as their improved academic achievement, behaviour and social competence. Better social and behavioural outcomes were similarly reported by Sylva *et al.* (2003) in settings where staff 'showed warmth and were responsive' (p. 4). This also mirrors Laevers' extensive research (1994, 2000) which highlights the significance in children's academic and cognitive achievement of their emotional well-being and their needs for attention, affection, social recognition and support in feeling competent being met (Fig. 7.1). These findings are further supported by Hyson (2003), Richburg and Fletcher (2002), Ulich and Mayr (2002), Pollard and Davidson (2001).

While Moyles *et al.* (2002) did indeed find that educators invested 'much time and energy in developing relationships' with children (p. 131), sadly there was a distinct 'continuum of effectiveness' (p. 130).

Creating respectful, reciprocal and responsive relationships is important with all children and parents, but can be additionally so in relation to cultural diversity. Culture is deemed 'a pervasive and dynamic process that influences every aspect of how we perceive and interact with others', and includes 'beliefs, languages, behaviours' (Barrera and Corso, 2002, p. 104). Barrera and Corso's approach to inter-cultural understanding requires the three attributes of respect, reciprocity and responsiveness. These enable compassionate acceptance of varied perspectives and advocate reconciling

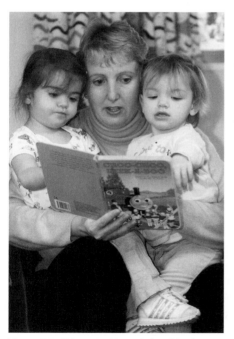

Figure 7.1 Warm positive relationships have many benefits for children.

differing viewpoints before decisions are taken and actions planned. The approach, apparently tried and tested, could be particularly useful in meeting the challenge of diversity in ECEC settings and Article 2 of the UN Convention on the Rights of the

Child: children should be treated 'without discrimination of any kind, irrespective of the child's or his or her parents or legal guardian's race, colour, sex, language, religion, political or other opinion, national, ethnic or social origin, property, disability, birth or other status' (UNICEF, 2003) – a sentiment which is endorsed in all UK government and UN policy/advice documents (see websites).

To be effective, early years educators must be fully cognisant of this fundamental right. They must recognize and respond to the typical childhood and the additional needs of 'children of different developmental possibilities, abilities and individual needs' as well as their family, social and cultural contexts (Wunschel, 2003, p. 30/31). For example:

- children experiencing poverty and disadvantage;
- children with disabilities/special needs;
- children with family responsibilities/chores;
- children from minority ethnic groups;
- refugee children;
- immigrant children;
- children who have experienced trauma/war/family breakdown/abuse;
- children who are chronically/long-term sick.

There does seem to be evidence of educators demonstrating positive attitudes to cultural pluralism, inclusion and variations in child-rearing practices (Bhavnagri, 2001) and fully intending to address diversity (Falconer and Byrnes, 2003; Burriss, 2000). Unfortunately, however, amongst instances of good practice, gaps are apparent between intentions and actual practice, as well as misconceptions on the part of educators (Falconer and Byrnes, 2003; Pattnaik, 2003; Ennals, 2002; Soodak et al., 2002; McCay and Keyes, 2001; Burriss, 2000). For example, inconsistency in the support for special needs children in England is regularly noted (Smith, 2004a,b; Ennals, 2002) and Ulich and Mayr (2002, p. 140) identified 'unequal development chances' in kindergarten activities leading to gender differences and disadvantage to younger and minority ethnic children. Likewise, marginalization of some ethnic groups can emanate from low expectations of them (Bhavnagri, 2001). Most people would accept that prejudicial and discriminatory practices impact negatively on children who are victims, but they are also harmful to non-target children. For example, it is well-recognized that young children make discriminatory and stereotypic statements after absorbing the attitudes of those whom they observe and with whom they interact (ECF, 2003; Vakil et al., 2003; McCay and Keyes, 2001; Van Ausdale and Feagin, 2001; Lane, 1999; Derman-Sparkes, 1993).

Equality of opportunity is not about treating all children exactly the same; rather, it reflects our holistic approach of sensitive, responsive and, as far as possible, individualized ECEC according to need. It is about entitlement and social justice. All children must feel they are being treated fairly and equitably. Early years are, after all, the years when discriminatory concepts, attitudes, images, language develop (ECF, 2003; Pattnaik, 2003; Vakil et al., 2003; Rhedding-Jones, 2002; Van Ausdale and Feagin, 2001; Lane, 1999). Consequently, early childhood must be a crucial period for supporting children in developing positive self-concepts and bias-free attitudes, unlearning prejudiced views and behaviour and learning effective ways to challenge discrimination and counter the distorted realities associated with prejudice. ECEC educators must facilitate intercultural and inclusionary understanding and, as Pattnaik suggests, create an ethos of 'living diversity rather than just doing diversity' (2003, p. 205).

Naturally it is essential that early years educators understand fully their own attitudes towards racism, sexism, disability and other differences and are able to confront instances of discrimination firmly, but tactfully. Of especial significance for educators in pursuit of equality of opportunity is the context-sensitive ecological model of ECEC (e.g. Bronfenbrenner, 1979) illustrating how we cannot understand a child's needs in isolation from one another or from his/her family, culture, community, group, society, etc. The holistic approach and collaboration with parents and communities are, therefore, essential (e.g. Aytch *et al.*, 2004; Johnson *et al.*, 2003; Pattnaik, 2003; Vakil *et al.*, 2003; Puri, 2002; Bhavnagri, 2001).

Knowledge, understanding, skills and attitudes needed by educators

It is important to consider the knowledge, understanding, skills and attitudes which are known to enable educators to interact and work effectively with young children and provide a range of appropriate and challenging learning activities.

Educator knowledge, understanding, skills and attitudes

Moyles *et al.*'s (2002) *Study of Pedagogical Effectiveness* provides an extremely comprehensive set of guidance statements on the role of, and the skills, values, knowledge and personal qualities required by, effective early years educators (pp. 50–58). These relate to supporting children's learning and play; promoting the development of children's thinking and communication skills, attitudes and behaviour patterns; creating a positive, safe, pleasant and stimulating environment; establishing relations with stakeholders and parents; planning assessment and evaluation; ensuring children's entitlements; teaching and learning practices. It is a worthy reference document derived from the team's careful research.

To this we might usefully add UNESCO's (2001) *Framework for Action on Values Education in Early Childhood*. This includes a set of guiding principles for action offering helpful advice for educators on underpinning values; effecting successful relationships between children and adults, creating a respectful, child-friendly learning environment; implementing the integrated approach; maximizing the significance of children's families; and developing a broad values-based curriculum.

The Reggio Emilia experience can also assist. Educators work on the underpinning principle of reciprocity which necessitates them being partners, co-learners, guides and facilitators in the learning process, able to collaborate effectively with colleagues and children's parents. They are also encouraged to undertake research, so must possess or acquire the necessary skills – for example, reflecting on their practice, observing and listening to children and collecting, analysing, evaluating and utilizing data for the enhancement of that practice.

Siraj-Blatchford *et al.* (2002), in their *Researching Effective Pedagogy in the Early Years*, conclude that good outcomes for children are linked to educators ensuring adult–child interactions involve sustained shared thinking and open-ended questioning, having sound knowledge of the ECEC curriculum and child development, and developing shared aims with parents. Providing formative feedback to children during activities and having clearly thought-out behaviour policies also had positive effects.

Guidelines for implementing the English Foundation Stage Curriculum can be found in the guidance document (QCA/DfEE, 2000).

Particularly important for educators is understanding how young children learn, referring naturally to an holistic view of learning relating to all aspects of development – for example, intellectual, linguistic, emotional, social, cultural, gender-related, moral and spiritual. Vygotsky (1978) advocated that educators encourage children's learning via social interaction and apprenticeship-type relationships with a more cognitively skilled other, and also through play, instruction, first-hand experience, observation, imitation and practice (see Chapter 6 for an in-depth discussion of this approach).

Planning and organizing for holistic and educative play is another essential and exciting – but never easy – aspect of the educator's role, even though it may appear quite effortless in the hands of a skilled practitioner.

In general, there is widespread acceptance of the benefits of play for children and, more recently, also for society (Smith, 2004b; Curtis and O'Hagan, 2003; Kapasi, 2001; Vygotsky, 1978; also see Chapter 6). Lillemyr *et al.* (2001) succinctly summarize the benefits of play from a global perspective, reminding us that play is a natural childhood instinct and that children's right to play is embedded in Article 31 of the UN Convention on the Rights of the Child (UNICEF, 2003) (Fig. 7.2).

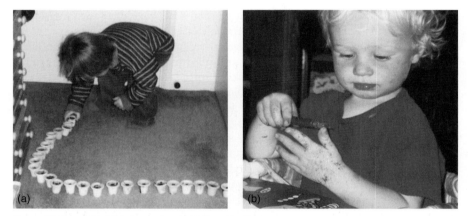

(a)   (b)

Figure 7.2 (a and b)   Play is a natural childhood instinct.

Interestingly, Moyles *et al.* (2002) found that, although play was at the root of practitioners' thinking and principles, adult engagement in children's play was not well understood or much utilized as a vehicle for learning. Also, the Association of Teachers and Lecturers have published research claiming play needs to be 'given a higher priority across the foundation stage' (Smith, 2004b, p. 19).

Educator–child interaction

Much research data confirm the importance of 'talk' in children's learning, with the quality and quantity of interaction between adults and children being crucial. Sadly, much talk occurring in nursery settings is used for organizational purposes and is not particularly advantageous to the development of children's learning and development. Sustained meaningful conversations between one adult and one child are apparently rare (Pianto and La Paro, 2003).

Sensitive interaction with children was highlighted in almost all of our quality frameworks. It occurs when the educator responds appropriately to a child's needs, questions, requests or interests, allows opportunities for choice and discussion and avoids being negative and restrictive (Landry, 2002).

Katz (2003) argues that, since interactions can lead to rich, meaningful and valuable learning experiences and long-term beneficial outcomes for children, they should be the main focus of educators' energies. Wylie and Thompson (2003), Landry (2002) and Ramey and Ramey (2002) endorse the effectiveness and pivotal nature of interactions in children's learning and also educators being a vital source of stimulation. Through the process of scaffolding, children's interest, cognitive and social development, reasoning skills and emotional well-being can be promoted. Scaffolding, according to Coltman *et al.* (2002), is children learning 'more effectively through carefully structured joint activity (involving verbal interaction) with experienced others' (p. 48); this takes them to the limit of their zone of proximal development, much as Vygotsky advocated (see Chapter 6, p. 103).

Wylie and Thompson (2003) identify different educator–child interactions that have shown positive correlations with children's enhanced competences. These are:

- Being responsive to individual children.
- Asking open-ended questions.
- Guiding children in their activities and thinking.
- Joining in children's play.
- Providing children with learning experiences that involve interaction with peers.

It is also worth returning to the 'sustained shared thinking' of Siraj-Blatchford *et al.* (2002, p. 3) to help us further understand educator–child interactions. They found that the 'cognitive construction' involved in the interactions is mutual; each party engages with the understanding of the other, and learning is achieved through a process of 'reflexive co-construction'. For learning to occur, both parties must be

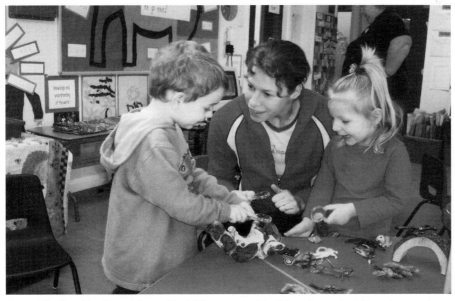

Figure 7.3 Sensitive interactions with children can lead to rich and meaningful learning experiences.

involved, and there must be some element of instruction as well as 'sustained shared thinking'. Responding to and extending child-initiated interactions were found important, as were open-ended questions that stimulate debate, higher-level thinking, problem-solving and questions from the child. Discussions, debating stories, adults answering 'why' questions, explaining how things work, helping children explore their thoughts and feelings, co-operative play, adult modelling and one-to-one situations were also identified as beneficial in terms of children's cognitive development. For Espinosa (2002), reciprocity or balance in any adult–child interaction, with each taking turns at listening and talking, is additionally vital (Fig. 7.3).

Appropriate and challenging learning activities

We have examined how we might work and interact effectively with young children; now, we must consider what the children will actually learn.

Bertram and Pascal (2002) and Mooney *et al.* (2003) established from international surveys that many countries have curriculum guidelines for children from 3 years until school age. While the content varies somewhat, common learning areas were apparent – for example, social, emotional, cultural, aesthetic, creative, physical, environmental with a few countries including language, literacy and numeracy. By way of example, we will consider three quite different 'curricula' from Italy, New Zealand and England.

There is no formally specified curriculum in Reggio Emilia. Learning activities derive from the emphases on the child as rich and competent, the stimulating environment, the multiple forms of representation, and the aims to develop children's critical thinking and abilities to enable them to contribute fully to a democratic society. The strong social-constructivist standpoint of starting from the child's experiences, interests and understanding is also significant.

The much-applauded Te Whariki, a progressive socio-cultural early years curriculum developed in New Zealand, provides guiding principles, aims and goals for learning and development, leaving educators to determine how the goals are actually achieved. The Maori weaving metaphor (Whariki) is a 'woven mat for all to stand on' allowing different perspectives 'to be woven into the fabric' (Carr and May, 2000, p. 59) with a 'spider web' rather than sequential curriculum model to accommodate the view of children's development as a 'tapestry of increasing complexity and richness' (p. 60). It has many strengths, including 'its bicultural nature, holistic and anti-racist approach' (Soler and Miller, 2003, p. 62) and the potential for rich developmental experiences, although Soler and Miller (2003) foresee possible difficulties in the child being the 'sole source of the curriculum' (p. 64).

The English foundation stage curriculum for children aged 3–5 years (a stage of the National Curriculum) is organized into six learning areas:

- personal, social and emotional;
- communication. language and literacy;
- mathematical development;
- knowledge and understanding of the world;
- physical development;
- creative development.

Each learning area has a set of early learning goals to be achieved by most children by the end of their reception year and formulated to inform planning, lay the foundations for future learning and aid transition into Key Stage One of the National Curriculum. To support practitioners, 'stepping stones' of progress towards the learning goals are identified in the guidance document (QCA/DfEE, 2000). These are deemed not to be age-related, but rather to indicate developing knowledge, understanding, attitudes and skills. Sets of aims and principles are provided to underpin practice and a constructivist approach, partnership with parents, a mixture of adult- and child-initiated pedagogic strategies and learning through play are encouraged (for more detail, see Chapter 8).

A group of illustrious early years professionals/academics wrote a letter to the TES (17/1/03, p. 28) entitled '*The foundation stage is solid*'; they referred to the warm welcome that the principles received. Drummond (2003) also acknowledges that enthusiastic welcome from practitioners, but laments its uncritical nature, while Ellis (2002) is concerned about the stage-based approach and difficulty of implementation in reception classes 'pitting early years ideals against school pressures' (p. 117). Soler and Miller (2003) feel that the early learning goals have been shaped predominantly to ensure smooth school entry, though Staggs (2004) argues they reflect the basic principles of learning. Lip service to play is of further concern to Soler and Miller (2003).

Any specified curriculum needs to be made personally relevant to individual children with their own experiences, natural interests and enthusiasms applied to the learning in an enjoyable and meaningful way. Quality learning must also be realistically challenging.

Laevers' (1994, 2000) experiential model can be useful in this endeavour with its involvement and deep-level learning characterized by the degree of concentration, persistence, motivation, fascination and intensity children demonstrate during activities. Ulich and Mayr (2002) and Pascal (undated) elaborate on Laevers' involvement, confirming its value in relation to the quality of children's activities and consequential benefits. Pianto and La Paro (2003) similarly found activities necessitating higher thinking and problem-solving skills important for ensuring children's academic success (Fig. 7.4).

Developmentally appropriate practice (DAP) has been influential in ECEC for several years – a largely Piagetian constructivist approach portraying the child learning through play in an environment tailored to his/her developmental stage needs. DAP sounded sensible and was intuitively appealing. Recently, how been challenged for its failure to take sufficient account of chil

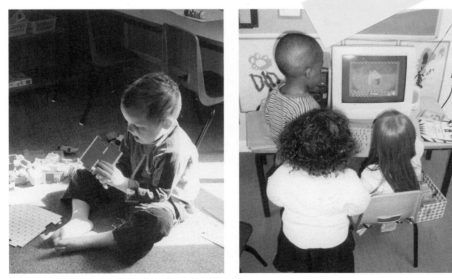

Figure 7.4 'Involvement' leads to deep-level learning.

cultural contexts and zone of potential development (ZPD) (e.g. Aldwinckle, 2001; Burriss, 2000). Even back in 1998, Woodhead advocated 'rejecting narrow, prescriptive, decontextualized views' of childhood development (DAP) in favour of 'a more open, holistic, context-specific approach' (p. 7). He acknowledged the existence of universal elements of development, but cited evidence illustrating the impact of multiple ecological factors. Consequently, he proposed practice/activities appropriate to the context of children's development which;

- are '*based on local variations in children's experiences of growth and change*';
- '*consider the age and individuality of children as well as the social context of their care*';
- '*are consistent with and complementary to children's learning experiences within family and community*'; and
- '*provide opportunities for children to learn in a variety of ways which suit their age and stage of development, the goals of their ECEC setting and the available resources*'.

(Adapted from Woodhead, 1998, p. 10/11)

More recently, Wunschel (2003) has endorsed the concept of contextually appropriate practice summarizing how educators might devise activities to promote quality learning and development. Activities might emanate from children's developmental needs and interests as well as from their familial, social and cultural environments. Knowing and observing children, carefully assessing their progress and discussions with their parents would naturally be crucial. Introducing topics worth knowing (negotiated with stakeholders, colleagues and studying research/policy) and using first-hand, real-life experiences are also recommended. Activities according with a legally specified curriculum would be necessary, as would provision of opportunities and experiences to allow children to experiment, ask questions and discover answers. To these, Siraj-Blatchford (2003) would add working within each child's area of proximal (next) development and extending children's thinking to ensure involvement and deep learning.

WORKING IN PARTNERSHIP WITH CHILDREN'S FAMILIES

A crucial aspect of our holistic philosophy and integrated approach was to consider and work with each child within the context of his/her family. What constitutes a family may vary greatly, but it is generally recognized as being the foremost influence on children's development. Knowing the family, especially parents or any person with legal responsibility for a child's care and upbringing, is considered advantageous to understanding and working with a child within a social-constructivist paradigm (Hamilton *et al.*, 2003; Wunschel, 2003; Barrera, 2001). See Chapters 5 and 9 for discussions on families.

The benefits to children of close collaboration between educators and families are now widely accepted (e.g. Hamilton *et al.*, 2003; Moore, 2003; Sylva *et al.*, 2003; Wunschel, 2003; Foot *et al.*, 2002; Hughes and McNaughton, 2002; Shpancer, 2002; Siraj-Blatchford *et al.*, 2002; Lillemyr *et al.*, 2001). Evidence indicates that effective home–nursery links can have a positive impact on children's achievement, development, behaviour, attitudes to school and continuity between home and nursery (Wherry, 2004; Foot *et al.*, 2002; McCullough, 2002; Shpancer, 2002; QCA/DfEE, 2000).

More recently, research has evinced additional benefits to parents/carers: increased confidence and self-esteem; greater insight into children's development and ECEC experiences; more positive moments with their children; an improved ability to handle their child's difficult behaviour; and appreciation for having a voice in their child's education (e.g. Wherry, 2004; Foot *et al.*, 2002; Hughes and McNaughton, 2002).

While early years professionals claim to value the role and contribution of parents (Moyles *et al.*, 2002) and accept that parents have rights (Foot *et al.*, 2002), many researchers have noted difficulties and tensions on the part of educators and parents (e.g. Blue-Banning *et al.*, 2004; Hughes and McNaughton, 2002; Keyes, 2002). Also, variation in the extent of parental participation in different ECEC settings has been observed, with very few demonstrating 'genuine partnership parity' (Foot *et al.*, 2002, p. 17). There is, however, general agreement that partnerships/collaboration might be developed and/or strengthened via:

- Professionals convincing parents that their involvement can be beneficial to their children's education and development.
- Respect for parents, their views, the role they play in children's lives, their home culture, religious beliefs, choices and decisions.
- Commitment to the partnership/working together and an obvious sense of equity.
- An atmosphere of trust with parents feeling valued and made to feel welcome in the ECEC setting.
- Shared educational aims and joint/negotiated planning, decision-making and setting of expectations whenever possible.
- Appreciation of and, when possible, response to, parents' suggestions and feedback.
- Respectful interactions, including responsive listening and endeavouring to understand parents' points of view.
- Sharing information on the child; for example, needs, health, welfare, development, progress, characteristics, special events/unfortunate happenings.
- Home visiting schemes, perhaps when children start nursery.
- Support for parents, such as books, leaflets, website, meetings, support groups, workshops.
- Recognition and utilization of parents' skills and expertise.
- Tactfully making explicit how parents may contribute actively to the ECEC setting, explaining their role and any necessary procedures.
- Opportunities for parents to support the ECEC setting (e.g. fundraising; play/help with children); assisting with visits/trips; invitations to special occasions; help with projects; social events.

(*Sources*: Blue-Banning *et al.*, 2004; Moore, 2003; Swick, 2003; Foot *et al.*, 2002; Hamilton *et al.*, 2002; Siraj-Blatchford *et al.*, 2002; QCA/DfEE, 2000; ECEF, 1998.)

There is also the important fact that the nursery stage is the optimum period in a child's education to establish, with children and families, the concept and practice of family–educator collaboration.

ENHANCING QUALITY IN ECEC SETTINGS

Evaluation is an essential aspect of quality in any ECEC programme – essential, that is, in enhancing provision and achieving high standards and best outcomes for children and their families. It is, however, a complex process and depends much on people's concepts of quality and ability 'to perceive, reflect and understand' (Yánez, 2001, p. 3).

First, we must note that the Office for Standards in Education (Ofsted) is now responsible for inspecting funded nursery provision for children aged 3 and 4 years, child-minding and day care. They have established formal criteria and processes for these inspections. The documents are publicly available, and early years professionals are obliged to pay careful attention to the specified requirements (see Ofsted and SureStart websites). Helpful as inspection can be, to achieve real quality within an inclusionary paradigm, we must go beyond these procedures.

Evaluation should be applied to all the dimensions of quality in any setting, and there is strong consensus that multiple perspectives, including children's views, are significant in the process (Clark *et al.*, 2003; Farrell *et al.*, 2002; Ilfeld, 2001; Yánez, 2001; Pascal and Bertram, 1994). Evaluation strategies might include:

- formal and informal observations;
- asking questions, informally or via interviews/questionnaires, of all participants to elicit views;
- listening carefully to children, parents, colleagues, inspectors, advisors, managers and headteachers;
- asking and answering questions of ourselves;
- comparing our provision and practice with that of others (via visits or reading);
- sharing views, discussing educational ideas and practice with others;
- asking a critical friend to observe and assess our practice;
- process evaluation:
  - observing day-to-day activities and evaluating particularly in terms of involvement; exploration; mental effort; challenges; matching child's capabilities; task orientation and engagement; quality of interactions.
- product evaluation:
  - evaluating the outcome of activities in terms of development, changes in children's awareness, attitudes, interests, understanding, knowledge, learning, behaviour, skills and competences.
- partnership evaluation:
  - how effective are partnerships with parents, stakeholders, other professionals, the community.
- using formal and standardized procedures for assessing children's experiences and learning outcomes (e.g. Laevers' (1994) Leuven Involvement Scale for Young Children (LIS-YC); the Early Childhood Environment Rating Scale (ECERS-R, ECERS-E) (Harms and Clifford, 1998).

Most crucially, just as with our observations in Chapter 1, we must act on the results of evaluative procedures, especially when we have identified an aspect of practice in need of improvement. Indeed, evaluation must be viewed as integral to our regular planning cycle. This 'reflective practice' requires us to reflect on our observations and evaluations; to discuss them with colleagues, other professionals, parents and children; and to study relevant research and so develop an informed action plan to improve elements of our provision in need of enhancement or enrichment. Through such a process, evaluation emerges as an extremely important strategy for working towards and improving quality in our ECEC provision.

Conclusion

We commenced this chapter by defining early childhood education and care. Identifying its benefits for children, families and society provided a sound rationale for its existence and promotion. We then considered several concepts of quality ECEC and explored the significant process variables from the resultant consensus framework. By studying dimensions of quality, debating them with relevant others and working towards an agreed concept of quality in our early years settings, we hope to come just a little closer to realizing the high standards that most of us seek.

Student activity

Remind yourself of the characteristics of Laevers' concept of 'involvement'. With a fellow student, observe a group of six to eight children engaged in a learning task, and identify the different levels of involvement amongst the children. Note any differences in outcomes. Discuss your findings with a colleague.

REFERENCES AND *FURTHER READING

Aldwinkle, M (2001): The DAP debate: Are we throwing the baby out with the bath water? *Australian Journal of Early Childhood Education*, **26**(2), 36–40.

Aytch, L, Castro, D, Cryer, D and Bailey, D (2004): *Quality Practices for Infants and Toddlers with Disabilities and their Families.* http://www.fpg.unc/~ncedl/.

Barrera, RM (2001): Bringing home to school. *Scholastic Early Childhood Today*, **16**(3), 44–56.

Barrera, I and Corso, RM (2002): Cultural competency as skilled dialogue. *Topics In Early Childhood Special Education*, **22**(2), 103–114.

Bernard van Leer (2004): *Bernard van Leer Foundation.* The Hague: Bernard van Leer Foundation.

Bertram, A and Pascal, C (2002): *Early Years: An International Perspective.* London: QCA.*

Bhavnagri, NP (2001): The global village. *Childhood Education*, **77**(5), 256–260.

Blue-Banning, M, Summers, JA, Frankland, HC, Nelson, LI and Beegle, G (2004): Dimensions of family and professional partnerships: constructive guidelines for collaboration. *Exceptional Children*, **70**(2), 167–184.

Bracey, GW and Stellar, A (2003): Long-term studies of pre-school: lasting benefits far outweigh costs. *Phi Delta Kappa*, **84**(19), 780–783, 797.

Bronfenbrenner, U (1979): *The Ecology of Human Development.* Cambridge, MA: Harvard University Press.

Burchinal, MR and Cryer, D (2003): Diversity, childcare quality, and developmental outcomes. *Early Childhood Research Quarterly*, **18**(4), 401–426.

Burriss, KG (2000): Research into practice. *Journal of Research in Childhood Education*, **14**(1), 118–122.

Carr, M and May, H (2000): Te Whariki: curriculum voices. In Penn, H (ed.), *Early Childhood Services: Theory, Policy and Practice.* Buckingham: Oxford University Press.*

Ceglowski, D and Bagalup, C (2002): Four perspectives on child care quality. *Early Childhood Education Journal*, **30**(2), 87–92.

Clark, A, McQuail, S and Moss, P (2003): *Exploring the Field of Listening to and Consulting Young Children.* London: DfES.*

Coltman, P, Petyaeva, D and Anghileri, J (2002): Scaffolding learning through meaningful tasks and adult interaction. *Early Years*, **22**(1), 39–49.

Curtis, A and O'Hagan, M (2003): *Care and Education in Early Childhood.* London: Routledge/Farmer.

Dahlberg, G (2000): Everything is a beginning and everything is dangerous. In Penn, H (ed.), *Early Childhood Services.* Buckingham: Oxford University Press.*

Dahlberg, G and Asen, G (1994): Evaluation and regulation: a question of empowerment. In Moss, P and Pence, A (eds), *Valuing Quality in Early Childhood Services.* London: Paul Chapman Publishing.

Derman-Sparkes, L (1993): Challenging bias in child care. *Coordinate*, **33**, 8–13.

DfES (2001): *Childcare and Early Education.* London: DfES.

Drummond, MJ (2003): Dangers of uncritical acceptance. *Times Educational Supplement*, 13 June, p. 25.

Early Childhood Education Forum (1998): *Quality in Diversity in Early Learning.* London: ECEF/NCB.

Early Childhood Forum (2003): *Consultation Response – Aim High: Raising the Achievement of Minority Ethnic Pupils.* ECF/NCB.

Edwards, C, Gandini, L and Forman, G (1998): *The Hundred Languages of Children*, 2nd edn. London: Ablex Publishing Corporation.*

Edwards, CP, Katz, LG and Clements, D (2002): The best-kept secret this side of Italy: Reggio Emilia has been an Italian success story ever since it was created 50 years ago. Learn how it can improve preschool education in the United States. *District Administration*, **38**(8), 38–40.

Ellis, N (2002): The Foundation Stage: a problem of competing philosophies. *Forum*, **44**(3), 117–120.

Ennals, P (2002): Together from the start. *Children Now*, Winter, 6–7.

Espinosa, LM (2002): High-quality preschool: why we need it and what it looks like. *Preschool Policy Matters*, **1**, 1–10.

Falconer, RC and Byrnes, DA (2003): When good intentions are not enough: a response to increasing diversity in an early childhood setting. *Journal of Research in Childhood Education*, **17**(2), 188–200.

Farrell, A, Taylor, C and Tennent, L (2002): Early childhood services: what children can tell us. *Australian Journal of Early Childhood*, **27**(3), 13–17.

Fleer, M (2002a): Research evidence with political currency: keeping early childhood on the international agenda. *Australian Journal of Early Childhood*, **27**(1), 1–7.

Fleer, M (2002b): Early childhood education: a public right and not a privilege. *Australian Journal of Early Childhood*, **27**(2), 1–7.

Foot, H, Howe, C, Cheyne, W, Terras, M and Rattray, C (2002): Parental participation and partnership in pre-school provision. *International Journal of Early Years Education*, **10**(1), 5–19.*

Froebel, F (1877): *Reminiscences* (translated by H. Mann). London: Cambridge Press.

Gammage, P (1994): In defence of children. In Laevers, F (ed.), *Defining and Assessing Quality in Early Childhood Education*. Leuven: University Press, pp. 3–12.

Goodfellow, J (2001): Wise practice: the need to move beyond best practice in early childhood education. *Australian Journal of Early Childhood*, **26**(3), 1–6.

Hamilton, ME, Roach, MA and Riley, DA (2003): Moving towards family-centered early care and education: the past, the present and a glimpse of the future. *Early Childhood Education Journal*, **30**(4), 225–232.*

Harms, T and Clifford, R (1998): *Early Childhood Environment Rating Scale* (revised edn). New York: Teachers College Press.

Hewett, VM (2001): Examining the Reggio Emilia approach to early childhood education. *Early Childhood Education Journal*, **29**(2), 95–100.

Heymann, J (2003): Role of early childhood care and education in ensuring equal opportunity. *UNESCO Policy Briefs on Early Childhood*, **18**, Nov–Dec, 1–2.*

Hicks, T (2003): Interim research indicates many head start benefits. *Education Daily*, **36**(133), 1–2.

Hughes, P and McNaughton, G (2002): Preparing early childhood professionals to work with parents: the challenges of diversity and dissensus. *Australian Journal of Early Childhood*, **27**(2), 14–20.

Hyson, M (2003): Putting early academics in their place. *Educational Leadership*, **60**(7), 20–23.

Ilfeld, EM (2001): Emerging maps of effectiveness. *Early Childhood Matters*, **99**, 6–13.

Johnson, DJ, Jaeger, E, Randolph, SM, Cauce, AM and Ward, J (2003): Studying the effects of early child care experiences on the development of children of color in the United States: towards a more inclusive research agenda. *Child Development*, **74**(5), 1227–1244.

Kapasi, H (2001): *Asian Children Play: Increasing Access to Play Provision for Asian Children*, 2nd edn. London: Playtrain.

Katz, LG (2003): The right of the child to develop and learn in quality environments. *International Journal of Early Childhood*, **35**(1,2), 13–22.*

Keyes, CR (2002): A way of thinking about parent/teacher partnerships for teachers. *International Journal of Early Childhood*, **10**(3), 177–191.

Laevers, F (1994): The innovative project: experiential education and the definition of quality in education. In Laevers, F (ed.), *Defining and Assessing Quality in Early Childhood Education*. Leuven: Leuven University Press, pp. 159–172.

Laevers, F (2000): Forward to basics: deep-level-learning and the experiential approach. *Early Years*, **20**(2), 20–29.*

Landry, SH (2002): *Supporting Cognitive Development in Early Childhood*. Report on conference held at Little Rock, Arkansas, 30 April.

Lane, J (1999): *Action for Racial Equality in the Early Years*. London: NEYN.*

Levin-Rozalis, M and Shafran, N (2003): *A Sense of Belonging*. The Hague: Bernard van Leer Foundation.

Lillemyr, OF, Fagerli, O and Sobstad, F (2001): *A Global Perspective on Early Childhood Care and Education*. Paris: UNESCO.

Martin, D (2004): Childcare tops the Labour agenda. *Childcare Now*, 14–20 July, pp. 12–13.

McCay, LO and Keyes, DW (2001): Developing social competence in the inclusive primary classroom: the ability to promote social competence in inclusive settings is a critical teacher competency for a developmentally appropriate early childhood program. *Childhood Education*, **78**(2), 70–78.

McCullough, N (2002): Literary liaison: sending literacy home and back to school. *Reading Horizons*, **42**(4), 293–306.

McGavin, H (2003): Italian style. *Times Educational Supplement*, 25 July, pp. 20–21.

Mitchell, L (2004): *Characteristics of Professional Development Linked to Enhanced Pedagogy and Children's Learning in Early Childhood Settings: A Best Evidence Synthesis (2002–2003).* Wellington: NZ Council for Educational Research.

Moll, LC (1990): *Vygotsky and Education.* Cambridge: Cambridge University Press.

Mooney, A and Blackburn, T (2003): *Children's Views on Childcare Quality.* London: DfES.*

Mooney, A, Cameron, C, Candappa, M, McQuail, S, Moss, P and Petrie, P (2003): *Early Years and Childcare International Evidence Project: Quality.* London: DfES.*

Moore, KB (2003): Making the home–school connection. *Scholastic Early Child Today*, **18**(1), 14–15.

Moss, P, Dahlberg, G and Pence, A (2000): Getting beyond the problem of quality. *European Early Childhood Education Research Journal*, **8**(2), 103–115.

Moyles, J, Adams, S and Musgrove, A (2002): *Study of Pedagogical Effectiveness in Early Learning.* London: DfES.*

Myers, R (2001): *Early Childhood Care and Development.* Paris: UNESCO.

New, R (2000): *Reggio Emilia: Catalyst for Change and Conversation.* ERIC/EECE Digest. http://www.ecap.crc.uiuc.edu/eecearchive/digests/2000/new00.html.

OECD (2001): *Starting Strong: Early Childhood Education and Care.* Paris: OECD.*

Ofsted (2001): *Sessional Day Care: Guidance to the National Standards.* Nottingham: DfEE (now DfES).

Papps, I and Dyson, A (2004): *The Costs and Benefits of Earlier Identification and Effective Intervention.* London: DfES.

Pascal, C (undated): *The Effective Early Learning Project: Achievements and Reflections.* http://www.ecdu.govt.nz/publications.

Pascal, C and Bertram, A (2001): Evaluating the costs and benefits of early childhood programmes. *European Early Childhood Education Research Journal*, **9**(2), 21–44.

Pattnaik, J (2003): Learning about the 'other': building a case for intercultural understanding among minority children. *Childhood Education*, **79**(4), 204–211.

Pianto, RC and La Paro, K (2003): Improving early school success. *Educational Leadership*, **60**(7), 24–29.

Pollard, EL and Davidson, L (2001): *Foundations of Child Well-being.* UNESCO Monograph 18. Paris: UNESCO.*

Prince, DL, Hare, RD and Howard, EM (2001): Longitudinal effects of kindergarten. *Journal of Research in Childhood Education*, **16**(1), 15–27.

Puri, S (2002): Promoting race equality through peer support. *Peer Support Forum Briefing Paper*, November 2002, 1–3.

QCA/DfEE (2000): *Curriculum Guidance for the Foundation Stage.* London: QCA.

Raban, B, Ure, C and Waniganayake, M (2003): Multiple perspectives: acknowledging the virtue of complexity in measuring quality. *Early Years*, **23**(1), 67–77.

Ramey, CT and Ramey, SL (2002): Early childhood education: from efficacy to improved practice. Conference report: *A Summit on Early Childhood Cognitive Development*, pp. 2–7.

Reynolds, A and Stevens, P (2002): Chicago longitudinal study. *Newsletter of the Chicago Longitudinal Study*, **2**, 1–4.

Rhedding-Jones, J (2002): An undoing of documents and other texts: towards a critical multiculturalism in early childhood education. *Contemporary Issues in Early Childhood*, **3**(1), 90–116.

Richburg, M and Fletcher, T (2002): Emotional intelligence: directing a child's emotional education. *Child Study Journal*, **32**(1), 31–38.

Rimm-Kaufman, SE, Voorhees, MD, Snell, ME and La Paro, KM (2003): Improving the sensitivity and responsiveness of preservice teachers toward young children with disabilities. *Topics in Early Childhood Special Education*, **23**(3), 151–153.

Schweinhart, LJ (2003): *Benefits, Costs, and Explanation of the High Scope Perry Preschool Program.* Paper presented at the Meeting of the Society for Research in Child Development, 26 April 2003.

Shpancer, N (2002): The home–daycare link: mapping children's new world order. *Early Childhood Research Quarterly*, **17**, 374–392.

Siraj-Blatchford, I (2003): Supporting children's learning: The EPPE Project. *Report of the Nottingham Early Years Conference*, September 2002, pp. 9–15.

Siraj-Blatchford, I, Sylva, K, Muttock, S, Gilden, R and Bell, D (2002): *Researching Effective Pedagogy in the Early Years.* London: DfES.*

Smith, R (2004a): Charities attack government strategy. *Children Now*, 18–24 February, p. 9.

Smith, R (2004b): Early years teaching. *Children Now*, 11–17 February, p. 19.

Soler, J and Miller, L (2003): The struggle for early childhood curricula: a comparison of the English Foundation Stage Curriculum, Te Whariki and Reggio Emilia. *International Journal of Early Years Education*, **11**(1), 58–67.

Soodak, LC, Erwin, EJ, Winton, P, Brotherson, MJ, Turnbull, AP, Hanson, MJ and Brault, LMJ (2002): Implementing inclusive early childhood education: a call for professional empowerment. *Topics in Early Childhood Special Education*, **22**(2), 91–102.

Staggs, L (2004): Solid support. *SureStart*, **1**, Winter 2003/04, 8–9.

Swick, KJ (2003): Communication concepts for strengthening family–school–community partnerships. *Early Childhood Education Journal*, **30**(4), 275–280.

Sylva, K, Melhuish, E, Sammons, P, Siraj-Blatchford, I, Taggart, B and Elliot, K (2003): *The Effective Provision of Pre-school Education (EPPE) Project: Findings from the Pre-school Period.* London: DfES.*

Ulich, M and Mayr, T (2002): Children's involvement profiles in daycare centres. *European Early Childhood Education Research Journal*, **10**(2), 127–143.

UNESCO (2001): *Framework for Action on Values Education in Early Childhood.* Paris: UNESCO.*

UNICEF (2000): *Education for All: No Excuses.* New York: UNICEF.

UNICEF (2003): *A World Fit for Children.* New York: UNICEF.*

Vakil, S, Freeman, R and Swim, TJ (2003): The Reggio Emilia approach and inclusive early childhood programs. *Early Childhood Education Journal*, **30**(3), 187–192.

Van Ausdale, D and Feagin, JR (2001): *The First R – How Children Learn Race and Racism.* Oxford: Rowman and Littlefield.

Vygotsky, LS (1978): *Mind in Society: The Development of Higher Psychological Processes.* Cambridge, MA: Harvard University Press.

Wherry, JH (2004): *Selected Parent Involvement Research.* http://www.parent-institute.com/educator/resources/research.

Woodhead, M (1998): 'Quality' in early childhood programmes – a contextually appropriate approach. *International Journal of Early Years Education*, **6**(1), 5–17.

Wunschel, G (2003): *From Car Park to Children's Park*. The Hague: Bernard van Leer Foundation.

Wylie, C and Thompson, J (2003): The long-term contribution of early childhood education to children's performance – evidence from New Zealand. *International Journal of Early Years Education*, **11**(1), 69–78.

Yanez, L (2001): The effectiveness initiative: first fruits. *Early Childhood Matters*, **99**, October, pp. 3–13.

Zietlow, R (2002): Education: early childhood efforts may save money in the long run. *State Government News*, **45**(5), p. 21.

WEBSITES

www.bernardvanleer.org
www.dfes.gov.uk
www.oecd.org
www.ofsted.gov.uk
www.qca.gov.uk
www.surestart.gov.uk
www.unesco.org
www.UNICEF.org

THE EARLY SCHOOL PATHWAY

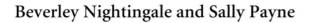

8

Beverley Nightingale and Sally Payne

> This chapter aims to:
>
> ■ contextualize early childhood education within an historical, legal and socio-cultural framework;
>
> ■ examine the early years of a child's statutory school 'journey' (from reception to the end of Key Stage One).
>
> The major (but not sole) focus is on the English education system.

INTRODUCTION

We shall commence this chapter by identifying aspects of the historical, legal and socio-cultural contexts of relevance to children's first years at school – mainly with reference to England. Then, we shall consider children's experiences as they start and progress through the earliest stages of their statutory school 'journey'.

HISTORICAL AND LEGAL FRAMEWORK

School starting age

There is sometimes uncertainty over exactly when children must start school. In England and Wales, a large number start when they are 4 years old, and others when they are 5 years old. Different Local Education Authorities (LEAs) have differing entry procedures. Some stagger entry to three points in the academic year – September, January and April – whilst others have one entry in September. Funding, budgets and size of cohort can also impact on decision making between and within counties year by year. In actual fact, children are legally required to begin their statutory schooling at the start of the term after their fifth birthday (unless parents decide to educate their child outside school). In Scotland, statutory education begins in the August after a child's fifth birthday, with only that one entry point in the year. The official school starting age in Northern Ireland is 4 years, with one start date in September. In other European countries compulsory schooling starts later, at 6 or 7 years. Typical school starting ages in several European countries are presented in Table 8.1.

Many European children do, of course, start their educational experience earlier in some form of pre-school setting; for example in the UK, in LEA nurseries, nursery classes or private or voluntary early years provision; in Belgium, kleuterschool/kindergarten/école maternelle; in Denmark, børnehaver; in France, école maternelle;

Table 8.1 School starting ages in European countries

Country	School starting age (years)
Belgium	6
Denmark	7
France	6
Germany	6
Greece	5½
Hungary	6
Ireland	6
Italy	6
Luxembourg	6
Netherlands	5
Norway	7
Portugal	6
Spain	6
Sweden	7
United Kingdom	
(England, Scotland, Wales)	5
(Northern Ireland)	4

Sources: www.eurydice.org/documents/preschool_n_primary/en/FrameSet.htm
and www.literacytrust.org.uk

and in Germany, kindergarten. Nurseries are also available in virtually all European countries for the youngest children (aged 0–3 years).

Early childhood education

For England and Wales, the Education Act 1944 established the primary phase of education (5–11 years) and the Education Reform Act 1988 established four key stages within the compulsory schooling period:

- Key Stage One: 5–7 years
- Key Stage Two: 7–11 years
- Key Stage Three: 11–14 years
- Key Stage Four: 14–16 years.

Early childhood education is usually perceived as starting at 3 years and, depending on perspective, lasting until 5, 7 or 8 years of age. For the purposes of this chapter, we take early childhood education as lasting from 3 years until the end of Key Stage One; we will focus on children's experiences in the school element of the foundation stage (4–5 years) and at Key Stage One (KS1).

In line with many governments around the world, since the 1990s early education in the UK has been taken seriously, and successive government initiatives have raised its profile and enhanced its quality and quantity, particularly for the under-fives – which provision had previously lacked co-ordination, focus and funding (Pugh, 1996). Information on recent UK policy developments relating to early childhood can be found in the Introduction of this book, and also in Chapter 10.

One significant early years legislative initiative that is important to consider early in this chapter is the introduction of the foundation stage and its curriculum, the result of much consultation with early years professionals and specialists. Its intention was to enhance and enable children's development and prepare them for entry into school and a successful start to the National Curriculum. It succeeded the controversial outcome-oriented curriculum presented in *Desirable Outcomes for Children's Learning on Entering Compulsory Education* (SCAA/DfEE, 1996) which was interpreted too prescriptively by many practitioners, thus often losing its play-based underpinning thread.

The foundation stage curriculum (QCA/DfEE, 1999) sets out the *early learning goals* to be achieved by the majority of children at the end of their foundation stage. In 2000, this was supplemented by *Curriculum Guidance for the Foundation Stage* (QCA/DfEE, 2000) which provided detailed and (many deemed) appropriate curriculum guidance for young children from 3 years, in a wide range of settings. Guidance notes were principled [the principles deriving from 'good and effective practice in early years settings' (QCA/DfEE, 2000, p. 11)], enabling a play-oriented approach and allowing teachers and practitioners creativity in its planning. All settings that offered this framework and worked to criteria set out by the Qualifications and Curriculum Authority (QCA) received grant funding for eligible children. This initiative was warmly endorsed by many – though not all – early years professionals and academics (see Chapter 7, p. 131).

The Education Act 2002 incorporated the foundation stage into the National Curriculum in England and, for the first time, there were statutory generic curriculum guidelines for young children's education. In September 2004, Wales commenced the pilot for its foundation stage for 3- to 7-year-olds with the Welsh version of the Desirable Outcomes curriculum to be phased out by 2008, when it is anticipated their foundation stage will be fully implemented. Northern Ireland's foundation stage will be finally agreed when the early years review, initiated in 2004, is complete; Scotland has its own non-statutory *Curriculum Framework for Children 3–5*.

The English foundation stage curriculum commences in pre-school settings with 3-year-olds, and continues until the end of the school (reception) year in which children reach the age of 5 (DfES, 2003). This means, before they commence KS1 of the National Curriculum, most children will have experienced the foundation stage curriculum in a reception class and also probably a nursery or maybe in a foundation stage unit which, in some schools with the available resources, are replacing separate nursery and reception classes. There does, however, seem to be differential practice as to when children finish the foundation stage curriculum and start KS1. For example, many reception teachers ensure that able children access KS1 when it is appropriate, whilst others present a watered-down version of KS1 to reception children. Additionally, split age classes, combining foundation stage and KS1 pupils, which exist in some schools for economic reasons, can intensify the dilemma over exactly which curriculum guidance to follow.

This situation is allied to the long-standing debate in the UK which has centred on the age at which a more formal style of teaching should be introduced to young children (e.g. David, 1999; Fearn, 1999). This has undoubtedly influenced the foundation stage curriculum which the guidance (QCA/DfEE, 2000) affirms is not intended to be formal, and indeed purports to mirror many aspects of the pre-schools of Europe which have an informal, play-based curriculum, ensuring that young children are primarily 'making sense' of the world in which they live. Recent emphases on literacy, numeracy and the raising of standards in primary education, however, have meant that many teachers – with the exception of the most confident, competent and creative – may be introducing formal learning too soon (Adams *et al.*, 2004). In addition, greater accountability and the pressure on teachers to meet targets have led, in some settings, to children's entitlement to a broad and balanced foundation stage curriculum being eroded. Fortunately this has the chance to change with the introduction of the DfES' (2003) *Excellence and Enjoyment: A Strategy for Primary Schools* which sets out to redress the balance of perceived constraints and gives schools and teachers greater freedom in their curriculum decision making.

Legislative requirements for schools

The Department for Education and Skills (DfES, previously the Department for Education and Science) and the Department of Education and Employment (DfEE) oversees education and training in England. [Equivalents are: The Department of Education, Northern Ireland (DENI); The Scottish Executive Education Department (SEED); The National Assembly, Learning Wales.]

The Qualifications and Curriculum Authority (QCA) is a non-departmental public statutory body formed in October 1997 to promote quality and coherence in education and training in England. The QCA's prime duty is to advise the Secretary of State for Education and Skills on matters affecting the school curriculum, pupil assessment and publicly funded qualifications offered in schools, colleges and workplaces. [Equivalents are: The Council for Curriculum, Examinations and Assessment (CCEA) in Northern Ireland; The Scottish Qualifications Authority (SQA); The Qualifications, Curriculum and Assessment Authority for Wales (ACCAC).]

The Office for Standards in Education (Ofsted) was set up in 1992 to help improve the quality and standards of education and child care in England through independent inspection and regulation, and to provide advice to the Secretary of State for Education and Skills. It is separate from the DfES. Ofsted is responsible for the management of the system of school inspection, and inspectors regularly visit primary schools to ensure that standards are acceptable. [Equivalents are: The Education and Training Inspectorate of Northern Ireland (ETI); Her Majesty's Inspectorate of Education in Scotland (HMIE); Her Majesty's Inspectorate for Education and Training in Wales (ESTYN).]

Though changes may come about as a result of the government's *Five-year strategy for children and learners* announced in July 2004 (see DfES website), central government currently shares responsibility with LEAs for the following:

- planning the supply of school places;
- making sure every child has access to a suitable school place, or has suitable provision made for him/her;
- supporting and challenging schools, in inverse proportion to their success, and intervening where a school is failing its pupils;
- allocating funding to schools.

Legislation affecting schools and education has been prolific in recent years, and this chapter can only cover some of the many reforms and changes that have impacted on schools. Currently, schools in England are legally required to have the following policies in place:

- Admissions Policy
- Charging Policy

- Child Protection Policy
- Curriculum Policy
- Health and Safety Policy
- Performance Management Policy
- Policy on Collective Worship
- Pupil Discipline (including anti-bullying) Policy
- Race Equality Policy
- Staff Appraisal Policy
- Sex Education Policy
- Special Educational Needs Policy.

In addition, schools must legally publish details of significant plans, reports and procedures; for example, an action plan following an Ofsted inspection, the governors' annual report to parents, home–school agreements, and a school prospectus. Helpfully, the DfES (2004a) has recently updated its guidance and regulations to schools, particularly for governors, to promote greater understanding of the formal requirements and their associated complexities. Further information on such elements of education in England, Northern Ireland, Scotland and Wales can be found on the relevant websites.

SOCIO-CULTURAL CONTEXTS

Schools and communities

Primary schools serve and, ideally, are closely integrated into their local communities, being conceived as a living part of the social fabric of that community. The more collaborative the endeavour between school and community, the greater are the benefits to children's development and learning (Anning *et al.*, 2004). Much emphasis in the 1990s was on developmentally appropriate practice (Kelly, 1994), but it is now acknowledged that the socio-cultural context is significant (Woodhead, 1996; Drury *et al.*, 2000). While this acknowledgement has been gathering momentum for some time (Bredekamp and Copple, 1997; MacNaughton, 2000), translation into practice can be time-consuming and requires effort, dialogue and partnership amongst all parties (see Chapter 7, pp. 124–133, for more details). Community-led decision making has shown its merits in such initiatives as the SureStart intervention programme (Drury *et al.*, 2000), and political shifts are seeing greater emphasis placed on working with parents and giving greater consideration to the local community, its history and children's socio-cultural needs. The UK is culturally diverse, and the idea of a 'one glove fits all' approach to education cannot be sustained in dynamic and evolving cultural contexts. Schools and communities need to engage and collaborate with one another to explore meanings and ensure that children's development and learning are rich in experiences and embedded in the social and cultural realities of their lives. It is also vital that, in this collaborative venture, the complementary roles of all participants are fully recognized and utilized.

Parents and schools

Working with parents or their primary carers is not new; Froebel placed great importance on parents as educators, and believed it was teachers who should promote and support this (e.g. Liebscher, 1992). The concept is implicit and explicit in the Children Act 2004 (see website) in its aim to improve and support children's all-round well-being. Successive governments have demanded closer working with parents, and thus enabled many parents to take a more active role in the education of their children. This directive is based on the premise that if a child realizes that his or her parents are enthusiastic about education, he or she is more likely to view his/her schooling in a positive light and be more receptive to learning. Parents determine a child's home environment; therefore, if the school and home work together, better understanding is likely, with accepted benefits for children.

Additionally, many parents very much want to be part of the process – supporting, enabling and facilitating their child's learning, whilst also increasing their own knowledge and skills. Some parents take an informal view of this role, others a more formal view – the continuum shows that, just as there are many types of parenting, there are many different types of parental involvement. Perspectives on, and definitions of, partnership are just as many and just as varied (Curtis and O'Hagan, 2003). It is, however, accepted by all early education experts that school–home links are central in developing the learning of young children (Bruce, 2004).

Early years professionals are well aware of the importance of building and maintaining relationships with parents. Schools and teachers who have invested time and resources in this endeavour recognize the many benefits to their work, to children's learning, to parents, and to the community. There must, however, be mutual respect in the building of any partnership and, again, the complementary roles of each participant must be seen as being of equal value and fully utilized. Issues of power relationships need to be considered and reframed where necessary – reflection, dialogue and action are naturally paramount in this process. (Chapter 7, pp. 132–133, includes further debate on this topic and additional strategies to encourage parent involvement and/or partnership.)

The wider team in the classroom

The effects of the funding formula in schools, inclusion and labelling are just some of the factors that may result in a variety of support staff and adults working alongside teachers in the classroom. Various degrees of assistance both professional and voluntary may come from:

- Nursery Nurses (they hold a Nursery Nursing qualification to work with children up to the age of 8 years).
- Teaching Assistants (they assist the teacher with many tasks, including working with small groups of children or individuals. They usually have had lots of practical experience with children and, increasingly, they hold the Teaching Assistant's qualification).
- Learning Support Assistants (they provide support for children with special needs).
- Other teachers in parallel or adjacent classes.
- Advisory teachers and advisers.
- Professionals from outside agencies such as speech and language therapists, educational psychologists.
- Headteacher or Deputy Headteacher.
- Volunteers such as parents/primary carers and other relatives (e.g. grandparents).
- Students on placement.

- Visitors.
- Governors.

Teachers organizing and managing the learning environment, working with other adults on a permanent or periodic basis, whilst ensuring the effective utilization of these human resources, need sound managerial skills and the ability to use their own and others' strengths to best advantage (Curtis and O'Hagan, 2003; Moyles, 1992). To benefit all those involved and especially the children, it is important there is:

- thorough planning;
- clear communication in a supportive environment;
- knowledge of the skills and interests of each person and the use of these to the learning environment – all to be valued and acknowledged;
- modelling of certain behaviours;
- constructive feedback given;
- monitoring and evaluation of the assistance.

Hayes (1999, p. 214) advocates that, since 'collaboration is at the heart of effective schooling', it needs to be developed with all adults in the classroom being clear about their own and others' roles and responsibilities. Additionally, ensuring that each team member understands policy and procedures, as well as the ethos and aims of the school, will further support this collaborative working and avoid the risk of any enterprise being a disheartening and unprofitable experience for all concerned.

Many support staff are closely involved in planning along with the teacher, a co-operative venture that benefits all concerned (Ofsted, 2002). The accompanying sharing of knowledge, skills and understanding will, of course, support the strategies employed in the process of children's learning and also the analysis and enhancement of practice. Regular team meetings will be necessary for such activities, and particularly important for disseminating learning, passing on significant information and sharing relevant matters of import and concern.

Multi-professional working

Abbott and Pugh (1998, p. 62) believe that '… the multi-disciplinary nature of the work of the early years teacher (and his/her team) has often been largely ignored'. Yet this is important in working to the holistic philosophy and in teachers' (and classroom colleagues') multi-professional work with outside agencies where the focus has to be on collaborative working. This inter-disciplinary practice received an increased emphasis under the Children Act 2004, which requires co-ordinated planning, commissioning and delivery of education, health and social welfare services for children and families. Accordingly, this integrated practice demands early years professionals and support workers who understand children's all-round needs and development as well as the complexities and socio-cultural contexts of their lives. These adults must also be capable of genuine co-operation with relevant others in the best interests of children's welfare and education.

Continuing professional training and development can be helpful in this endeavour for everyone working in any early years field in whatever capacity; they can be supported in acquiring or enhancing the necessary skills and knowledge, particularly as roles and responsibilities change and evolve in the early years environment. Attendance at multi-disciplinary training sessions (involving a range of relevant professionals) can, however, be particularly valuable for encouraging stronger and more effective inter-professional working with and for children and their families.

While Fisher (2002) firmly reinforces the idea that effective teamwork within a setting (including parents) is an indicator of high quality and of considerable benefit to children, we must remember that it is teachers who carry the ultimate responsibility for their classes and for standards. As an ideal, successful foundation stage and KS1 classrooms would exude co-operation from the harmony of the classroom environment and its planned curriculum to the inter-working and collaborative practices amongst the inhabitants, visitors and other relevant professionals.

THE EARLY YEARS OF THE SCHOOL 'JOURNEY'

The first days in school

'The morning came, without any warning, when my sisters surrounded me.... "What's this?" I said. "You're starting school today." They picked me up bodily, kicking and bawling, and carried me up the road'

(Lee, 1959, p. 43).

Let us now examine this all-important first stage of a child's 'journey' through the education system.

A child arrives in school. Is it a first experience of the setting? Has there been separation from mother before? Is the child ready? Many different questions may be posed – each child will have his/her own experiences, memories and feelings, but in Britain will have to go to school, at the latest, on the first day of term following his/her fifth birthday.

Starting school is experienced not only by the individual child but also by the parents and often other family members as well. 'Parents are children's first and most enduring educators' (QCA/DfEE, 2000, p. 9). They too will have had unique lives; nature and nurture affect all. The connections between the contexts of home and school need to be in place if the transition is to be a positive and untroubled experience. As we have already discussed, communication between participants is paramount. The relationship that is built must be based on mutual trust and respect and take into account contextual aspects of the individual family. Children must also have a feeling of confidence as learners when starting school and ideally this needs to be communicated by both school and home to enable the child to commence this 'journey' happily and successfully.

Schools vary with regard to preparation for new children. Their prospectus can be most helpful in informing parents of procedures and in supporting children's entry. Many have arrangements where the teacher goes to the child's home, or the child visits the school. Some children have older siblings and will be familiar with the environment. Playgroups and nurseries have visits from local reception teachers and also take their children on a visit to the school, perhaps to listen to a story, enjoy a creative activity or play a game. Intakes may be staggered with groups of new children starting on different days of the week or attending part-time for an initial period – perhaps going home after lunch. Good practice ensures that the environment immediately shows each child that he/she is valued. Pictures recording visits linking school and home are displayed to welcome new children. First languages and cultural artefacts are integral to the setting. Initial activities will recognize children's needs, interests and experiences linking to topics such as '*Ourselves*' and '*My family*' or '*Pets*'. Teachers, nursery nurses and teaching assistants will ensure that individuals are not excluded. Inclusion is paramount, with the school curriculum being only the starting point for meeting the additional needs of individual and groups of children. The Qualification and Curriculum Authority (QCA website, National Curriculum online, pp. 1–5) offers three underpinning principles (with useful accompanying guidance) for achieving inclusion in schools:

1. Setting suitable learning challenges.
2. Responding to pupils' diverse learning needs.
3. Overcoming potential barriers to learning and assessment for individuals and groups of pupils.

Also on the QCA website, under *Guidance for Teachers* (pp. 1–3) there is some helpful and fairly detailed advice on challenging stereotypes and racism and valuing diversity in schools by:

- using appropriate resources;
- presenting a broad and balanced curriculum;
- challenging assumptions;
- understanding globalization; and
- creating an open climate.

Anti-discriminatory and non-stereotypical practice (Fig. 8.1) should be the norm (see Chapter 7, pp. 124–127, for further discussion on this topic).

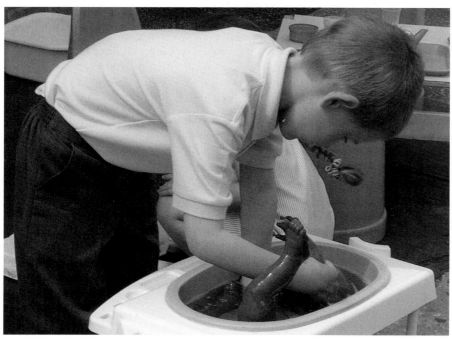

Figure 8.1   Non-stereotypical practice should be the norm.

Implementation of the foundation stage curriculum

The child is now a fully 'inducted' member of 'big school'. The wheels of the curriculum begin to turn. In England, the foundation stage curriculum provides the route for the child to travel (QCA/DfEE, 2000). It comprises six areas of learning:

- Personal, social and emotional development.
- Communication, language and literacy.
- Mathematical development.
- Knowledge and understanding of the world.
- Physical development.
- Creative development.

The early years curricula for Northern Ireland, Scotland and Wales can be found on the CCEA, SQA and ACCAC websites.

   In the reception year in England, the National Literacy and National Numeracy Strategies must also be introduced. (See DfEE, 2000a,b for guidance on implementation in the reception year.) These strategies are intended to be consistent with the relevant elements of the foundation stage early learning goals and provide a bridge to English and Mathematics in the National Curriculum.

Table 8.2   **The six areas of learning with sample stepping stones and early learning goals**

Area of learning	Example of a first stepping stone	Example of an early learning goal (ELG)
Personal, social and emotional development	Have a positive approach to new experiences	Continue to be interested, excited and motivated to learn
Communication, language and literacy	Listen to favourite nursery rhymes, stories and songs. Join in with repeated refrains, anticipating key events and important phrases	Listen with enjoyment, and respond to stories, songs and other music, rhymes and poems and make up their own stories, songs, rhymes and poems
Mathematical development	Enjoy joining in with number rhymes and songs	Say and use number names in order in familiar contexts
Knowledge and understanding of the world	Show curiosity and interest by facial expression, movement or sound	Investigate objects and materials by using all of their senses as appropriate
Physical development	Respond to rhythm, music and story by means of gesture and movement	Move with confidence, imagination and safety
Creative development	Join in favourite songs, respond to sound with body movement	Recognize and explore how sounds can be changed, sing simple songs from memory, recognize repeated sounds and sound patterns and match movements to music

Source: Information taken from QCA/DfEE (2000).

Each of the foundation stage six learning areas includes a pathway of stepping stones progressing to early learning goals to be achieved by most children by the end of the foundation stage. Table 8.2 provides examples of early stepping stones in each of the six learning areas and the early learning goals to which they are leading.

Much emphasis has been placed on the development of personal, social and emotional aspects in the early years (see Chapter 4 for further discussion). Figure 8.2 illustrates one pathway through the personal, social and emotional map from an initial stepping stone to the corresponding early learning goal – echoing the emphasis on children developing a sense of community and the importance of respecting others.

Although Table 8.2 and Figure 8.2 indicate how the foundation stage curriculum is presented and may be interpreted, there is no substitute for continually referring to it in its entirety. The examples provided in the curriculum guidance document (QCA/DfEE, 2000, pp. 26–127) of what children may do and what the practitioner needs to do have been found by teachers to be invaluable in informing good practice.

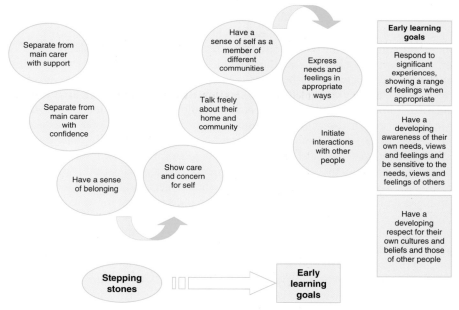

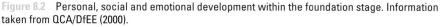

Figure 8.2 Personal, social and emotional development within the foundation stage. Information taken from QCA/DfEE (2000).

Planning the foundation stage 'journey'

The route must be planned using the specified map (e.g. foundation stage curriculum) to give the general direction. It is also vital to identify where each child is on that map in order to ascertain his/her starting point and thus select the most appropriate route.

'Plan–do–review' is the simple version of the planning cycle. This becomes more complex but more meaningful when it includes assessment, reflection and evaluation with the planning cycle as an ongoing or rolling process and the all-important observation of children informing each aspect (see Fig. 8.3).

As we noted earlier, many pupils will have commenced their 'journeys' in some form of pre-school provision. Several will have travelled far, others less far, and some will just be beginning – the teacher must take each child forward by building on the child's current level of knowledge, understanding and abilities.

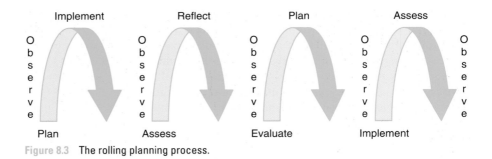

Implement	Reflect	Plan	Assess

Observe   Observe   Observe   Observe   Observe

Plan	Assess	Evaluate	Implement

Figure 8.3   The rolling planning process.

Documentation may well have accompanied a child from a previous setting, and this may be useful in assessing where he or she is on the map and, therefore, where he/she will start the next stage of his/her 'journey'. There is little doubt, however, that observation and knowing each child and his/her family are the key tools to ensuring the planned (and hopefully delivered) curriculum meets individual needs. (Do refer back to Chapter 1, which provides guidance on the process of observation.)

The responsibility for planning each child's 'journey' lies with the teacher, often in consultation with the whole foundation team and using the foundation stage or other relevant pre-school curriculum guidance. Planning consists of long-, medium- and short-term plans (see Fisher, 2002; QCA/DfES, 2001). The long-term or yearly plans ensure that the child will follow a carefully structured route of breadth and balance according to the aims of the relevant curriculum, and also of the establishment. Medium-term or half-termly plans (sometimes planned on a two-year cycle to allow for classes of two-year groups) enable resources and topics to be organized and monitored. Short-term plans deal with the detail, outlining the rich, stimulating and challenging activities that children will experience over a short period (e.g. a week or fortnight). They will identify the planned learning objectives, teaching and learning strategies and resources – all cross-referenced to the stepping stones and early learning goals or equivalent. The whole foundation team must be familiar with these plans and be sure of the learning outcomes which they are responsible for helping children achieve. Differentiation (taking account of children's different starting points and varying needs) will be indicated – demonstrating the specific provision for groups of children and inclusion for individual needs (Smidt, 2002). Cross-curricular planning is desirable because it encourages pathways through the curriculum to visit more than one area of learning, accommodating the fact that children's learning is holistic rather than compartmentalized (see Bruce, 1997, and the Introduction to this book).

While support for planning is available in many forms (e.g. websites, books, journals), professional expertise is essential when decisions are taken, for example what to include, omit or amend; how to implement plans to maximize the opportunity for each child in terms of benefit and achieving his/her potential; how to individualize each child's journey (QCA/DfEE, 2000); how to enthuse children and encourage their involvement and interest.

It is, of course, also vital that professionals understand how children think and learn. Educators will naturally pose questions derived from theories of learning, for example:

- How do I organize the children?
- Does this activity need children to work together to maximize their zone of proximal development?
- What is the role of the adult?
- Is scaffolding required to provide suitable steps to achievement?
- Does the activity need modelling, or will that stifle creativity?

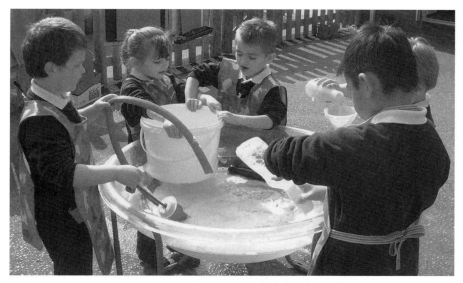

Figure 8.4 Teaching and learning styles appropriate to the child and the activity: for example, during water play children can be developing mathematical, scientific, linguistic and social skills.

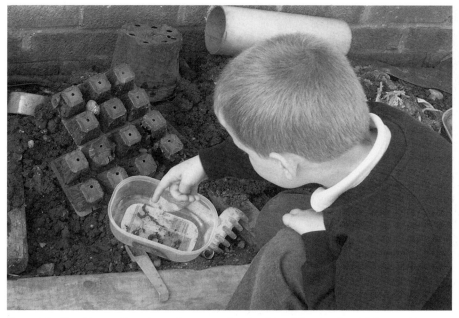

Figure 8.5 Teaching and learning styles appropriate for the child and to the activity.

- Are appropriate resources provided with which the child might experiment?
- Is there space to work?
- Is there time to listen and encourage?
- Are there opportunities for the child to make decisions and help him or her become an independent learner?
- Are the teaching and learning styles appropriate for the child/children and to the activity (see Figs 8.4 and 8.5)?
- Will each child be involved, motivated and interested by the activity?

Readers can helpfully revisit Chapter 6, in which learning is discussed at some depth (particularly Piaget, Vygotsky and Bruner), and Chapter 7, which examines additional aspects of early years teaching and learning. It must also be noted that children learn from the offered curriculum, which is wider than the legally prescribed curriculum, encompassing all of a child's school experiences – intellectual, creative, physical, emotional, social and spiritual – and all decisions made by associated adults. The offered curriculum in turn may be different from the received curriculum – that is, what the children actually learn from the provision (Whitebread, 2003) and including the hidden curriculum which is all that is learned by the children that was not planned or part of the designated curriculum.

The classroom environment

This is an important aspect of the offered curriculum, and must be devised to promote and support children's all-round development and learning. Children learn from their environment by taking an active and independent role which will give them the confidence to assume and seek further knowledge. Figure 8.6 illustrates the prominence of choice within and between activities in order to foster a child's independence.

Of course the teaching team must make certain that children participate in a wide range of planned activities to ensure their development and learning are holistic and the full statutory curriculum is covered – sound reasons for organizing activities that are stimulating and enticing!

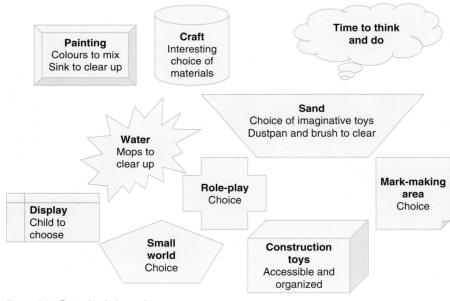

Figure 8.6   Fostering independence.

The outdoor environment

Whatever can be learnt indoors can also be learnt outdoors (Drake, 2001); the curriculum can be enriched and children's holistic learning enhanced by a carefully planned outdoor environment. In addition, traditional playground games, hop-scotch,

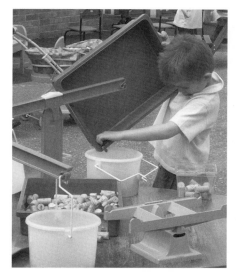

sand/water trays, climbing frames, role-play areas, water-mark making on a hot sunny day, environmental art, wheeled bikes and toys can contribute to an exciting outdoor extension to the curriculum and classroom environment – given appropriate organization and resourcing. The outdoors also allows children 'to learn by working on a larger, more active scale than is (often) possible indoors' (QCA/DfEE, 2000, p. 15) (Fig. 8.7).

Assessment to inform individual journeys

Individual 'journeys' are in progress; the child is at school; he or she steps on the stones placed and adjusted by the adults; gains a firm footing and moves on.

Figure 8.7   Whatever can be learnt indoors can be learnt outdoors.

Assessment, as demonstrated in the rolling planning process (see Fig. 8.3), is integral to a successful 'journey'. This assessment may be *formative*, to inform the next step, *diagnostic* to determine specialist requirements, or *summative* to take stock of children's attainment at the end of their reception year as well as inform planning for them in Year 1. Limited or speedy progress may indicate the need for specialist provision. This may take the form of Special Educational Needs (SEN) or membership of 'gifted and talented' groups. Debates about 'respectful' assessment, appropriate timing and accountability rage; Drummond (2003) and Nutbrown (1999) present comprehensive discussions.

The Foundation Stage Profile (see website) was introduced in England in 2002 as a means of assessing and summing up children's progress towards the early learning goals (or beyond) at the end of their foundation stage; it also identifies their learning needs in readiness for them commencing KS1. The profile, based on children's achievement in their day-to-day activities, is completed throughout their first (reception) year in school. A statutory requirement is for data from the profiles to be sent to the LEA to inform national trends. Although there are, at the time of writing, no plans to publish performance tables, schools can monitor their own statistics against national figures.

While potentially useful to parents and KS1 teachers, these profiles are not without their critics; for example, Goveas (2004) reports their rejection at the National Union of Teachers' Conference in 2004, and Ofsted (2004) notes that teachers have not found them especially helpful in supporting children's entry into KS1. The lack of detail and focus, the impersonal tick boxes, unclear questions and workload implications for teachers are all cited.

Transition to Key Stage One

It is expected that most children will complete the stepping stones and achieve the early learning goals by the end of the reception year; some will have gone beyond, others may still have some way to travel. Children moving from reception to Year 1 might experience a change in environment and ethos – perhaps even an 'abrupt transition' (Ofsted, 2004, p. 2). The meticulously planned play approach of many reception classes may be entirely or largely replaced by the all sit and 'work' approach of a teacher who finds himself/herself alone with up to 30 children. There may be the necessity for children to learn as a whole class for inappropriate periods of time. In practice, and as an ideal, the experienced professional in the enlightened and sufficiently resourced school maintains a smooth transition over whatever time is needed to prepare children for the less play-oriented approach of subsequent primary school years.

THE NATIONAL CURRICULUM

The National Curriculum for England for education in maintained (not independent) schools provides a statutory framework outlining what must be taught and specifying attainment targets for children's learning at each of the four key stages (noted earlier in this chapter); it also identifies how and when children's achievement will be assessed and reported. The National Curriculum has four main purposes:

1. To establish an entitlement for every pupil (irrespective of social background, culture, race, gender, differences in ability and disabilities).
2. To establish standards.
3. To promote continuity and coherence.
4. To promote public understanding.

Source: DfEE/QCA, 1999, p. 13 and QCA website, 'Why have a National Curriculum?'.

Members of the school community (including governors, teachers, parents, children and representatives from relevant local organizations) contribute to decisions about the actual curriculum offered to each child within the statutory requirements. This resulting school curriculum (which is broader than the National Curriculum) must:

■ ensure that pupils become confident, creative and independent learners with a broad knowledge base, a good range of skills (particularly literacy, numeracy, ICT and physical) and able to solve problems, understand and integrate into our diverse society and be effective citizens of the future;

Table 8.3   Key Stage One subjects of the National Curriculum

Status	Subjects
Core subjects	English, Mathematics, Science
Non-core foundation subjects	Design and technology (DT), Information and communication technology (ICT), history, geography, art and design, music, physical education (PE)
Additional statutory area	Religious education (RE)
Non-statutory area	Personal, social and health education (PSHE)
General teaching requirements	Inclusion, Use of language and ICT across the curriculum; Health & safety

Source: Information taken from DfEE/QCA 1999.

■ encourage intercultural understanding, development of values, integrity, self-esteem and emotional well-being, equality of opportunity, respect for the environment, themselves and others and responding actively to opportunities and challenges.

(Adapted from QCA website, *About the school curriculum.*)

Primary schools essentially cover Key Stage One (5–7 years) and Key Stage Two (7–11 years). Details of Key Stage One (KS1) of the National Curriculum are provided in Table 8.3.

Programmes of Study specify what should be taught within each subject at each key stage, while the *attainment targets* set out the knowledge, skills and understanding pupils must achieve in each subject by the end of each key stage. Four general teaching requirements are required to permeate all subjects: inclusion, language, ICT, health and safety and pupils' all-round development and key skills are to be promoted right across the curriculum.

The English National Curriculum has been criticized for being too prescriptive and assessment-driven, for the arbitrariness of the attainment targets, and for its potential detriment to pupils' motivation (e.g. Rodd, 2002), although Boutwell (2001) felt it sufficiently worthy to advocate its adoption in the USA.

Additionally, an accumulation of inspection, research and test evidence pointing to a 'need to improve standards of literacy and numeracy' (DfEE/QCA, 1999, p. 2) resulted in the introduction in England of the National Literacy Strategy in 1998 (DfEE, 1998) and the Numeracy Strategy in 1999 (DfEE, 1999) to raise standards and complement the National Curriculum. Each strategy framework contains a set of yearly teaching programmes with key objectives that are central to pupils' achievements (www.dfes.gov.uk). Structured daily lessons have been implemented in schools (see Tables 8.4 and 8.5).

Table 8.4 The structure of the National Literacy Strategy (Key Stage One)

Whole class	Whole class	Group and independent work	Whole class
15 min approx.	15 min approx.	20 min approx.	10 min approx.
Shared text work A balance of reading and writing	Focused word work	Independent reading, writing or word work Teacher working with at least one group	Reviewing, reflecting, consolidating teaching points, and presenting work covered in the lesson

Source: Information taken from DfEE 1999.

Table 8.5 The structure of the National Numeracy Strategy (Key Stage One)

Whole class	Whole class, group, and independent work	Whole class
5–10 min approx.	30–40 min approx.	10–15 min approx.
Oral work and mental calculation	Main teaching activity Input and pupil activities	Plenary to round off the lesson

Source: Information taken from DfEE 2000.

Subsequently, a set of objectives for speaking and listening have been developed for Years 1 to 6 in response to a perceived need by teachers (DfES, 2004b).

The national curricula for Northern Ireland, Wales (statutory) and Scotland (non-statutory) and their literacy and numeracy initiatives can be found on the CCEA, ACCAC and LTS websites.

Planning within the National Curriculum

A thorough and considered planning process is equally crucial at KS1 of the National Curriculum. Teacher assessment continues throughout Years 1 and 2 with observation and record keeping, supported by examples of children's work, providing evidence of their progress and informing the planning process. Targets (derived from the scheme of work) are often shared with children so that they know what is expected and feel involved and empowered. This can encourage development of responsibility, reflection and evaluation on their part. The whole assessment process, which helps to pinpoint children's progress and developing levels of knowledge, understanding and competence, together with attention to the demands of the National Curriculum (the programmes of study, attainment targets and general teaching requirements), knowing children and their families and professional expertise, all enable planning for, and provision of, an appropriate curriculum for groups of children and individuals (see Fig. 8.8).

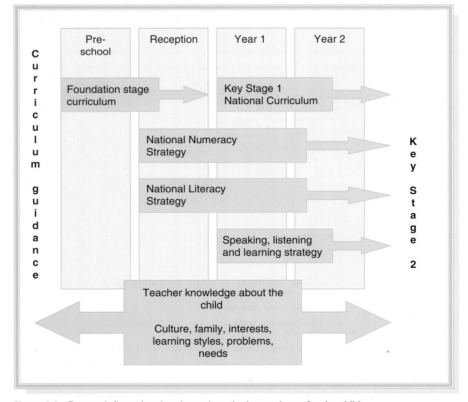

Figure 8.8   Factors influencing the planned curriculum pathway for the child.

STANDARD ATTAINMENT TASKS (SATs)

At the end of KS1 in England, Standard Attainment Tasks (SATs) appear for the purpose of summatively assessing children's attainment. This has been via a combination of statutory tests and tasks in English and Mathematics. There were, however, considerable criticisms of this early testing as in some instances it led to inappropriate formal teaching and 'drilling' to improve test results; it also decreased children's enthusiasm for learning. In 2003, Charles Clarke, the Education Secretary, announced a change to a more flexible approach giving greater emphasis to teacher assessment at KS1 (DfES, 2003). This was trialled in 2004 and will probably be implemented in 2005. Northern Ireland and Wales use teacher assessment at this early stage, but Scotland uses nationally set assessments to confirm teacher evaluations.

FUTURE DEVELOPMENTS

The guidance for the education of young children is continually developing as a result of reflection by professionals, politicians and parents and the advent of new technology – the rolling planning process or reflective practice on a grander scale.

For example, some schools have introduced changes to the structure of the school day, lengthening mornings and reducing afternoons. The introduction of four terms within the school year and extended schools (open from 8:00 am until 6:00 pm and weekends, offering for example a range of clubs, services, study support and family learning) are being piloted. Also, new problems and issues emerge; for example, there has been a great deal in the media about children not being sufficiently fit and healthy, with blame being attributed to an unhealthy diet and sitting too much in front of TVs or computer screens. Such issues lead to new initiatives, for example a stronger emphasis on physical activity in curricula. Carson (2004) provides a brief account of intentions in this subject area.

Importantly, a greater recognition of the need for local authorities, relevant agencies, organizations and practitioners to collaborate (to provide an integrated service for young children and families) is much emphasized in the Children Act 2004. The primary school may even become the base for a multi-professional workforce (health, education and social care) that can better ensure holistic and optimum provision to promote young children's all-round development and well-being and support their families, thus giving our children the best possible start in life.

Conclusion

This chapter has introduced some of the main historical legal and socio-cultural factors that form the landscape against which a child's early years 'journey' is set. It is a very significant and certainly not simple journey that each child makes during their first years of schooling. National initiatives, planned in response to observations of societal trends, create transitions. Professionals strive to locate appropriate routes for each child through the network of possibilities. The fraternity of the child, parents, school and community is paramount for the journey to be expedient. Children have the right to follow the best pathways in today's landscape to ensure a positive and enjoyable experience for them, to optimize their development, opportunities and talents and to enable them to be of benefit to society in general.

'They said: "You're Laurie Lee, ain't you? Well you just sit there for the present." I sat there all day but I never got it. I ain't going back there again! But after a week I felt like a veteran ...'

(Lee, 1959, p. 44)

Student task

Find out about the following early childhood pioneers: Margaret McMillan, Friedrich Froebel, Maria Montessori, Robert Owen, Susan Isaacs and Johann Heinrich Pestalozzi.
   Identify similarities and differences:

■ in their backgrounds;
■ in their theories of education (e.g. role of play; involvement of parents);
■ in the application of their theories to early years settings;
■ with early childhood education today.

Share your findings with a fellow student/peer.

REFERENCES AND *FURTHER READING

Abbott, L and Pugh, G (eds) (1998): *Training To Work in the Early Years.* Buckingham: Open University Press.

Adams, S, Alexander, E, Drummond, MJ and Moyles, J (2004): *Inside the Foundation Stage: Recreating the Reception Year.* London: Association of Teachers and Lecturers.

Anning, A, Cullen, J and Fleer, M (eds) (2004): *Early Childhood Education: Society and Culture.* London: Sage Publications.*

Boutwell, JS (2001) A case of unconstitutional immigration: the importation of England's national curriculum to the United States. *Vanderbilt Journal of Transitional Law,* **34**(2), 133–400.

Bredekamp, S and Copple, S (eds) (1997): *Developmentally Appropriate Practice in Early Childhood Programs* (revised edition). Washington DC: National Association for the Education of Young Children.

Bruce, T (1997): *Early Childhood Education,* 2nd edn. London: Hodder and Stoughton.

Bruce, T (2004): *Developing Learning in Early Childhood.* London: Paul Chapman Publishing.*

Carson, G (2004): Inspiration to boost perspiration. *Children Now*, 23–29 June, p. 11.

Curtis, A and O'Hagan, M (2003): *Care and Education in Early Childhood.* London: Routledge-Falmer.

David, T (ed.) (1999): *Teaching Young Children.* London: Paul Chapman.

Department for Education and Employment (1998): *The National Literacy Strategy Framework for Teaching.* London: DfEE.

Department for Education and Employment (1999): *The National Numeracy Strategy.* London: DfEE.

Department for Education and Employment (2000a): *Guidance on the Organisation of the Daily Mathematics Lesson in Reception Classes.* London: DfEE.*

Department for Education and Employment (2000b): *Guidance on the Organisation of the National Literacy Strategy in Reception Classes.* London: DfEE.*

Department for Education and Employment/Qualifications and Curriculum Authority (1999) *The National Curriculum.* London: DfEE/QCA.**

Department for Education and Skills (2003): *Excellence and Enjoyment: a Strategy for Primary Schools.* London: DfES.

Department for Education and Skills (2004a): *A Guide to the Law for School Governors*, 2nd edn. London: DfES.

Department for Education and Skills (2004b): *Speaking, Listening, Learning: Working with Children in Key Stages 1 and 2.* London: DfES.*

Drake, J (2001): *Planning Children's Play and Learning in the Foundation Stage.* London: David Fulton Publishers.*

Drummond, MJ (2003): *Assessing Children's Learning,* 2nd edn. London: David Fulton Publishers.*

Drury, R, Miller, L and Campbell, R (eds) (2000): *Looking at Early Years Education and Care.* London: David Fulton Publishers.

Fearn, A (1999): Let formal lessons start at three says Ofsted. *The Times*, 23 June, p. 12.

Fisher, J (2002): *Starting from the Child,* 2nd edn. Buckingham: Open University Press.*

Goveas, A (2004): School transition. *Children Now*, 2–8 June, p. 17.

Hayes, D (1999): *Foundations of Primary Teaching,* 2nd edn. London: David Fulton Publishers.

Kelly, V (1994): A high quality curriculum for the early years. *Early Years*, **15**(1), 6–12.

Lee, L (1959): *Cider With Rosie.* London: Penguin.

Liebscher, J (1992): *A Child's Work.* Cambridge: Lutterworth Press.

MacNaughton, G (2000): *Rethinking Gender in Early Childhood Education.* London: Paul Chapman Publishing.*

Moyles, JR (1992): *Organizing for Learning in the Primary Classroom.* Buckingham: Open University Press.

Nutbrown, C (1999): *Threads of Thinking,* 2nd edn. London: Paul Chapman Publishing.

Office for Standards in Education (2002): *The Curriculum in Successful Primary Schools.* London: Office for Standards in Education.*

Office for Standards in Education (2004): *Transition from the Reception Year to Year 1: An evaluation by HMI.* At www.ofsted.gov.uk under 2004 Publications.

Pugh, G (ed.) (1996): *Contemporary Issues in the Early Years,* 2nd edn. London: Paul Chapman.

Qualifications and Curriculum Authority/Department for Education and Employment (2000): *Curriculum Guidance for the Foundation Stage.* London: QCA.*

Qualifications and Curriculum Authority/Department for Education and Employment (1999): *Early Learning Goals.* London: QCA.

Qualifications and Curriculum Authority/Department for Education and Science (2001): *Planning for Learning in the Foundation Stage.* London: QCA.*

Rodd, J (2002): A perspective from England. *Childhood Education*, **78**(6), 334.

SCAA/Department for Education and Employment (1996): *Desirable Outcomes for Children's Learning.* SCAA/DfEE.

Smidt, S (2002): *A Guide to Early Years Practice,* 2nd edn. London: Routledge-Falmer.

Whitebread, D (ed.) (2003): *Teaching and Learning in the Early Years,* 2nd edn. London: Routledge-Falmer.*

Woodhead, M (1996): *In Search of the Rainbow.* Netherlands: Bernard van Leer Foundation.*

WEBSITES

Children Act 2004 – www.legislation.hmso.gov.uk/acts/acts2004/20040031.htm
Foundation Stage Profile – www.qca.org.uk/ages3-14/foundation/163.html
National Curriculum – www.nc.uk.net
National Association for Special Educational Needs – www.nasen.org.uk
Department for Education and Skills – www.dfes.gov.uk
Department for Education, Northern Ireland – www.deni.gov.uk
Scottish Executive, Education Department – www.seed.gov.uk
National Assembly, Learning Wales – www.learningwales.gov.uk
Qualifications and Curriculum Authority – www.qca.org.u
Council for Curriculum, Examinations and Assessment Northern Ireland – www.ccea.org.uk
Scottish Qualifications Authority – www.sqa.org.uk
Qualifications, Curriculum and Assessment Authority for Wales – www.accac.org.uk
Office for Standards in Education – www.ofsted.gov.uk
Northern Ireland Education and Training Inspectorate – www.deni.gov.uk/inspection_services.htm
Her Majesty's Inspectorate of Education in Scotland – www.hmie.gov.uk
Her Majesty's Inspectorate for Education and Training in Wales – www.estyn.gov.uk

THE CHILD IN SOCIETY

Val Thurtle

This chapter aims to:

- introduce the four major sociological perspectives;
- examine childhood as a social construct;
- investigate the child within society and within the family.

INTRODUCTION

Students of early childhood very often have a wealth of experience and ideas. While these can be wisely used to enrich practice, some individuals may take their own background as the norm against which others are compared. Using sociological perspectives is one way to counteract such a tendency, encourage academic questioning of beliefs and values that seem common sense or natural, and give consideration to the social influences acting upon children, so viewing them within the context of their social setting. Psychologists have traditionally focussed upon the individual child while the sociological concept of the child is rooted in an exploration of the wider social world.

WHAT IS A SOCIOLOGICAL PERSPECTIVE?

Many sociology texts start with the question 'What is sociology?'. For Giddens (2001), 'sociology is the study of human social life, groups and societies' (p. 2). It used to be said that sociology was the 'science of society', but this gives the impression of a discipline that uses the positivistic methods of the natural sciences. Sociology goes further – in a sense it is a way of thinking. Abercrombie *et al.* (2000), following Runciman, claim it is four distinct activities: reporting; explanation; description; and evaluation. In doing this it can be seen as a process from which there may not be fixed or agreed outcomes.

Sociology is deemed a critical activity, asking questions about the state of society and about the forces that support institutions and preserve social order. In other words, sociology is a discipline that asks awkward questions in a systematic manner. Such an approach will develop the 'sociological imagination' (Mills, 1971), cultivating the ability to think beyond the mundane and familiar, and take new viewpoints from which to examine and, hopefully, understand people's everyday lives.

SOCIOLOGICAL PERSPECTIVES

Any contact with sociological texts will soon throw up the terms *functionalism*, *Marxism*, *feminism* and *social interactionism*. Theorists from different backgrounds will take different views of the social world, so one cannot say that there is 'a' sociological perspective; rather there exist a variety of different outlooks.

Describing these stances at a purely introductory level, structural functionalists would see society as being composed of various systems that work together. Each part of the social system performs a certain function that contributes to the well-being and continuity of society. Beliefs and values are shared, leading to harmonious co-operation. This perspective dates back to Emile Durkheim, and was expounded by sociologists such as Parsons and Merton. The approach was much used in the 1950s and 1960s, particularly with regard to the family, but it has less of a following in the early twenty-first century. Such a view may not seem appropriate today, but is frequently held up as an ideal by politicians discussing the family or education system.

Marxists find their origins in the work of Karl Marx and Friedrich Engels, but these have been reinterpreted and refined. There are, therefore, many kinds of Marxists. They see the world in terms of conflict, such conflict being found particularly between those who control the means of production and those who do not. This control influences all sections of a given society – the education system, the media and the health services. While functionalists would see conflict as dysfunctional, the Marxist views conflict as having positive outcomes and indeed as being 'normal'.

Feminists, too, can be seen as viewing the world in terms of conflict, discord between women and men, or discord between women and patriarchal structures. Feminist writing is particularly important to those concerned with the care, health and education of children, as these areas have often been ignored by mainstream sociology and taken up by feminist researchers.

These three views have largely been concerned with the system or infrastructure. Interactionists have been far more interested in the small-scale or micro level, investigating the meanings that actors give to any social situation. Looking at the work of symbolic interactionists and ethnomethodologists, the reader may find it difficult to decide where sociology ends and psychology begins, demonstrating that traditional subject divides may not always be appropriate when dealing with something as complex as childhood – hence the evolution of Early Childhood Studies which takes an holistic perspective, recognizing that the clear focus of concern should be upon the child and not the subject discipline!

Such an overview is incredibly condensed, but it makes the point that a variety of viewpoints exist within sociology. The critical reader, therefore, needs to ask where any writer is coming from, and through which world view they are interpreting their findings. Additionally, given that all of us have our own past experiences and dearly held beliefs, the issue is raised whether sociology or indeed any study can be truly value free.

We must also be aware that what happens in the wider society can impinge upon the child. For example, a particular political party may come to power and follow a policy which leads to the child's parents becoming redundant, which in turn changes the economic status of the family, consequently impacting on the child. The reporting in the media of the murder of a child and the conviction of another may well influence carers' attitudes and styles of discipline.

This chapter further develops concepts raised earlier. It reflects on how we define a child, looking at how the child has been perceived over a historical period, and considering the family and the place of the child within it. This can only be an introduction to the subject, and further studies are required to examine how children are integrated into wider society and to delve deeper into the interrelating issues of class, ethnicity, gender and poverty.

WHAT IS A CHILD?

We could take a simple definition based on age to define a child, as indeed the United Nations Convention on the Rights of the Child does. This internationally agreed definition sees childhood as the period from birth to 18 years of age, yet worldwide, throughout the United Kingdom and even in our own localities, there are differences in how children and young people are viewed and treated and in what is expected of them. Concern with these perspectives underpins social constructivism, which draws attention to the influence of culture, history and social processes on the way people make sense of the world (Stainton Rogers, 2003). Sociologists have used discourse analysis, taking a close examination of how a particular cluster of ideas is applied to a particular construct or concept. This could be relevant to 'community', 'parenthood' or in our case, the child or childhood. With our socially constructed view of childhood, taken from our own attitudes, expectations and understandings there is no benchmark or underpinning truth that tells what children are (Stainton Rogers, 2001). How then should we consider a child or childhood? A child could be defined in terms of physical growth or developmental maturity, but our own parents may never see us as mature, and always regard us as a child in need of emotional and practical support. Financial independence may mark the end of childhood; for some that will be at 16 years of age, while others will be well into their twenties or beyond. Clearly there is no obvious cut-off point. Alternatively, we could define the end of childhood in terms of activities that our particular social world permits us to engage in – for example, to drive a car, vote, buy alcohol, or get married. Any discussion will soon identify national and social differences in definitions of the end of childhood in the twenty-first century.

Childhood, then, is not an objective entity. Various social groups at different times have defined children in a myriad of ways. A brainstorm of current views in Western society might come up with some of the following.

Children are innocent and in need of care and protection, whilst others see them as 'devils' needing controls and strict discipline. The James Bulger case, which has become part of the United Kingdom collective memory, represented these two views, often in the same news report. In February 1993, a 2-year-old boy, James Bulger, was taken from a shopping centre and murdered on a railway siding in north Liverpool by two 10-year-old boys. The murdered child was presented as the former, while the perpetrators, only a few years older than him, were seen as the latter. Goldson (2001) argues that we hold these two concepts of childhood in tandem. Children are seen as innocent and vulnerable, but those who are thought to have moved beyond the limits of what is deemed acceptable are classified as 'threats', 'problems' and different. For others, children are regarded as investments in the future, necessitating the sacrifice of parents, a reduction in holidays to pay private school fees or a regular contribution of parents' weekly spending money throughout the year into the Christmas fund for children's presents. The state is expected to contribute to their health, welfare and education so that they grow up to be effective members of the work force of the future. Children might be seen as 'products' requiring careful monitoring during their production. 'Standard Assessment Tasks and Attainment Targets' in the National Curriculum and monitoring by health visitor and school nurse teams could be seen in this light. A look at the media might provide the picture of the child as a designer accessory, something the well-turned-out woman (and man) must acquire.

A review of television advertisements in the months leading up to Christmas demonstrates that children represent a potential market in their own right. They are the ones who will buy or demand the current plastic craze or drag their parents to the 'in' fast-food outlets after the Christmas shopping. For most of the time, Western society perceives children as being different, and worthy of their childhood. Certainly a view of children presented by books such as this is that they are of sufficient interest to merit dedicated in-depth study and have whole curricula devised around them.

As discussed in the Introduction of this book, these views of childhood are not necessarily those of other cultures and different historical times. For example, in a developing country, children as young as 5 years of age might have defined tasks within and outside the family contributing to its economic stability (see Chapter 15 for further discussion). Our twenty-first century view of childhood, therefore, is a relatively new socially constructed phenomenon.

SOCIOLOGICAL PERSPECTIVES ON THE CHILD

How would the different sociological perspectives view the child? Functionalists would see children as being socialized into future roles, the family being the primary agent, with institutions such as the school and peer group being involved in secondary socialization. For functionalists, the firm guidance of vulnerable or difficult children is necessary if society is to survive and prosper.

Marxists would also be concerned with preparation for future life, but would see it as rather more controlled, with those in power ensuring that the majority were equipped for their lives as powerless workers. Hartley (1993) argues that this process is evident in the structure and organization of the nursery school, where children learn to fit into a regimented timetable – preparation for the factory of the future? According to this mode of thinking children are said to be inculcated with the values of the private property system, and obedience to authority is acquired, as are prejudices, including those of a racial and sexual nature. Indeed it is such value systems and practices which are reputed to keep the oppressed majority divided and therefore not a threat to the ruling classes.

Feminists have been much concerned with the gender roles that children learn or acquire at an early stage. Grabrucker's (1988) reflective diary of her parenting of her young daughter gives a very readable insight into this.

Interactionists would be concerned with the relationships and activities between children. While they would be unlikely to attach this label to themselves, preferring to be seen as anthropologists, *Children's Games in Street and Playground* (Opie and Opie, 1969) does just this.

While different sociological perspectives can be identified, the study of childhood traditionally was largely left to the psychologists, psychiatrists and educationists, influenced by the 1960s work of Piaget. Sociologists became interested in childhood in the 1970s and 1980s, moving from concern with the development of the individual to a focus on children as a social group, albeit one of low status and power. The concept of childhood was seen as socially created, influenced by gender, race, status and other factors and evolving in different ways. They tended not to see children as deficient in adult capabilities but having behaviour, thinking and culture that could be judged and valued in its own right. This social group was not just being moulded by the adults who were bringing them up; rather, they were active participants in their own socialization (Hill and Tisdall, 1997).

It is not a case of choosing a psychological approach (hinging on development) *or* a sociological approach (evaluating groups and social influences), as the interaction of both approaches and different ways of thinking can give a broader and richer view of the diversity of children and childhood.

CHILDREN IN HISTORY

The medieval period and the Enlightenment

Thinking about children in history, we are dependent on the material left behind, and we need to consider its reliability. If children were not very significant in medieval and earlier times, were they worth writing about, and was there a written record? If they were not important to those who had the skills and means to write, does this imply they were unimportant to others, particularly close family? Also our information may be distorted by Hollywood movies and television period dramas perhaps giving the reconstructed childhood of the past a rosy glow or inaccurate twist.

Aries (1962), who has been questioned on his historical accuracy and interpretation of material using contemporary ideas, argues that there was no concept of childhood prior to the medieval period. Children were viewed as property, but then so were wives. Child mortality in the eighteenth century was high, with two out of three children dying before their fifth birthday. Infanticide has probably been practised in all societies (Trainor, 1988), despite being prohibited as early as Roman times (Shahar, 1990). The level of care was low, with accounts of poor hygiene and wet-nursing by dubious mother substitutes. Children lived in the adult world, they were dressed in the same clothing as adults from an early age, shared the same entertainment despite its bawdy nature, and were sometimes apprenticed away from home by the age of 7 years. In contrast to Aries' view, Shahar (1990) argues that childhood did exist in the central and late medieval periods. Children were not idealized as later, but there were traditional child-care practices, as well as emotional and material investment in children. The medical and educational theories might be very different from those of today, but they did exist.

It is often argued that there was little emotional involvement until survival was assured. Montaigne's famous sixteenth-century remark would bear this out: 'I have lost two or three children, not without regret but without great sorrow'. However, Pollack (1983) shows that the loss of young children left some parents distraught with grief. The poverty of the fifteenth and sixteenth centuries meant that many parents could not afford to prolong childhood, sending older children to work while infants were coddled. Parents who lived and worked in servility were used to harsh treatment themselves, and meted this out to their children. Comparison of the methods of child management used by these parents with those of the twenty-first century parent does not mean that their affection and concern for their offspring were any less.

The sixteenth to the eighteenth centuries were times of great change – economic, religious and political. The ideas of the Enlightenment portrayed children as being different from adults and needing care and protection. Rousseau viewed children as individuals to be valued; they were deemed to be working through various stages of development but were essentially romantic innocents. Locke saw them as empty slates (*tabula rasa*, Latin for blank slate) ready for learning and education. In the same period, those of a puritan or Calvinistic persuasion – perhaps influenced by a fear of revolution and certainly in line with their theological stance of original sin – saw children as inherently sinful and therefore in need of harsh discipline. These ideas were the start of significant trends in educational thinking.

Aries (1962) demonstrates the increasing importance of children in art, reflecting their growing importance in society. Starting with funereal art, he shows how children were initially portrayed as small adult effigies, but over a period of time they were depicted within the family, and later alone in individual portraits. To commission an expensive portrait of a child indicated that the child had been noticed and valued. Of course only the most affluent would have used resources in this fashion, and the views of the rather less well-off might have been quite different.

The coming of the Industrial Revolution meant that some children found work in the factories and mines, contributing to our picture of the 'dark satanic mills', but children had always been involved in families' work or on their land. Describing New Zealand colonial life in the mid-nineteenth century, Graham (1993) states that children's 'labour was essential to the functioning and economic viability of the family enterprise' (p. 67). The same must have been true of farms and smallholdings throughout the Western world and beyond. There might be gender differences in the work that was expected of girls and boys, but both were expected to work.

The nineteenth century

The nineteenth century saw controls on child labour through the Mines Act of 1842 and the Factory Acts of 1844, 1850 and 1853. Humphries *et al.* (1988) point out that, until the 1920s, children in Britain commenced their working lives while still as young as 12 years.

Until well into the nineteenth century there was no expectation that any family member would have a separate identity. Macdonald (1990) draws attention to the fact that, in pioneering New Zealand, it was common for the names of a deceased child to be used for a subsequent child (family historians can also testify to this happening in the UK). Only later was it seen as morbid, and the practice ceased.

Throughout the nineteenth century children were increasingly idealized and seen in a rather sentimental light. Class differences were evident, with the children of the affluent being pampered and educated, while those of the poor might well be working on the land, in factories or as chimney-sweeps. Whilst class differences were evident, child mortality was much reduced ensuring that each child born had a greater chance of reaching adulthood.

Change was under way as a result of stratified diffusion, by which the ideas of the upper classes today became those of the working classes tomorrow. One can speculate about the part played by the Royal Family in this process. Queen Victoria's large and apparently happy family may, for example, have increased the prestige of family life and contributed to the status of the child.

Industrialization went hand in hand with the smaller nuclear family, facilitating movement to the industrial centres. Within the smaller family, the focus was increasingly on the child, who became a source of entertainment as well as concern.

Interest in the welfare and control of the child was evident in wider society. Compulsory elementary education was introduced in Britain in 1870, and hospitals for children were opened around the same time. Schools, orphanages and reformatories were all devised as 'character factories' turning out obedient and dutiful citizens (Humphries *et al.*, 1988). It has been argued that there was little altruism involved in compulsory education, but rather that it was a way of making the child more civilized and self-disciplined to become suitable factory fodder (Rose, 1991). At the end of the nineteenth century this was done by an authoritarian regime, which wielded power in inward-looking institutions. The regimes were not dissimilar, whether they were orphanages for the poor and abandoned, reformatories for the apparently criminal, or preparatory schools for the children of the rich. Hopkins' (1994) view of universal education is far more optimistic, seeing childhood transformed as it became centred upon schools, which led to improvements in health, nutrition and leisure opportunities.

Ideas of the child as 'father of the man' became widespread in the early twentieth century through the works of Freud and others. At the same time it became obvious that children had a culture of their own, with their own toys and games, manufactured for the rich and devised at home for the poor.

Using such material and much else, Hill and Tisdall (1997) present different constructions of childhood suggesting, for example, that childhood could be labelled romantic or sinful, or children seen as the factory child, the school child, the psycho-medical child.

To the present day

Ideas that had their origins in the nineteenth century came to fruition at the beginning of the twentieth century. Families shrank in size, with the small number of children being highly valued and the time and resources of the family becoming increasingly child-centred.

The control and surveillance of children affected just about every child, but in a less repressive way. Services for children were started and developed. The Notification of Births Act in 1907 led to health visiting services (started in 1862) being offered to all mothers and their babies. The advent of the School Health Service may have been triggered by the poor health of army recruits and a fear that the empire could not be adequately defended, but it led to health surveillance and treatment being far more freely available to children, and the introduction of school meals made a real difference to the nutritional status of many children.

With the increased influence of psychologists and physicians, all child-orientated services became psycho-medical in nature. Children were increasingly under the clinical gaze of experts. Functionalists might argue that such an approach, and the ensuing interventions, were for the good of the child and his or her wider community, while Marxists would argue that apparent concern, whether expressed in terms of health or education, was merely a means of giving capitalism a human face.

The twentieth century had seen no shortage of experts ready to advise parents on children's upbringing and education. The development of the mass media meant that their influence has been far-reaching and such experts have had considerable effect on the confidence of many parents in their child-rearing abilities. For example, the work of Dr Truby King reached beyond New Zealand where he had advocated breastfeeding by a strictly structured and disciplined regime. In 1917, his first Mothercraft Society was set up in Earls Court, London and thousands of infants were reared with the help of his book, *Mothercraft*, raising child-rearing to the status of 'scientific motherhood'.

Criticism of the Truby King method followed in the 1950s, with fears that such a rigid approach would harm the child. Liberal theories gained ascendance, with children being encouraged to be creative and to explore their environment. King was replaced by Benjamin Spock's *Common Sense Book of Baby and Child Care* in 1946. This fitted well with the work of the Swiss psychologist Jean Piaget, who argued that children were moving through a variety of stages which could be facilitated by appropriate stimulation from parents and carers. The twenty-first century sees other authorities, including doctors, psychologists and media stars such as Bob Geldof, writing about fathers, and J.K. Rowling, writing about lone parents (a visit to the child-care section of any high-street bookshop will identify the current guru).

What then can we say about the child in history? Clearly there have been a variety of approaches, and our twenty-first-century views are undoubtedly derived from them. Both in history and at the present time there is not one view of childhood, but a variety influenced by class, gender, ethnicity, affluence and the very thinking of the time (see also the Introduction and Chapter 13).

THE CHILD IN THE FAMILY

Most people have lived in a family at some point in their lives, and undoubtedly there are many views of the family. There is the nuclear family with mum, dad and two, possibly three, children often depicted beaming at each other from the cereal packet (Leach, 1986). An Irish student drew me the most detailed family tree, with third, fourth and fifth cousins carefully named. Did she, I asked, consider them all to be 'family' to the extent that she would entertain them if they visited her in England? Of course she did, she replied, as she looked at me pityingly, who only sends a Christmas card to my rarely-seen first cousins. If folks live away from their aunts and uncles, are they any less family? Does family depend on residence? Is it still a family if there is only one parent? Is a lesbian couple rearing a child a family? Do families have to be based on blood ties, or is a kibbutz an extended family of sorts? Once we start, the variety of permutations is immense. While we consider the variety in family structure, we need to think about the impact that such variations might have on children.

Defining the family

A 'common-sense' starting point for discussions of the family is that of the functionalists, much used in theoretical discussions of the family throughout the 1950s and 1960s. Murdock, writing in 1949 (cited in Haralambos and Holborn, 2000), defined the family as:

> '… *a social group characterised by common residence, economic co-operation and reproduction. It includes adults of both sexes, at least two of which maintain a socially approved sexual relationship and one or more children, own or adopted of the sexually cohabiting adults*'.

Reading this today we may have doubts about the importance of the common residence, and difficulties in defining a socially approved sexual relationship. Some of the 'families' mentioned in the last section do not fit Murdock's description. For him, the family is universal, with different family forms being variations on the basic family structure.

Clearly functionalist in nature, this definition identifies the functions of the family. A favourite debate of the 1970s centred around the question 'Is the family losing its functions?' The family (in whatever form) is still much concerned with sexual activity and reproduction. While it may no longer be a unit of economic production, it is a significant unit of consumption – look at any advertising on the television to see who is being encouraged to purchase a three-piece suite, family car or particular sorts of food. For many, its religious functions are not significant but it provides the majority of health care. In some societies it marks out an individual's niche in society and gives a place where people can play, experiment or even regress. Parsons (1956) collects some of these ideas together, discussing the functions of the family in terms of the primary socialization of children and the stabilization of adult personalities.

Social welfare systems may be the safety net for those who fall on hard times, but kin still provide material help for each other (Finch, 1989), whether in the form of child care, financial loans or gifts, though the felt need to do so varies enormously from family to family. The British Social Attitude Study of 1995 (McGlone *et al.*, 1998) asked people who they would go to for help with household and gardening jobs, support during illness and borrowing money. Husband, wife or partner was the first choice, with other relatives coming next. Those with a child under 16 who had been given a loan or gift of money had received it from a parent or in-law. McGlone *et al.* (1998) concluded that family remains an important source of practical help, being more important than friends or neighbours. We know too that a high proportion of illness episodes are handled in the home without recourse to healthcare workers and, in the same way, the family is frequently seen as the initial educator of young children. Successive governments have promoted the role of the family, and it remains important, with the onus being on health, social care and education services, particularly, working in partnership with the family to achieve the best outcomes for each family member. It may seem then that, far from the family losing its functions, it has sustained and developed its many roles. A glance at the popular press may suggest that the family has taken over responsibility or blame for the 'problems' of society. Certainly, when any young person or young adult is convicted of a distressing or person-focussed crime, their family background and early years are well examined.

If we prefer not to define the family in terms of function, perhaps we should turn to residence. The term 'family' is often confused with household – that is, those sharing common housekeeping. If blood ties are important in the definition of the family, a household of students sharing common housekeeping is not a family, but religious sisters may see themselves as such. The concept of household may be useful if we are looking at patterns of consumption or social interaction, but it is not the same as a family. Families may extend beyond a single household, or one household might include more than one family, or indeed none at all.

The definition of family therefore proves difficult and, like childhood, we can argue that it is socially constructed in different places and across time. As a working definition we could use Giddens' (2001) definition: 'A group of individuals related to one another by blood ties, marriage or adoption, who form an economic unit, the adult members of which are responsible for the upbringing of children' (p. 689).

We may criticize this definition because it places emphasis on marriage rather than long-term relationships. It does not allow for interactions of neighbours and friends, which might be as significant as kin ties, and it assumes the presence of children. However, it does enable us to focus on families with young children.

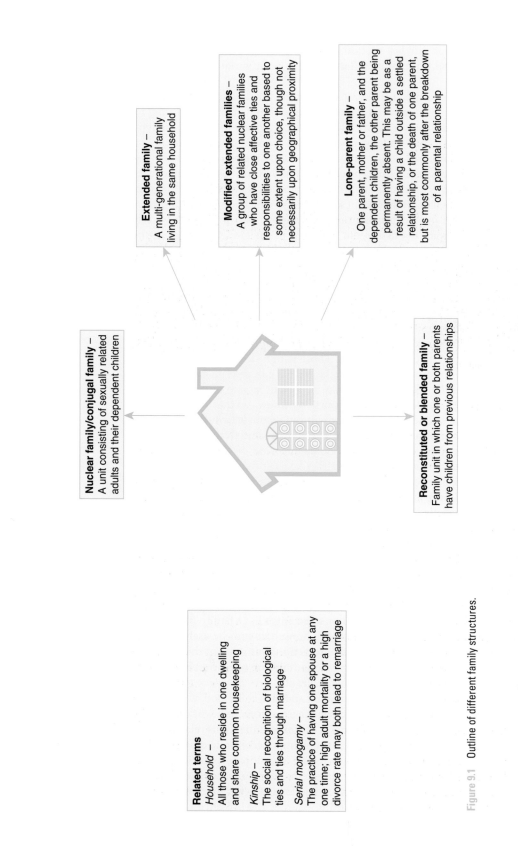

Related terms

Household –
All those who reside in one dwelling and share common housekeeping

Kinship –
The social recognition of biological ties and ties through marriage

Serial monogamy –
The practice of having one spouse at any one time; high adult mortality or a high divorce rate may both lead to remarriage

Nuclear family/conjugal family –
A unit consisting of sexually related adults and their dependent children

Extended family –
A multi-generational family living in the same household

Modified extended families –
A group of related nuclear families who have close affective ties and responsibilities to one another based to some extent upon choice, though not necessarily upon geographical proximity

Lone-parent family –
One parent, mother or father, and the dependent children, the other parent being permanently absent. This may be as a result of having a child outside a settled relationship, or the death of one parent, but is most commonly after the breakdown of a parental relationship

Reconstituted or blended family –
Family unit in which one or both parents have children from previous relationships

Figure 9.1   Outline of different family structures.

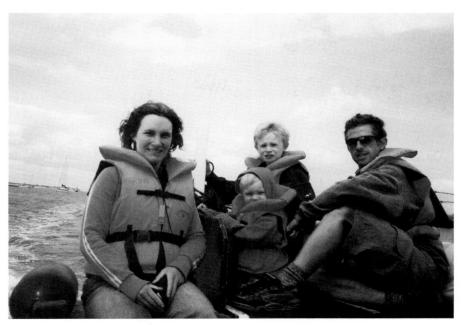

Figure 9.2   Nuclear family.

Diversity in family structures

Such a definition as cited above allows for a variety of family structures, some of which have already been mentioned. Figure 9.1 gives an outline of terms used in relations to different types of families and related definitions.

When reading magazines, watching television and perhaps even watching a children's play, we may gain the impression that the typical family in the UK and other Western societies is the nuclear family. Is the nuclear family statistically typical, or is it an ideal of how families 'should' be? (See Fig. 9.2.)

Government statistics (see Table 9.1) demonstrate that between 1971 and 1997 the number of one-person households doubled potentially as a result of relationship breakdown, the gradual increase in those of pensionable age who live alone, and other adults who choose to do so. Between 1971 and 2003, the proportion of households consisting of a couple with dependent children has declined from 35 per cent to 22 per cent. Clearly we do not all live in the 'cereal-packet-style' family! How then do children live?

Focussing on families with children, Table 9.1 shows the percentage of children living in different types of family, demonstrating changes over a 30-year period. The majority of children do live with an adult couple, but these are not necessarily both their biological parents, some of these couples with children may be some type of stepfamily (see also Chapter 5).

A minority of children may live in collective or communal settings reflected in the multi-family figures, but the numbers of these are difficult to estimate, and it seems that few children stay in such settings for all of their childhood. Indeed, many children live their childhood in changing circumstances. They perhaps commence life in a two-parent home, and when the relationship breaks down they live for a while in a lone-parent setting, and when the parent forms a new relationship they live in a two-parent household with the new step-parent.

Table 9.1   Changes in the proportion of different households in recent years

Households: by type of household and family

Great Britain	Percentages				
	1971	1981	1991	2001[1]	2003[1]
One person					
Under state pension age	6	8	11	14	15
Over state pension age	12	14	16	15	14
Two or more unrelated adults	4	5	3	8	8
One-family households					
Couple[2]					
No children	27	26	28	28	28
1–2 dependent children[3]	26	25	20	19	18
3 or more dependent children[3]	9	6	5	4	4
Non-dependent children only	8	8	8	6	6
Lone parent[2]					
Dependent children[3]	3	5	6	5	5
Non-dependent children only	4	4	4	3	3
Multi-family households	1	1	1	1	1
All households (=100%) (millions)	18.6	20.2	22.4	24.2	24.5

1. At spring. These estimates are not seasonally adjusted and have not been adjusted to take account of the Census 2001 results.
2. Other individuals who were not family members may also be included.
3. May also include non-dependent children.

Source: Census, Labour Force Survey, Office for National Statistics in Social Trends 2004.

The number of children being brought up in lone-parent households has been of much concern to policy-makers, educationalists and church-leaders alike. Table 9.1 demonstrates that the proportion of children living in a lone-parent family at any one time increased, and now seems to have stabilized. Yet this is a high proportion of dependent children. The 2001 census (National Statistics Online, 2003) revealed that at the census point, nearly one in four (or 22%) children lived in one-parent families, with more than 90 per cent of these being headed by a mother. Such figures cannot describe the way in which each family has reached this point – it may be through death, divorce or separation, breakdown of co-habitation, parents who never married, and/or adoption. We can hardly treat lone parents as an homogeneous group. Nor can such figures show the amount of time a child spends in a lone-parent household. For some it may be a transitory period, as children go on to become part of a blended family, with different children leaving blended or other family situations to live in a one-parent family (see Fig. 9.2 for depictions of different family structures).

The media frequently presents the child from the lone-parent family as disadvantaged, but it is difficult to analyse the issues, influenced as we are by media and political hype. Being a lone parent is often linked with socio-economic disadvantage and poverty, particularly as the majority of lone parents are women, who are likely to be in a less advantageous position in the workplace and who, because of their child dependants, may take less well-paid forms of employment. Whilst the number of children living in poverty – however we choose to define poverty – seems to have decreased in recent years (see Table 9.3 on p. 180) and while not all children from lone parents are in these figures, they are very probably over-represented statistically within the data. It can be argued that it is preferable for a child to be in a stable, lone-parent family than in an emotionally charged two-parent household, but we have noted the transitory nature of many lone-parent families that reform as blended families, which necessitates further readjustments. How should we measure the outcomes of lone-parent families? Perhaps this can be done by reviewing the educational achievements of the child, or by comparing the crime statistics of children from one- or two-parent homes. The children's own 'success' in marriage may be relevant, or their mental health in adult life. All of these measures are problematic, involving other confounding variables and taking years to complete.

Unfortunately, Table 9.1 does not show the proportion of children in the UK that are being reared in an extended family. Some of the 'couple'-style families may be part of larger families living together, or couples where parts of the extended family live in the very close vicinity. Classical extended families such as Arensburg and Kimball's (1968) *Family and Community in Ireland* may now be quite rare. Young and Willmott (1973) have shown that traditional communities as described in their *Family and Kinship in East London* (Young and Willmott, 1957) have moved and changed. It seems likely that extended families all living under one roof are not common, although they may be more the norm within some ethnic groups. We need to beware of viewing our stereotypes as the way things will remain. Among families from the Indian subcontinent (itself too wide a generalization), kin networks may be strong, arranged marriages may occur and the kin links may tie in with business, yet increasingly women are working outside the home, kin networks are strained by geographical distance, and smaller domestic units are formed because of the limited size of available housing. For any group the family, whether extended or nuclear, is not a fixed entity.

The typical UK family is no longer a classical extended family, if indeed it ever was (Laslett, 1965), nor is the nuclear family or lone parent raising children generally isolated from the wider kin group. We have already noted that some families will look to the wider kin group for practical help of both a material and a financial nature. This may be most obvious when part of the family is coping with very young children and dependent elderly members. However, there may be significant differences in the amount of help that can be expected from different cultural groups in society. Kin links are not only about the exchange of services. You might like to consider to which members of your family you send Christmas cards, or whom you would invite to a celebration. Whilst most of us do not live with our kin, we have links with them, although the 'rules' about with whom we maintain contact seem to be haphazard and ill-defined. Allan (1985) found that the parent–child link was the central bond, whilst siblings were generally less involved in each other's lives. It seems likely that cousins and more distant relatives will, with a few exceptions, be even less involved. Litwak (1965), describing a modified extended family, believes that there is some degree of obligation in the links that are maintained and the family help that is given. For Allan, with his 'modified elementary family', more choice is involved. This choice will be influenced by geographical proximity as well as by how much individuals enjoy each other's company.

An issue that is still largely unexplored is how these kinship links are maintained in blended families. How do they work when children have five or six grandparent figures in their lives? Can one look to one's ex-sister-in-law for baby-sitting services, or does it come down even more to questions of choice?

It is clear that children are being brought up within a diversity of family structures, and even if these structures are apparently self-contained they are likely to have links with other kin members. Whatever is the norm in our own experience may seem very strange to others. The nuclear family is often presented as the ideal and, while numerically most common, it is itself a relatively new form of the family, having become more numerous at the time of industrialization because it allowed easier movement of labour (itself supporting a capitalist enterprise). It may be that the nuclear family seen in the UK in the early twenty-first century is quite different in its structure and function to that experienced in the 1960s where many of the key texts and ideas on the subject originate.

DIVERSITY IN THE WAYS IN WHICH FAMILIES WORK

If there are variations in family structures, there are probably even more differences in what goes on within families. This is a very private area and not one that most of us feel enthusiastic about exposing to interested researchers.

The aspects which we could discuss are again vast, so the following section focusses upon the increase in the number of women in the work force, the division of labour within the family, and the child-centred nature of the family.

Women in the workplace

To say that women who stay at home do not work is likely to bring down a hail of abuse from feminists and anyone, male or female, who has spent any length of time at home with small children. Women have always worked in the family business, on the land or in the home just as, until the last century, most children did. The twentieth century saw a marked increase in the number of women working outside the home in paid employment, particularly since the Second World War (Summerfield and Babb, 2003). Working-age women with dependent children are marginally less likely (68%) to be economically active than those without (76%). The age of the youngest child impacts on economic activity, with 55 per cent of women with their youngest child being under 5 years working compared to 73 per cent of those whose youngest child was between 5–10 years, and 80 per cent of those whose youngest was aged 11–15 (National Statistics Online, 2004). Women are more likely than men to work part-time, which in turn is likely to affect their earning power as part-time workers are often working in less-skilled positions and have weak bargaining power. They may well choose part-time work because of their dependent children, which accords with the information that women spend more time than men caring for children. That said, parents who work part-time and full-time are likely to be profoundly interested in increased quality child care (see Chapter 7).

Who then is caring for the children? Role reversal occurs less often than is supposed, but the family is providing much of the care, with fathers working different hours and other family members providing child-care services (Hewison and Dowswell, 1994). This of course reinforces the idea that the nuclear family is not an isolated entity. Other children will be attending pre-school services – the variety of which is

Table 9.2 Changes in the types of early years provision in recent years (in England, Wales and Northern Ireland)

Day care places (thousands) for children[1]	1987	1992	1999	2000	2001
Day nurseries					
Local authority provided[2]	29	24	16	18	19
Registered	32	98	235	261	282
Non-registered[3]	1	1	12	2	2
All day nursery places[4]	62	123	262	281	304
Child-minders					
Local authority provided[2]	2	2	9	3	3
Other registered person	159	275	360	349	331
All child-minder places[4]	161	277	369	353	338
Playgroups					
Local authority provided	4	2	3	2	7
Registered	434	450	383	391	347
Non-registered[2]	7	3	3	1	1
All playgroup places[4]	444	455	389	394	369
Out of school clubs[5]	–	–	119	153	165

1. Under the age of 8 in England and Wales. Under the age of 12 in Northern Ireland.
2. England and Wales only.
3. England only before 2000; England and Wales only from 2000.
4. Figures do not add to totals. Total figures for England include an imputed figure for missing values.
5. For children aged 5 to 7 in England and Wales. In Northern Ireland for children aged 4 to 8.

Source: Department for Education and Skills; National Assembly for Wales; Department of Health, Social Services and Public Safety, Northern Ireland. In Social Trends 2003.

shown in Table 9.2 – allowing parents to participate in the workplace, giving carers relief and of course, benefiting the children themselves (see Chapter 7). Attendance at pre-school, therefore, means that, for some children from a very early age, the nuclear family may not be the primary agent of socialization. Table 9.2 shows how the provision of day care has changed over recent years. There has been an increase in nursery provision; most of this is privately run, registered provision, although the number of places provided by child-minders and in playgroups has decreased. Playgroups, of course, never sought to provide day-care provision for working parents, and perhaps they should not be considered in this discussion on women in work. Yet the closing of playgroups in some areas may have a huge impact on the early stimulation of some children (e.g. those whose parents find it difficult to travel out of the immediate area) and on the community life of a village or isolated locality.

Do women and their families benefit according to whether they are in the home or in the workplace? Emotions run high on this issue, and good arguments can be put forward on both sides. Material from the National Child Development Survey (Joshi and

Verropoulou, 1999), a longitudinal study which used a sample of children born in a particular week in 1958, was used to look at the effect of return to work when the child was less than a year old. This work suggested that later on in life the children of working mothers were better adjusted, less anxious and more socially mature compared to children whose mothers did not work. Generalizations, however, are difficult to make from such data, and what was true in the 1950s might not be true in subsequent decades. Some mothers may feel that they could not contemplate leaving a child with carers at such a young age, and the role of early years practitioners is to support parental choice and not to be judgemental of it. For some families the discussion is purely academic, as the mother's income is a vital part of the family budget. We know that many families do successfully manage to combine work and family life, and this is made easier in many situations today by family-friendly workplaces with flexitime, job shares, home working with computer support, and parental leave.

Division of labour within the family

Marxists have traditionally seen the family, or at least the wife, as being there to service the worker, to allow him to go off to work each day knowing that his domestic needs will be met and that he will be greeted at the end of the day by the knowledge that in his home, if not in the workplace, he is valued and loved. It is worth considering if the whole family in the Western world would be involved in this. Woodhead (2003) points out that in many cultures the children will be involved in domestic chores, caring for siblings and even trading in the market. He points out that little is known about the effect of this on their development. It is probable that children providing labour within the family is variable, with some children carrying a heavy burden and far more contributing very little. In the traditional view the father goes to work and the mother stays at home. Such a view lingers in our stereotype of the nuclear family. Oakley (1974) found that women saw housework as monotonous, fragmented, lonely and not regarded as real work. Feminists have long claimed that the family oppresses women, forcing them into a powerless position where they continue to work longer hours than their spouses (Oakley, 1974). Hochschild (1989) asks whether, with the increase in the number of women in the work-force, particularly those with young children, domestic labour has been more equally shared, or whether the working mum is now working the 'second shift'.

Young and Willmott (1973), describing the symmetrical family, suggested that the family was becoming more centred on the home, wider kin were of less significance, and the roles of men and women were less segregated. They might not contribute the same domestic labour, but the roles were more flexible, and both would contribute a similar amount to the home. More recently Delphy and Leonard (1992), considering domestic work with child care, concluded that men undertook some child care but the amount of time spent by women on domestic work was twice that of their male partners. The women, even if they were in paid employment, took the responsibility for the care of children, the sick and the elderly. Ferri and Smith (1996), using material from the previously mentioned longitudinal study, found it was rare for fathers to take prime responsibility for children, and the increased employment of mothers outside the home had little impact on the contribution of the male partner to child care. Following this feminist approach, Purdy (1997) argued that women with children are disadvantaged and exploited in the family, largely as a result of their child-care responsibilities. This long-term commitment to child care was particularly an added burden to those who were financially poor.

If we do not agree with this feminist view, we may like to think that the division of labour has become more equitable, with an exchange system in operation – for example, while mum cooks all of the meals, dad does all of the home maintenance. Reviewing evidence from both the UK and the USA, Morris (1990) suggests that there has been little significant change in established roles, although there are some signs of flexibility in domestic tasks. In the UK, husbands do engage in child care while their wives work, and men do increase their domestic input if there are young children and the wife is working. However, if the wife is not working outside the home, the spouse is likely to decrease his domestic input and spend more time at his paid work. Unemployed men were found to be unlikely to take over a housewifely role, and married women's employment did not prompt a significant rise in domestic involvement by their spouses. Overall, Morris concludes that the traditional female responsibility for household work has not been eroded, and while male input may have increased, it is insufficient to compensate for the increased number of female hours in the workplace.

To come up with one picture of how families divide labour is, however, problematic. Bond and Sales (2001), while researching household work, decided the household circumstances and the characteristics of the man and woman were influential factors, perhaps including time spent in paid employment, economic power, attitudes, social class and the presence of children.

What impact does this have on the child in the family? If the family is the powerful agent of socialization that most sociological perspectives maintain, the picture can be regarded as rather depressing. A process of imitation, identification, role learning and conditioning is passing on stereotyped roles. This apparent maintenance of the status quo needs to be balanced by the fact that change has occurred, and ultimately children are socialized – not programmed. Choice is therefore possible.

Poverty

If there are more mothers working, we might expect this to reduce the number of children living in poverty, with the move to a two-income family being caught up with the desire to provide extra or even the bare necessities for the children.

Discussions of poverty are huge and complex, and frequently start with what is meant by poverty. The debate often hinges on 'absolute' poverty in comparison to 'relative' poverty. Absolute definitions focus on the idea of subsistence when even the basic survival needs, namely water, food and shelter, are absent. Relative poverty considers the standard in a particular society at a particular time. A family who cannot afford (rather than choose not to have) a fridge, car, television or holiday may be seen and see themselves as poor in some social settings, but not in others. Both definitions of poverty rely on someone to decide what the criteria are for labelling an individual or family as poor. Official bodies and those studying poverty have to do this, and in any study on rising or falling poverty it is worth considering the definition used and checking that the same view has been used at different points in time. Rather than setting a particular figure, the two most frequently used approaches are counting those on income support or below the average income with a check to ascertain if this is before or after the deduction of housing costs. These are, however, measures that are relative to rising costs and inflation and allow comparison of some kind. Table 9.3 shows the percentage of children in the UK living in households earning below 60 per cent of the median income. While we may debate how the table was constructed, it indicates that the number of children living in these circumstances rose between 1979 and the early 1990s and stabilized in the late 1990s. The Department of Work and

The child in society

Table 9.3 Are children of today better off than in the past? The percentage of children living in households earning below 60% of the median income

Children living in households earning below 60% of median income[1]

Great Britain	Percentages	
	Before housing costs	After housing costs
1979	12	14
1980		
1981	18	20
1982		
1983		
1984		
1985		
1986		
1987	21	25
1988–89	23	26
1989–90		
1990–1	26	31
1991–2	27	32
1992–3	27	33
1993/94	25	32
1994/95	23	32
1995/96	21	32
1996/97	25	34
1997/98	25	33
1998/99	24	33
1999/00	23	32
2000/01	21	31
2001/02	21	30

1. Equivalized household disposable income.
Data not available for 1980 and 1982–1986.
Data from 1979 to 1993/94 are for UK from the Family Expenditure Survey.
FES figures are single calendar years from 1979 to 1987, two combined calendar years from 1988–9 to 1992–3, and two financial years combined from 1993/94. From 1994/95 onwards, data are for single financial years from the Family Resources Survey for Great Britain.

Source: Households Below Average Income, Department for Work and Pensions. In Social Trends 2004.

Pensions (2004) notes that numbers of children living in low-income households fell by 600 000 (after housing costs were deducted) or 500 000 (before housing costs were deducted) – not quite meeting government targets at the time. They currently claim that steady progress is being made towards the government target for 2004/05 (a reduction to 3.1 million children living in families earning below 60% of the median income).

For children to grow up in poverty hurts our sense of morality and makes us feel uncomfortable. There is a vast literature that indicates its effects are not positive; for example, children living in economically disadvantaged circumstances have poorer health in terms of infant mortality rates, childhood accidents and mental health problems (Acheson, 1998). They may have a more limited education or be less able to make use of the educational opportunities offered to them, leading to poorer outcomes in terms of literacy and qualifications. A poor environment in terms of housing and play facilities may impact on the quality of life. Behavioural problems are often seen as more evident amongst those living in poverty, along with lack of parental support, increased likelihood of domestic violence and child abuse. Of course it is often said that families from more advantaged backgrounds are better able to cover up their difficulties, or have the funds to seek help.

We cannot say that trends will apply to all. It is easy to find examples of those who grew up in economically challenged circumstances but achieved a great deal and stayed healthy throughout their childhood and adult life. Yet there is concern that, for many children and their families, poverty is another factor that can impinge negatively on their lives. The majority of parents from whatever background and living in various types of families want to do the best for their children, though they may have different ideas on what is 'best'.

The child-centred family

The family is regarded as having become far more child-centred in its approach in recent years, reflecting a growing interest in children in Western society as a whole. As noted previously, the symmetrical family was centred on the home, especially when children were small, the inward focus putting the child centre-stage with s/he perhaps the *raison d'être* of the family. Families today tend to be smaller than those of the nineteenth century, with much higher expectations that each child will reach maturity. Children are healthier and spend far longer in formal education, making them financially dependent upon their families for an extended period. Increased affluence for some has meant that there are more resources to spend on children, and the decrease in the number of working hours can allow more time to be spent with children and in families, although this does not necessarily apply to every Western child at the beginning of the twenty-first century.

Returning to the loss-of-functions argument, Fletcher (1988) argues that the family is centrally concerned with the upbringing of children – its prime function as demonstrated by an increased recognition by governments and other agencies of the importance and responsibility of families particularly in the lives of young children and adolescents (e.g. The Children Act 2004).

Conclusion

Diversity and variety are the watchwords in terms of sociological perspectives, views of childhood, and structures of families and how they operate. The student of the child in society needs to observe critically, look beyond common sense, and take nothing at face value!

Student activity

Select a view of children in history. It may come from a book (e.g. *The Railway Children* by E. Nesbit; *Oliver Twist* by Charles Dickens).

■ Find out what you can about children's lives during your chosen period, and identify whether all or a group of children would have lived this way.
■ Apply the four sociological perspectives outlined above to your setting.

Discuss your findings with a fellow student/ colleague.

REFERENCES

Abercrombie, N, Warde, A, Deem, R, Penna, S, Soothill, K, Urry, J, Sayer, A and Walby, S (2000): *Contemporary British Society,* 2nd edn. Cambridge: Polity Press.

Acheson, D (chair) (1998): *Independent Inquiry into Inequalities in Health.* London: Stationery Office.

Allan, G (1985): *Family Life.* Oxford: Basil Blackwell.

Arensburg, CM and Kimball, ST (1968): *Family and Community in Ireland,* 2nd edn. Cambridge, MA: Harvard University Press.

Aries, P (1962): *The Centuries of Childhood.* London: Cape.

Bond, S and Sales, J (2001): Household work in the UK: an analysis of the British Household Panel Survey 1994. *Work, Employment and Society,* **15**(2), 233–250.

Delphy, C and Leonard, D (1992): *Familiar Exploitation.* Cambridge: Polity Press.

Department of Work and Pensions (2004): *Reducing Child Poverty – PSA target 1 – Progress in 2003/04.* http://www.dwp.gov.uk/publications/dwp/2004/psa-targets/ child-poverty/progress.asp.

Ferri, E and Smith, K (1996): *Parenting in the 1990s.* London: Family Policy Studies Centre.

Finch, J (1989): *Family Obligations and Social Change.* Cambridge: Polity Press.

Fletcher, R (1988): *The Shaking of the Foundations: Family and Society.* London: Routledge and Kegan Paul.

Giddens, A with the assistance of Karen Birdsall (2001): *Sociology,* 4th edn. Cambridge: Polity Press.

Goldson, B (2001): The demonization of children: From the symbolic to the institutional. In Foley, P, Roche, J and Tucker, S (eds), *Children in Society.* Basingstoke: Open University, pp. 34–41.

Grabrucker, M (1988): *There's a Good Girl. Gender Stereotyping in the First Three Years of Life. A Diary.* London: The Women's Press.

Graham, J (1993): The pioneers. In Sinclair, K (ed.), *The Oxford Illustrated History of New Zealand.* Auckland: Oxford University Press, pp. 49–74.

Haralambos, M and Holborn M (2000): *Sociology Themes and Perspectives,* 5th edn. London: Collins Educational.

Hartley, D (1993): *Understanding the Nursery School.* London: Cassell.

Hewison, J and Dowswell, T (1994): *Child Health Care and the Working Mother: The Juggling Act*. London: Chapman & Hall.

Hill, M and Tisdall, K (1997) *Children and Society*. Essex: Addison Wesley Long.

Hochschild, A (1989): *The Second Shift. Working Parents and the Revolution at Home*. New York: Viking Penguin.

Hopkins, E (1994): *Childhood Transformed: Working Class Children in 19th-century England*. Manchester: Manchester University Press.

Humphries, S, Mack, J and Perks, R (1988): *A Century of Childhood*. London: Sidgwick and Jackson.

Joshi, H and Verropoulou, G (1999): *Maternal Employment and Child Outcomes*. London: Smith Institute.

Laslett, P (1965): *The World We Have Lost*. London: Methuen.

Leach, E (1986): The Cereal Packet Norm. *The Guardian*, 29 January.

Litwak, E (1965): Extended kin relations in an industrial democratic society. In Shanes, E and Streib, GF (eds), *Social Structure and the Family: Generational Relations*. Englewood Cliffs, NJ: Prentice-Hall, pp. 290–323.

Macdonald, C (1990): *A Woman of Good Character*. Wellington: Allen and Unwin.

McGlone, F, Park, A and Smith, K (1998): *Families and Kinship*. London: Family Policies Centre.

Mills, CW (1971): *The Sociological Imagination*. Harmondsworth: Penguin.

Morris, L (1990): *The Workings of the Household*. Cambridge: Polity Press.

National Statistics Online (2003): *Census 2001*. http://www.statistics.gov.uk/CCI.

National Statistics Online (2004): *Work and Family*. http://www.statistics.gov. uk/CCI.

Oakley, A (1974): *The Sociology of Housework*. Oxford: Martin Robertson.

Opie, I and Opie, P (1969): *Children's Games in Street and Playground*. Oxford: Oxford University Press.

Parsons, T (1956): The American family: its relation to personality and the social structure. In Parsons, T and Bales, RF (eds), *Family Socialization and Interaction Process*. New York: Free Press.

Pollack, L (1983): *Forgotten Children*. Cambridge. Cambridge University Press.

Purdy, LM (1997): Babystrike. In Marsh, HL (ed.), *Feminism and Families*. New York: Routledge.

Rose, L (1991): *The Erosion of Childhood: Child Oppression in Britain 1860–1918*. London: Routledge.

Shahar, S (1990): *Childhood in the Middle Ages*. London: Routledge.

Spock, B (1946): *Common Sense Book of Baby and Child Care*. New York: Duell Sloan.

Stainton Rogers, W (2001): Constructing childhood, constructing child concern. In Foley, P, Roche, J and Tucker, S (eds), *Children in Society*. Basingstoke: Open University, pp. 26–33.

Stainton Rogers, W (2003): What is a child? In Woodhead, M and Montgomery, H (eds), *Understanding Childhood: An Interdisciplinary Approach*. Chichester: John Wiley & Sons/Open University, pp. 1–44.

Summerfield, C and Babb, P (2003): *Social Trends*. London: The Stationery Office.

Trainor B (1988): Having and not having babies. What power do women have? *Women's Studies Journal*, **3**, 44–72.

United Nations (1989): *The Convention on the Rights of the Child*. http://www.unicef. org/crc/crc.htm.

Woodhead, M (2003): The child's development. In Woodhead, M and Montgomery, H (eds), *Understanding Childhood: An Interdisciplinary Approach*. Chichester: John Wiley & Sons/Open University.

Young, M and Willmott, P (1957): *Family and Kinship in East London*. London: Routledge and Kegan Paul.

Young, M and Willmott, P (1973): *The Symmetrical Family*. London: Routledge and Kegan Paul.

FURTHER READING

Abercrombie, N, Warde, A, Deem, R, Penna, S, Soothill, K, Urry, J, Sayer, A and Walby, S (2000): *Contemporary British Society*, 2nd edn. Cambridge: Polity Press.

Foley, P, Roche, J and Tucker, S (2001): *Children in Society*. Basingstoke: Open University.

Haralambos, M and Holborn M (2000): *Sociology Themes and Perspectives*, 5th edn. London: Collins Educational.

Woodhead, M and Montgomery, H (eds) (2003): *Understanding Childhood: An Interdisciplinary Approach*. Chichester: John Wiley & Sons/Open University.

SOCIAL POLICY: THE STATE, THE FAMILY AND YOUNG CHILDREN

Erica Joslyn, Christine Such and Emma Bond

The aims of this chapter are to:

- explore briefly the legacies of past policy and legislation;

- examine ways in which contemporary policy directs help and assistance to families with young children;

- discuss contemporary developments in relation to children's rights;

- consider some children's services that fall under the umbrella of child care policy.

The discussion focusses on the UK context.

INTRODUCTION

The welfare of children has always attracted a great deal of social and political support. The needs of young children and their families are addressed via a range of general policies, including health, education, social security and social care as well as specifically formulated policies such as the Children Act 1989 and the Children Act 2004, and the 10-year children's strategy *The National Service Framework for Children, Young People and Maternity Services 2004*. As society has developed, so have its perceptions of what constitutes and contributes to the welfare of children and families.

This chapter begins with an initial analysis of influential policy and legislation from the early nineteenth century, exploring the legacies that form the foundation of current policy and examining the principles and concepts that continue to be used in contemporary child care policy. It also identifies new areas of development and explores initiatives to improve the health and well-being of children and reduce poverty in families with children in need. National and local initiatives form an important part of policy activities and provide the framework for much that is available for young children and families in need.

The concept of children's rights – a significant social and moral development in modern society – has proved influential in shaping current social policies. The nature of children's rights as they relate to current child care policy is, therefore, considered. The chapter also examines a number of services for children, acknowledging the current political emphasis on the integration of these services and the promotion of voluntary responsibilities.

FOUNDATIONS OF CHILD CARE POLICY

During the past 200 years, child care policy has, on the one hand, sought the identification of children's needs as a point of intervention and investment for the future (Prout, 2003), whilst at the same time emphasizing the separateness of the family from the state (Fox Harding, 1997). Historically, concern for the welfare of children has been balanced by the principle that the power of the state should not result in unwarranted intervention into the private and domestic lives of families. As a consequence, the focus of nineteenth, twentieth and early twenty-first century policy has been less about the welfare of children within the family setting and more about living and working conditions, health and education. In addition, it is also significant that child care policy has been, and continues to be, subject to similar values and ideas that operate in policy in general.

One of the most influential pieces of early legislation was the New Poor Law of 1834. In order to promote a fuller understanding of the nature of welfare and policy it is essential to understand the motivation and philosophy of the Poor Law Report 1834. Broadly, the historical value of this legislation rests with its three conceptual planks:

- the principle of 'less eligibility';
- the notion of the workhouse test; and
- the introduction of administrative centralization and uniformity.

All three continue to bear upon child care policy into the twenty-first century.

The concept of 'less eligibility' was influential in designing a system in which the poor would receive assistance only if they entered a workhouse, where conditions would be harder for them than for those who remained out of the workhouse and on low wages. In effect, the workhouse test became the preferred mechanism for implementing the principle of 'less eligibility', which is the influential forerunner of what we now know as means testing. The rationale behind 'less eligibility' – that those in work should always be better off than those on state benefits – has remained an important factor in the fashioning of twentieth century and twenty-first century policy strategy.

In the nineteenth century, the concept of 'workhouse testing' (and 'less eligibility') was not only applied to adults, but also to the care of children. As a consequence, improvement in conditions for children in workhouses was severely restrained in order to ensure that workhouse children did not have better conditions than the children of the employed poor (Eekelaar and Dingwall, 1990). Provision under the New Poor Law legislation of 1834 included care for an increasing number of children who had been orphaned, deserted, or abandoned to the workhouses. First, this legislation introduced an enforceable legal duty upon parents to provide for children who would otherwise be left destitute. Second, it also empowered civil parish authorities to set to work or compulsorily apprentice those children whose parents could not help them. The emphasis of care services was on making productive use of children as cheap labour and ensuring their contribution to the improvement of the economy. The workhouse and parish authority assistance provided a harsh alternative to self-help, and was offered to the prospective pauper on the assumption that he or she would accept only if truly destitute. In essence, the emphasis of this legislation was to deter pauperism rather than to reduce poverty. Recently, however, policy and legislation have been more focussed on reducing child poverty, and some of the latest strategies will be explored later in this chapter.

In this New Poor Law legislation of 1834, civil parish authorities became the first administrative organizations to be given responsibilities for implementing this policy

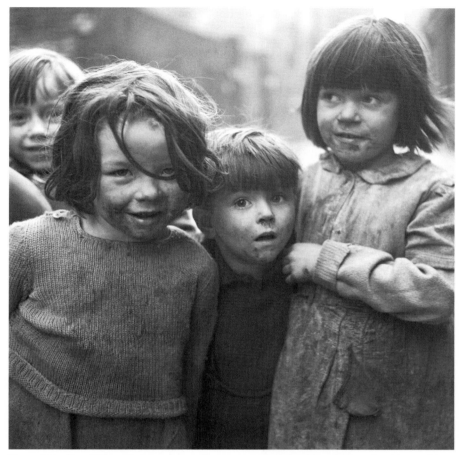

Figure 10.1 For children, the experience of poverty produces health and educational inequalities affecting their future life chances. © Hulton-Deutsch Collection/CORBIS.

and legislation. Current child care policy continues to assign responsibility for implementation to central, regional or local organizations.

Concern for children and their environment was a primary issue for the philanthropists of the nineteenth century who sought to establish alternatives to the workhouse (Fig. 10.1). Philanthropists promoted a number of different schemes, including boarding out, care in a scattered home or voluntary home, or emigration. The influence of these philanthropic ideas is reflected in the Poor Law Amendment Act 1889, which provided the first framework for the legal adoption of children and for taking children into the care of the authorities. The 1889 Amendment gave local authorities the power to transfer all parental rights for a child from their natural parent or parents to a guardian. In 1899, this power was extended to include orphans and the children of those who were considered 'unfit' to be parents. Such intervention into family life by the state was not particularly popular and Eekelaar and Dingwall (1990) suggest that it was probably only tolerated because these were the families of the 'disreputable' poor.

As a result of emerging concerns about mortality rates and the physical degradation of the working class in the early nineteenth century, efforts were also made to improve basic conditions for poor families through separate legislation. The Education Act of 1870 had created local education authorities that had responsibility for providing, for the first time, elementary school education for all children. The Public Health Act of 1847 facilitated the development of community health services aimed almost exclusively at improving environmental conditions and therefore improving health. Responsibility for these new services were given to local authorities who were already responsible for the provision of child care under the Poor Law and its amendments. Cumulatively, legislation for health and education services was making improvements to the lives of many children and families.

Our current understanding of child care services was established following the Second World War, and the notion of uniform provision has become well established since 1945. Local authorities have continued to hold overall responsibility for a wide range of services, including social services, child care and (decreasingly) education though, during the 1990s, policies encouraged local authorities to develop more pluralistic systems, with a variety of public, private and voluntary agencies working alongside them. Although local authorities are now no longer seen as the main providers, they continue to have a key role in ensuring that there is adequate provision to meet needs. We shall explore these roles and responsibilities later in the chapter.

Nineteenth-century legislation has, therefore, not only laid the foundation for many of the features which can be found in current legislation, but it can also be used to demonstrate the influence of changing social values and their impact on policy. In more recent times, for example, contemporary social policy has been subjected to a number of evolving developments such as the modern notion of children's rights. Children's rights, with their emphasis on the child's participation and perspective and child-centred care, have become embedded in a range of health, education and social care legislation.

Another feature of contemporary policy is greater recognition of the importance of diversity and inclusion in society and these concepts are also integral aspects of late twentieth and early twenty-first century policy making. Current child care and education policies are designed to be much more child-centred and inclusive, and to take proper account of the views and interests of children (Foley *et al.*, 2003). This is in contrast to early twentieth-century policy where the power of professionals dictated both the process and outcome of all social intervention. These developments reflect current perceptions of childhood and family life operating in twenty-first-century society, and we shall shortly consider them more fully.

In the study of child care policy, it is important to note that the principles of past policies can be seen to continue almost seamlessly into current policy and to provide a historical understanding of the concepts and ideas that underpin contemporary social policy. At the same time, policy and social thinking can be seen to evolve as a consequence of changing values and dimensions in society, and an analysis of policy can provide an understanding of how legislation can support changing social and moral factors in society. Thus, our understanding of current policy draws as much from our understanding of past legislation as from our understanding of contemporary society.

HEALTH CARE POLICY AND CHILDREN

The National Health Service Act 1948 remains the guiding legislation for contemporary comprehensive healthcare provision, free of charge, to all children under 16 years of age. The legislation provides for a tripartite system of:

- hospital services;
- primary care family practitioner services;

■ community services including maternity and child welfare clinics, vaccination and immunization, midwifery and health visitor services.

Paralleled by rising living standards, Daniel and Ivatts (1998, p. 76) suggest that the National Health Service Act 1948 achieved 'more for the health of women and children than any previous measure of health reform' and resulted in improving standards of health during the twentieth century.

According to Malin *et al.* (2002, p. 18), debates and definitions of risk are fundamental to understanding the purposes and functions of health polices as risk relates to decision making on national scales and 'at the level of personal and intimate behaviours'. In order to minimize the risk of ill health, health policy aims to encourage better heath as well as minister to illness. Alcock (2003) suggests that the primary care-led approach implemented during the late 1990s was committed to reducing mortality and morbidity rates through the provision of new forms of service response. Figures available from the National Statistics Office show that stillbirths, infant deaths and childhood deaths under 15 have, between 1980 and 2001, fallen steadily (National Statistics Online, 2004b).

In spite of this overall improvement in health status, there are, however, significant geographic, ethnic, social and occupational variations in health in the UK, and large social class divides and inequalities remain. Infants and children born into social class V are twice as likely to die than infants and children born into social class 1 (National Statistics Online, 2004b); Bradshaw (2003a) suggests that the incidence of low birth weight, morbidity and poorer child mental health are all much higher for children living in poverty. Health inequality is compounded by the availability of good medical care varying inversely with the needs of the population it serves (Tudor Hart, 1971), and poor families are most affected by restricted access to health services (Reading, 1997). Giddens (1991) argues that regular and detailed monitoring of health risks provides excellent examples of routine reflexivity and the interaction between expert systems and lay behaviour in relation to extrinsic risk. The relationship between poverty and ill health is well documented, and reducing the inequalities in infant mortality remains a government target. Health inequalities, high on the policy agenda, have led to interventions targeted to the more vulnerable groups of children. For example, the introduction of Health Action Zones in the late 1990s were designed to combat poverty (Alcock, 2003), and more recently the SureStart initiative was developed to achieve better outcomes for children from disadvantaged areas and improve their health, education and emotional development by supporting their parents and by the joint working of the 'existing local authority and community and primary health care services' (Malin *et al.*, 2002, p. 162). Additionally, the Public Health Minister, Yvette Cooper, announced in April 2004 that the government would be spending £40 million to tackle child poverty and health in rural areas through extending the services and support currently provided by SureStart. This, and a broader range of service developments, are outlined in the 10-year strategy for children *The National Service Framework for Children, Young People and Maternity Services* (DH/DfES, 2004).

Whilst policies aimed at tackling health inequalities are targeted to the poorer groups of the population, health-promotion strategies aimed at improving children's health across the population are becoming more prominent in government health policies. As Hill and Tisdall (1997, p. 138) observe:

'Childhood is the key site for attempts to influence behaviour, since this is the time when it is thought many habits are formed that have far-reaching health consequences.

Hence health promotion strategies directed at children often have as goals the prevention of poor health in adulthood'.

Shifting towards prevention, the Children Act (2004) makes children's well-being and physical and mental health central to policy and sets out to improve them via the co-ordination of all relevant services for children and families.

The importance of prevention is not, however, new in relation to children, and a number of services have traditionally been provided to ensure early identification of health-related problems. The health centre is the main vehicle through which a wide range of primary health care is provided by a multi-professional health team, delivering the primary care services, specifically general practitioners with a focus on early diagnosis and referral, and midwives and health visitors who have a statutory duty to care for babies and young children in the community. Health centres (usually run by general practitioners) provide a range of services, which normally include general practitioner surgeries, child health clinics including developmental surveillance, immunizations and antenatal clinics. The range of services being offered at health centres has been on the increase, with some health centres – in conjunction with community children's nursing teams – also providing care for children with chronic illness being cared for at home.

Healthcare is sought by parents and carers on behalf of children but, as Culpitt, (1999) suggests, questions about risks and hazards feature increasingly in public discussion. Conceptions of risk as reflected in the media can be highly influential in healthcare decisions that parents make on behalf of their children. Today's risks derive from internal decisions depending on simultaneous scientific and social construction (Beck, 1992), with Giddens (1999) highlighting the mobile character of science in the context of conflicting and changeable scientific information. Additionally, Hardy (2001) comments on the apparent increase in public dissatisfaction with the medical profession, portrayed through the media. A powerful example is the rise in the number of legal challenges by parents on the treatment of their children, also the level of concern over the controversial measles, mumps and rubella (MMR) immunization, with parents opting not to have their children vaccinated. The incidence of most major infectious diseases (e.g. measles, poliomyelitis, tuberculosis, diphtheria) is low, and in the UK the national childhood immunization programme had achieved 90 per cent coverage by 1991. Since parents have become increasingly concerned about the possible side effects of immunization, the immunization rates for the MMR vaccine have declined from 90 per cent in 1991 to 84 per cent in 2001, and between 1995 and 2001 there were 665 confirmed cases of measles in England and Wales (National Statistics Online, 2004b). Furthermore, Maconachie and Lewendon (2004) found that, out of 88 principal immunizers, one-third were concerned about at least one of the immunizations given to children. This is unfortunate because the principal immunizer's role 'in providing parents with advice and information is crucial in a voluntary programme' (Maconachie and Lewendon, 2004, p. 47).

Whilst the NHS Act and Community Care Act 1990 emphasized the role of parents and families as users of the health services, current government policy appears to be taking a more child-centred approach. The need for change was highlighted by the Bristol Royal Infirmary Inquiry, and led to the *National Service Framework for Children, Young People and Maternity Service 2004* which developed new national standards across the National Health Service and Social Services to improve the quality of, and access to, healthcare for children and reduce localized inequalities in provision. Daniel and Ivatts (1998, p. 75), however, point out 'even the best health care provision is only likely to ensure good health if other circumstances of life provide an environment conducive to this'. For example, whilst Ireland banned smoking in public places in March 2004, many children in the UK remain exposed to the health risks from passive smoking. Although the government is emphasizing the importance of national standards of care, any failure to address the fundamental problems of child poverty and provide adequate resources to improve nutrition and access to local services would continue to exclude poorer children from the benefits to be gained.

REDUCING CHILD POVERTY

It has been shown that children are more vulnerable and more at risk of experiencing poverty than others in society. The way in which poverty is defined affects the numbers identified as poor, and also perceptions of what it is like to live in poverty. Our understanding of children's experiences of poverty is often filtered through an adult perspective based on family and household circumstances as the key source of evidence. The dependency of children on adults to provide economic support and care renders them a group requiring special assistance. In Britain, it is estimated that one in three children are living in households with below half the average income; thus they are defined as poor (Novak, 2002). Cohen and Long (1998, p. 75) describe how the impact of unemployment and low pay over the previous 30 years, together with inadequate social security benefits and a regressive taxation system, increased the risks of poverty for families with children. Bradshaw (2003b) further illustrates that child poverty is concentrated in certain types of household, for example lone parent and certain minority ethnic groups. Child poverty is also coupled with other risk factors such as households without paid work and those with children aged under 5 years. The concept of social exclusion has been used to describe the way in which the poor become marginalized and to some extent set apart from others in society. For children, the experience of poverty has been charted as a series of risks producing health and educational inequalities affecting children's future life chances (Howard *et al.*, 2001).

It is recognized that governments have an interest in the well-being of children: to invest in the child is to invest in society's future, and this duty is encapsulated in the UN Convention on the Rights of the Child (UNCRC). In 1999, the UK government made a bold commitment to eradicate child poverty within a generation (Bradshaw, 2003b). Whereas the anti-poverty strategies of the early 1990s were focused on making local services more accessible to poor people and fostering social inclusion, more recent strategies (e.g. the SureStart initiative) have incorporated a more explicit child focus. This represents an important turning point because the focus of support and intervention is the child and the child's family in disadvantaged areas. The strategy, with its emphasis on integrated services, includes providing high-quality education and additional help in the early years to promote the holistic development of young children.

The government has increased benefit rates and introduced a more seamless tax and benefits system coupled with the use of child tax credit and working tax credit to support families with children. The use of means-tested or income-related support measures directed at support for children has continued to be a key part of the strategy. Children, and not just families, are now a more important focus of support and government intervention. At the same time, the value of child benefit as a method of support has declined from a high of 79 per cent in 1979 to 42 per cent in 2003 (Adam and Brewer, 2004). The amount of child-contingent aid a family receives depends on their circumstances, although the costs of raising a child are not easily calculated. The changes to taxation, with the Inland Revenue now playing a greater part in delivering child-contingent support, is a new development. Recent evidence suggests that families close to the poverty line have seen more of an improvement in their status than those in chronic poverty (Institute of Fiscal Studies, 2003). Any gains, however, may be eroded by changes to local employment conditions and job security, since part of the success of the strategy relies on continued economic growth. The social security system is complex and the ongoing use of means-testing for assessing eligibility for benefits may inhibit families from making claims. The position of unemployed or workless households in chronic poverty appears more impervious to change despite the push to promote the take-up of work as a route out of poverty. All parents, including lone parents, have been encouraged to take up paid work through the vigorous promotion of employment opportunities and child care support coupled with the policing of benefit use.

CHILDREN'S RIGHTS IN SOCIAL POLICY

The principle of protecting the rights and interests of the child was included in Acts such as the Children Act of 1948, the Children and Young Persons Act of 1969, the Children Act 1989 and the Children Act 2004. Lansdown and Lancaster (2004, p. 17), however, point out that 'children's interests are frequently disregarded in the public policy sphere in favour of more powerful groups', and they are critical of the welfare approach suggesting that, to promote children's welfare, a rights-based approach needs to be taken. The widespread changes in recent British social policy reflect the increasingly recognized influence of children's rights (as enshrined in the UNCRC), and Hill and Tisdall (1997) suggest that understanding current debates on children's rights relies on two concepts – 'Childhood' and 'Rights'.

Clarke and Cochrane (1998) note the importance of adopting a 'constructionist' perspective rather than a 'realist' perspective. Childhood, constructed as a time of innocence, vulnerability and dependence (Jenks, 1996), is vulnerable to changing definitions of what is normal and acceptable (Smith, 2000). The representations of childhood and images of children as either threat, victim or investment (Hendrick, 1994, 1997), influenced by media representations (Franklin, 2002), are significant to understanding societal responses and social policies directed towards children (Daniel and Ivatts, 1998; Prout, 2003). British social policy has been previously dominated by the ideology of the 'family':

> 'No other factor is as significant in explaining British social policy towards children as the nature of the relationship between the family and the state. This claim is more than a simple recognition that children spend most of their childhood within families: it is based on the view that children are virtually "invisible" within the family unit, and they have almost no separate social policy identity.'

(Daniel and Ivatts, 1998, p. 6).

The importance of the child seems to be growing, however, and the recent considerable increase in the study of children has resulted in children becoming a more central feature within social science (James *et al.*, 1998). Furthermore, there is a burgeoning interest in children's rights in social policy literature (see Chapters 1 and 15 for more details on children's rights).

Children's rights as granted in recent legislation can be summarized as the '4Ps Approach': provision for growth and development; prevention of harm; protection

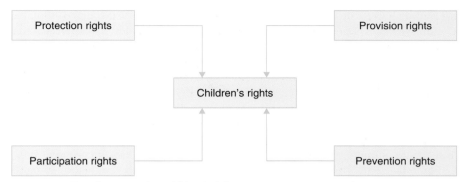

Figure 10.2   The 4Ps approach to children's rights.

against exploitation; and participation in decisions made on their behalf (Burr and Montgomery, 2003) (Fig. 10.2).

How rights are understood will have an impact on how they are supported. According to Franklin (2002, p. 21), children are often denied rights which adults 'take for granted' – mainly the right to make decisions about matters that concern them – from public policy to the private sphere of the home and family life. The 'participation' category can be problematic and controversial; for example, Burr and Montgomery (2003) outline two perspectives on children's rights:

1. *Protectionist*: philosophies that view children as needing adult protection and help, where adults make decisions on behalf of the child.
2. *Participatory*: philosophies that view children as needing empowering, where children make decisions on their own behalf.

The controversy between protectionist and participatory perspectives on children's rights centres on the issue of children's competence, but as Alderson (2002, pp. 158–159) observes:

> '*It is not a question as to whether or not 2-year-olds can understand, because they are interpreting and making sense of their experiences all the time. The question is how skilled and respectful are the adults in listening to the child and ensuring that clear relevant information is exchanged with them.*'

Also, in adopting a rights-based approach, assumptions about childhood and what Prout (2003, p. 22) describes as the 'unhelpful stereotypes of children that dominate public discussion' can be challenged. Furthermore, adults do not always act in children's best interests and 'have been responsible for decisions, policies and actions that have been inappropriate or even harmful to children, while claiming to be acting to promote their welfare' (Lansdown and Lancaster, 2004, p. 15). According to Beck (1992), society must become reflexive in order to evolve, and Prout (2003) suggests that hearing the voices of children is a result of such reflexivity and this has been influential in children being viewed as having something valuable to say. Listening to children's views is gaining importance in contemporary social work practice (Holland, 2004), as well as in health and education provision, and can have an impact on power relationships, challenging the assumption that adults know best. Empowerment 'as a mechanism or process through which needs may be met and rights satisfied' (Drake, 2001, p. 83) is a key principle of the Children Act 2004 and the *National Service Framework for Children, Young People and Maternity Services 2004*, ensuring a voice for children, even at national level, and driving the work of the new Children's Commissioner. Thomas (2001, p. 110) suggests that 'when children have an effective voice, services can be delivered more effectively, and the foundations are being laid for a better, more democratic society in the future'.

It is important, however, to bear in mind that any discussion of children's rights would be meaningless without considering the reality of children's lived experiences. With 4.3 million children living in poverty in 1999/2001 (Howard *et al.*, 2001), 17 per cent of girls and 19 per cent of boys with a long-standing illness or disability in 2000 (National Statistics Online, 2004a) and legislation failing to give children the same rights as adults to absolute protection from deliberate assault i.e. smacking (Newell, 2002; Children Bill, 2004), there clearly remains a vast divide between the rhetoric of rights and the reality of being a child. This has yet to be addressed through policy initiatives.

An understanding of all aspects of children's rights, including protection, prevention and respect for participation and children's autonomy is fundamental to early childhood studies and should underpin any discussion or debate on young children and childhood. A more child-centred approach to social policy can be achieved in striving for empowerment for children through advocacy and research (e.g. the Mosaic approach of Clark and Moss, 2001) which effectively challenges notions of dependency and listens to children's views and experiences.

EARLY CHILDHOOD SERVICES

For many years UK public policy relating to childhood was influenced by competing perspectives drawn from family support, health, child protection, education and care (Statham *et al.*, 2000) but, in the past few years, there has been a move to encourage greater co-ordination at a local and national level in the provision of early childhood services. This has included the establishment of early years partnerships, with joint working amongst providers and with users of services in order to promote children's holistic development (DfEE, 1998). Such partnerships consist of representatives from a range of services including local education, social services, health, employers, training agencies and parents. Local authorities were required to draw up Early Years Development and Childcare Plans from 1998 onwards, and these documents constituted an invaluable source of information on existing services and local intentions for future development. Government policy from 1997 to the present time has sought to promote reform to encourage the development of a more coherent and less fragmented early childhood service for children aged from birth to 7 years. The Children Act 2004 and *The National Service Framework for Children, Young People and Maternity Services*, driven by the philosophy that early co-ordinated intervention will make a positive impact on children's lives, now provide respectively the statutory framework and cohesive strategy, which, in future years, will hopefully see the creation of an integrated, or at least a much more joined-up, comprehensive and child-focussed service. Multi-professional children's centres, intended to play a key role in supporting groups of children who are disadvantaged/at risk, as well as measures to integrate planning, commissioning and delivery of mainstream child care, health, education and family support services feature in the recent Children Act.

Penn (2000) described three strands of existing policy for young children in the provision of care and education in the UK – nursery education, child care, and welfare care – but changes are occurring and these strands are certainly merging. This is a result of much research (see the Introduction of this book) and the government's increasing emphasis on, and promotion of, integrated education and care with education as the guiding principle of organization, in preference to care. We shall, therefore, consider the first two strands together.

Education and child care

The provision of child care was, for a long time, highly dependent on variables such as local access to services and parents' ability to pay (Pugh, 1996). Young children attended (and still do) a variety of different settings before starting full-time school; these include pre-school playgroups, day nurseries, childminders, nursery schools and nursery classes in primary schools. Attendance could be (and again still can be) full-time in some settings, but part-time in others, with some children attending more than one group or facility at any time. Pugh (1996) describes how the lack of an integrated national policy on child care and education, coupled with limited public financial support for the delivery of effective high-quality provision, has hampered the development of integrated education and care. It has been argued that the absence of policy was due in part to the government's hesitancy to intervene in day care because it was considered to be a private matter for families to provide (Pringle, 1998). The separate provision of nursery schooling for 3- to 6-year-olds on a full-time basis with a clear ethos and culture, well established in other European countries, failed to emerge in the UK and this too may have weakened the commitment to setting a comprehensive national policy (Anning, 2003). Quite some time ago now, the *Rumbold Report* (DES, 1990) expounded the principle that care and education for the under-fives are complementary and ought to be inseparable. Today, this is a strongly endorsed principle of good practice, clearly evident in the increasing use of the term *education and care* (Statham *et al.*, 2000; Martin, 2004; see also Chapter 7). At the time of publication of this book, every 3- and 4-year-old in the UK has the right to a free part-time early education place in a setting of their parents' choice (Fig. 10.3) (to be extended to 2-year-olds), with the Labour government keen to promote early learning both as a means to develop individual potential and as a strategy for preparing children for formal schooling (Anning, 2003).

The change may also amplify a strand of government educational policy which focusses on raising standards of performance and measuring achievement with early years learning providing the foundation for subsequent development and attainment (Tomlinson, 2003). The value of early intervention has also been promoted to address social exclusion. Thus, the welfare needs of children may still frame access to services, including early education, but there is a concern that the most vulnerable children at risk may be overlooked within this strategy.

The Education Act 2002 promoted a wider role for schools in the promotion of care, as well as the education, of young children and this, coupled with proposals to develop integrated teams of health and educational professionals, social workers and other child care workers based in schools as well as children's centres, will extend links between education and care (pilot schemes commenced in 2004). Responsibility for the setting of day care standards shifted from health to education. Prior to that, in 2001 an integrated inspection service for all early years was established under the direction of the Office for Standards in Education (OFSTED) to promote a common framework between the different providers, although four different regulatory regimes continue to co-exist (Pugh, 2003). The introduction in 2000 of a foundation stage curriculum for 3- to 5-year-olds in pre-school settings and reception classes in primary schools created a national curriculum appropriate to the early years. (More details

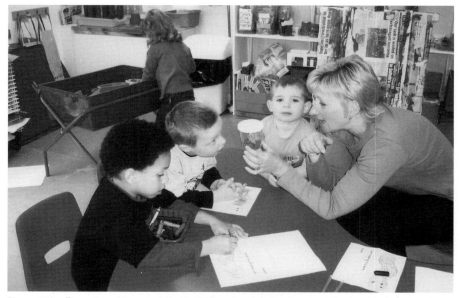

Figure 10.3 Every 3- and 4-year-old in the UK has the right to a free part-time early education place.

on this curriculum are provided in Chapters 7 and 8.) It may further highlight the differences in provision for children aged 3 and above, where there is public support and commitment to provide services based on early education, compared with services for children under 3, where there remains scope for expansion with the focus perhaps more on care rather than education. The recent development of a framework to support effective holistic practice with children from birth to 3 years should, however, be noted as a significant government initiative (DfES/SureStart, 2003b).

The Education Reform Act of 1998 introduced a number of changes to schools in England and Wales, which continue to shape existing provision and children's experiences of school. The introduction of a National Curriculum for pupils aged 5 to 16 in all maintained schools provided a common framework and increased the authority of central government over local educational authorities in England and Wales. Attainment targets were established for core subjects at the ages of 7, 11, 14 and 16 to monitor and regulate performance. Linked to these targets and associated statutory assessments, league tables were introduced in 1993 to enable comparisons between individual schools and ultimately to derive measures of school performance and effectiveness. Tomlinson (2003) highlights how the emphasis by government on raising educational attainment continues to dominate the culture of individual schools.

Demand for what has been termed child care is seen as fuelled by the needs of working parents; thus, we have employment-led reforms of child care. Morgan (1996, p. 2) argues that this has added to the drive for 'accessible, available, affordable, quality child care' in order to provide for working parents. She notes the institutionalized regimes of day care and the setting of a child care industry. The link between employment and demand for day care is a further public expression of investment in the child. During the 1990s there was a four-fold increase in private nurseries, and just over a double increase in child-minders (Scott, 1998). The increase in private provision may be fuelled by the demands of working parents, but it also raises issues to do with creating viable alternative strategies such as family-friendly employment policies to enable parents and their children to live in ways harmonious to balancing family and paid work commitments. The employment policies of the UK have been historically based on the experiences of the male wage earner with child care being perceived, over the years, as a private matter for the family (Williams, 1989). Given the assumption that the mother stayed at home to care for her children, public provision of child care was seen as unnecessary except in times when women's paid labour was required. The use of initiatives such as extending parental leave and more employers being encouraged by government to offer flexible working arrangements for parents/carers may help families to better manage the boundaries of work and care.

WELFARE CARE

In the 1990s in the UK there was a growing commitment to welfare-to-work (workfare) or work-oriented welfare reform. Child care subsidies for low-income working parents, meeting up to 70 per cent of their child care costs, were introduced in the UK to encourage parents to work rather than live on welfare (National Childcare Strategy: DfEE, 1998). Long-term dependency on welfare has been deemed to sap personal responsibility and initiative, resulting in a culture of poverty that passes from one generation to the next. Furthermore, the impact of poverty in early childhood has implications for children's development, health and education, which results in disadvantages continuing in some cases into early adulthood (Howard *et al.*, 2001). Thus the Labour government's commitment to end child poverty in the next 20 years has focused on policies that: ensure all children obtain a high-quality pre-school education; combat family poverty and social exclusion; and support vulnerable young people (Mullett, 2000). Extending day care and early years provision has obvious implications for the children of working parents, or prospective working parents.

VOLUNTARY SERVICES

No account of British social policy in relation to children could fail to acknowledge the major contribution of the voluntary and community sector in promoting children's rights, supporting their welfare and meeting their needs. From local parent and toddler groups, befriending, support and advisory services such as Home-Start to large international organizations such as Save the Children, the voluntary sector in Britain has grown extensively. Now an essential part of society, the voluntary sector is taking on more and more roles previously confined to the state, especially in providing services to the most vulnerable children: for example, those living in poverty; with special needs; having been or likely to be abused; or who are 'looked after'. The importance of the functions and responsibilities of the voluntary sector are well documented, and the Wolfenden Report 1978 viewed the voluntary sector as one of the four sets of institutions through which social needs are met, the others being the state/public sector, the private sector and the informal sector (families, households, friends, etc.) (Harris *et al.*, 2001). Daniel and Ivatts (1998), however, argue that it is the fragmentation between these sectors that led to the lack of 'effective and coherent policies, especially in relation to the early years'.

As a substantial provider in a mixed economy of welfare, charitable organizations also play an important role in identifying and highlighting social problems, and Harris *et al.* (2001) explore the diverse and dynamic role of voluntary organizations in both the formulation and implementation of social policy. Alcock (2003) discusses the complex nature of the relationship between the voluntary sector and the state, categorizing voluntary organizations into four areas: protective, representative, campaigning, and service organizations. In relation to children's services these areas are often interrelated and can overlap, as has been demonstrated in the contribution of the National Society for the Prevention of Cruelty to Children (NSPCC) to the neglect and abuse of children. They provide services to children directly, fulfil an advocacy role in relation to children's rights, and are responsible for national campaigns to raise public awareness. Also in a position to draw attention to areas where the state is deemed to be falling short, the work of pressure groups such as the Child Poverty Action Group play an essential role in disseminating information about the welfare of children, and in ensuring that the rights of children remain on the political agenda.

Malin *et al.* (2002) suggest that, under the Conservative government between 1979 and 1997, economic developments made voluntary work problematic, whereas the New Labour approach promotes voluntary activity with a stronger community orientation. The voluntary sector has a distinctive culture, which Kellock Hay *et al.* (2002) suggest is based on the unique characteristics of commitment to organizational values; lack of market mechanism; difficult to measure objectives; limited resources and diverse stakeholder objectives. Within any voluntary organization, the volunteers constitute its most important resource (Dunn and Mathews, 2001), and there is an ongoing need to recruit suitable volunteers, disseminate information and ensure that adequate resources and funds are raised. Voluntary organizations also have to fit in alongside the new wave of providers of services, either through new ventures such as the provision of playgroup facilities, or as adjuncts to official machinery such as advice centres or family service units. Voluntary services are needed to seal the gaps left by the financial and legislative restrictions upon statutory services. It is recognized by professionals and experts that there are insufficient funds to meet all needs, and that statutory care services can sometimes be somewhat insensitive and inflexible. Hence, voluntary services continue to flourish but, as Rochester (2001) points out, recent changes in legislation associated with the Children Act (DoH, 1989) have had an impact on the type of service that voluntary agencies can provide. The less formal drop-in provision (e.g. summer play schemes and out-of-school activities) are having to operate along similar lines to more formal types of organizations, and the 'informality and flexibility for which voluntary and community sector organizations have been valued are under serious threat' (Rochester, 2001, p. 73).

'Social policy expectations of voluntary organizations and the voluntary sector have undergone a dramatic transformation' (Harris *et al.*, 2001, p. 4). These recent major changes in the provision of services for children are reflected in the Children Act 2004, which provides a statutory basis for partnership working that involves the voluntary and community sector. They will contribute to the design and delivery of new services for children including the proposed new children's trusts.

Conclusion

Child care policy has moved from being, in the early nineteenth century, an adjunct to adult social policy to, in the late twentieth and early twenty-first century, deservingly attracting social and political attention in its own right. While much of child care policy and provision is still encompassed within traditional boundaries of the NHS, schools and social security, a number of initiatives and social developments have been influential in establishing a child care context that is now firmly recognized as an important feature of our social policy system.

Modern challenging ideas on the position and nature of childhood in society have played an important role in shaping and driving social policy towards a more child-centred approach. In addition, the nature of child care issues has driven social policy towards recognizing the value of partnership and joint working between agencies, demonstrated through the number and range of recent and current national and local initiatives.

This is not to suggest that child care policy is clear and comprehensive, but to argue that there has been some attempt in social policy to bridge the gaps between traditional service boundaries and professional groups in the interest of developing services that are more appropriate to the complex needs of young children and families. It also remains significant that child care policy continues to be limited by political objectives that ensure that family responsibilities remain paramount and prime in relation to meeting the needs of the young child.

Student activity

Find out about living conditions in the workhouse in the nineteenth century, and identify two philanthropists who worked for the benefit of children and families.

Ascertain how these philanthropists sought to establish alternatives for families with young children identified as being in need.

Discuss your findings with a fellow student/colleague.

REFERENCES

Adam, S and Brewer, M (2004): *Supporting Families. The Financial Costs and Benefits of Children Since 1975*. Bristol: Policy Press.

Alcock, P (2003): *Social Policy in Britain*, 2nd edn. Basingstoke: Palgrave Macmillan.

Alderson, P (2002): Young children's health care rights and consent. In Frankin, B (ed.), *The New Handbook of Children's Rights: Comparative Policy and Practice*. London: Routledge.

Anning, A (2003): Curriculum in the early years. *Highlight* 197, London: National Children's Bureau.

Beck, U (1992): *Risk Society: Towards a New Modernity*. London: Sage.

Bradshaw, J (2003a): Child poverty and child health in international perspective. In Hallett, C and Pout, A (eds), *Hearing the Voices of Children: Social Policy for a New Century*. London: Routledge Falmer.

Bradshaw, J (2003b): Poor children. *Children and Society*, **17**, 162–172.

Burr, R and Montgomery, H (2003): Children and rights. In Woodhead, M and Montgomery, H (eds), *Understanding Childhood: An Interdisciplinary Approach*. Chichester: Open University/John Wiley & Sons Ltd.

Clark, A and Moss, P (2001): *Listening to Young Children: The Mosaic Approach*. London: National Children's Bureau.

Clarke, J and Cochrane, A (1998): The social construction of social problems. In Sarage, E (ed.), *Embodying the Social Constructions of Difference*. London: Routledge and Open University Press.

Cohen, R and Long, G (1998): Children and anti-poverty strategies. *Children and Society*, 12, 73–85.

Culpitt, I (1999): *Social Policy and Risk*. London: Sage.

Daniel, P and Ivatts, J (1998): *Children and Social Policy*. Basingstoke: Macmillan Press Ltd.

Department of Education and Employment (1998): *Meeting the Childcare Challenge*. London: DfEE.

Department of Education and Science (1990): *Starting with Quality: Report of the Committee of Inquiry into the Educational Experiences Offered to Three- and Four-Year Olds (Rumbold Report)*. London: HMSO.

Department for Education and Skills (2003a): *Every Child Matters: Next Steps* Nottingham: DfES Publications.

Department for Education and Skills/SureStart (2003b): *Birth to Three Matters*. Nottingham: DfES Publications.

Department of Health/Department for Education and Skills (2004): *The National Service Framework for Children, Young People and Maternity Services*. London: DoH.

Department of Social Security (1989): *The Children Act*. London: HMSO.

Drake, RF (2001): *The Principles of Social Policy*. Basingstoke: Palgrave.

Dunn, B and Mathews, S (2001): The pursuit of excellence is not optional in the voluntary sector, it is essential. *International Journal of Health Quality Assurance*, **14**(3), 121–125.

Eekelaar, J and Dingwall, R (1990): *The Reform of Child Care Law: A Practical Guide to the Children Act 1989*. London: Routledge.

Foley, P, *et al.* (2003): Contradictory and convergent trends in law and policy affecting children in England. In Hallet, C and Prout, A (eds), *Hearing the Voices of Children: Social Policy for a New Century*. London: Routledge.

Fox Harding, L (1991): *Perspectives in Child Care Policy*. Harlow: Longman.

Franklin, B (2002): Children's rights and media wrongs. In Frankin, B. (ed.), *The New Handbook of Children's Rights: Comparative Policy and Practice*. London: Routledge.

Giddens, A (1991): *Modernity and Self-Identity: Self and Society in the Late Modern Age*. Cambridge: Polity Press.

Giddens, A (1999): *Runaway World: How Globalisation is Shaping Our Lives*. London: Profile Books Ltd.

Hardy, A (2001): *Health and Medicine in Britain since 1860*. Basingstoke: Palgrave.

Harris, M, Rochester, C and Halfpenny, P (2001): Voluntary organisations and social policy: twenty years of change. In Harris, M and Rochester, C (eds), *Voluntary Organisations and Social Policy in Britain: Perspectives on Change and Choice*. Basingstoke: Palgrave.

Hendrick, H (1994): *Child Welfare: 1870–1979*. London: Routledge.

Hendrick, H (1997): *Children, Childhood and English Society*. Cambridge: Cambridge University Press.

Hill, M and Tisdall, K (1997): *Children and Society*. Harlow: Prentice-Hall.

Holland, S (2004): *Child and Family Assessment in Social Work Practice*. London: Sage.

Howard, M, Garnham, A, Fimister, G and Veit-Wilson, J (2001): *Poverty: The Facts*. [online] Available from www.cpag.org.uk; accessed on 16 April 2004.

Institute of Fiscal Studies (2003): *How has Child Poverty Changed under the Labour Government: an Update*. London: IFS. Http://www.ifs.org.uk/inequality/bn32.pdf.

James, A, Jenks, C and Prout, A (1998): *Theorising Childhood*. Cambridge: Polity Press.

Jenks, C (1996): *Childhood*. London: Routledge.

Kellock Hay, G, Beattie, RS, Livingstone, R and Munro, P (2001): Change, HRM and the voluntary sector. *Employee Relations*, **23**(3), 240–255.

Landsdown, G and Lancaster, YP (2004): Promoting children's welfare by respecting their rights. In Miller, L and Devereux, J (eds), *Supporting Children's Learning in the Early Years*. London: David Fulton in association with the Open University.

Maconachie, M and Lewendon, G (2004): Immunising children in primary care in the UK – What are the concerns of primary immunisers? *Health Education Journal*, **63**(1), 40–49.

Malin, N, Wilmot, S and Manthorpe, J (2002): *Key Concepts and Debates in Health and Social Policy*. Buckingham: Open University Press.

Martin, D (2004): Childcare tops the Labour agenda. *Children Now*, 14–20 July, 12–13.

Morgan, P (1996): *Who Needs Parents?* London, ILEA.

Mullett, D (2000): Poverty to end: official. *Co-ordinate*, March 2000, 4–6.

National Statistics Online (2004a): *Disability: More boys than girls with disability* [online]. Available from http://www.statistics.gov.uk/cci/nugget.asp?id+795; accessed 15 April 2004.

National Statistics Online (2004b): *Infectious Diseases: Preventable infections on the increase* [online]. Available from http://www.statistics.gov.uk/cci/ugget.asp?id=720; accessed 14 April 2004.

Newell, P (2002): Global progress towards giving up the habit of hitting children. In Franklin, B (ed.), *The New Handbook of Children's Rights: Comparative Policy and Practice*. London: Routledge.

Novak, T (2002): Rich children, poor children. In Goldson, B, Lavalette, M and McKechnie, J (eds), *Children, Welfare and the State*. London: Sage.

Penn, H (2000): Policy and practice in childcare and nursery education. *Journal of Social Policy*, **29**(1), 37–54.

Pringle, K (1998): *Children and Social Welfare in Europe*. Buckingham: Open University Press.

Prout, A (2003): Participation, policy and childhood. In Hallett, C and Prout, A (eds), *Hearing the Voices of Children: Social Policy for a New Century*. London: Routledge-Falmer.

Pugh, G (ed.) (1996): *Contemporary Issues in the Early Years*. London: Paul Chapman.

Pugh, G (2003): Early childhood services. *Children and Society*, **17**, 184–194.

Reading, R (1997): Social disadvantage and infection in childhood. *Sociology of Health and Illness*, **19**, 395–414.

Rochester, C (2001): Regulation: the impact on local voluntary action. In Harris, M and Rochester, C (eds), *Voluntary Organisations and Social Policy in Britain: Perspectives on Change and Choice*. Basingstoke: Palgrave.

Scott, G (1998): Child-care: the changing boundaries of family, economy and state. *Critical Social Policy*, **57(4)**, 519–528.

Smith, R (2000): Order and disorder: the contradictions of childhood. *Children and Society*, **14**, 3–10.

Statham, J, Dillon, J and Moss, P (2000): Sponsored day care in a changing world. *Children and Society*, **14**, 23–36.

Thomas, N (2001): Listening to children. In Foley, P, Roche, J and Tucker, S (eds), *Children in Society: Contemporary Theory, Policy and Practice.* Basingstoke: Palgrave in association with the Open University.

Tomlinson, S (2003): New Labour and education. *Children and Society*, **17**, 195–204.

Tudor Hart, J (1971): The inverse care law. *Lancet*, **1**(7696), 405–412.

Williams, F (1989): *Social Policy: A Critical Introduction.* Cambridge, Polity Press.

FURTHER READING

Fawcett, B, Featherstone, B and Goddard, J (2004): *Contemporary Childcare: Policy and Practice.* Basingstoke: Palgrave.

WEBSITES

Children Act 2004 – www.legislation.hmso.gov.uk/acts/acts2004/20040031.htm
DfES – www.dfes.gov.uk
For information on policies relating to children – www.childpolicy.org.uk
National Children's Bureau – www.ncb.org.uk
For children's rights – www.unicef.org

CHILD PROTECTION, WELFARE AND THE LAW

Kevin Pettican

This chapter aims to:

■ discuss some of the professional challenges presented by child protection work;

■ consider legal and policy issues and developments in child protection and in safeguarding children;

■ identify the nature of physical, sexual and emotional abuse of children and child neglect in the context of multidisciplinary and multi-agency child protection work.

INTRODUCTION

Child protection is integral to child care policy and to good child care practice. It therefore forms an essential element of early childhood studies. The professional task of safeguarding children from abuse and helping those who may have already been abused, or significantly harmed, is both complex and emotionally demanding, and presents an enormous challenge to all those who have child care and child protection responsibilities and interests (Department of Health, 1999).

The challenge for professionals exists for several related reasons. It arises through the very nature of responding to painful situations in which children, who are dependent upon adults for their care and protection, may suffer significant harm, abuse or exploitation. Child protection work can be emotionally demanding and draining, however detached and objective the professional strives to remain. The professionals must guard consciously against over-identification with the child victim, but remain sensitive and empathic. They need to manage the powerful feelings of anger, sadness, frustration, helplessness and hopelessness that often emerge within them and can adversely colour perceptions, relationships and judgement-making. Managing one's feelings about a parent or carer who has harmed a child is also important, especially if one has a professional responsibility to provide ongoing services to the child and their family.

The professional challenge concerns the task of protecting the child in a sensitive yet effective manner, without destroying all the positive aspects of the child's family life. The child protection professional must remain child-focussed and supportive, consider the legitimate therapeutic interests of the child, but practice in a manner that does not undermine any legal and evidential processes that arise from an investigation.

These tasks and challenges are located within a professional and organizational context in which public expectations of what child protection workers should achieve are very high, where criticism is common, and where the wisdom of hindsight often leads the public and the media to believe it was obvious from the start what was needed. There is also a balance to strike between respecting a family's right to privacy and non-interference by the state, with regard to the way that parents/carers choose to bring up their children, and the state's legitimate responsibility to intervene and protect children against abuse and exploitation. Professionals often feel that they are damned when they do intervene, and damned when they do not.

Seden *et al.* (1996) have provided some encouraging evidence to support the contention that the complex process of reconciling state intervention in child protection situations with the need to preserve family autonomy can be achieved by child protection workers in a manner that is empowering both to the child and to the family, and which shows how well professionals can co-operate and work effectively together. The Children Act 1989, the Children Act 2004 and the *National Service Framework for Children, Young People and Maternity Services 2004* require child protection professionals to work in partnership with parents and fully involve them in child protection processes. The pattern of parental involvement in child protection processes has been well established for some time, and the benefits clearly outweigh the challenges (Thoburn *et al.*, 1995; DH/DfES, 2004).

Child abuse is an intensively private act, an act that usually occurs without witnesses and behind closed doors. The abuse may have been a one-off or series of abusive events, for example with sexual and physical abuse. Each single abusive event may be etched in the memory of the child. On the other hand, the abusive experience may have gone on over a long period of time, described as an abusive process. In such a situation it may be hard for the child to recall its beginning or the length of time for which it has been endured, as is often the case with emotional abuse and neglect. It could also be argued, of course, that, from the child's point of view, a series of abusive events amounts to an abusive process.

The private act of abusing a vulnerable and dependent child is also a matter for public interest and concern. Child abuse presents a direct and unwelcome challenge to society's most cherished values and beliefs about the care and safety of children, about the nature of parenthood and of family life (Parton, 1985). The frequent reporting of child deaths at the hands of parents, step-parents and carers leads to outpourings of moral outrage, public anger and a general sense of frustration and helplessness. It can also serve to generate a wider sense of unease and concern about the safety and welfare of children in society at large. The notion that families can, for some children, be dangerous places is something that society took a while to recognize (Dale, 1986). The culture of blame that surrounds the death of a child also tends to undermine public and political confidence in child protection services generally, and often leads professionals to feel that they are all tarred with the same brush for the apparent failures and incompetence of the few.

It could be argued that greater public awareness and disquiet shown by the media, about the abuse of children, has had a positive effect in society at large in that it has helped to create a visible public discourse about child abuse and child protection that simply did not exist in this form previously. In its wake have come many changes that we now take for granted. For instance, anyone who works with children will be well aware of all the checks that are made about them and the changes to child care practice that have occurred to ensure the safety and welfare of vulnerable children. In the early 1990s many of these routine practices simply did not exist.

Another crucial factor that has supported the public and professional discourse on child abuse and child protection has been the publication and discussion of a series of child abuse Inquiry Reports. Each Inquiry Report is important because it refers to an individual tragedy – the death of a child. It is also important in terms of public, political and professional accountability. But the impact of a Report's findings often seem to fade as media and public attention move on to other pressing matters of the day. For professionals, agencies and the government, however, there are general lessons that can be learned from each individual Inquiry Report, lessons that can inform professional and agency practice and help address weaknesses in practice and in the child protection system.

Of particular note in this context are the influential findings of the Laming Inquiry into the death of Victoria Climbié (January, 2003) which identified several aspects of poor child protection practice and systemic failures that required urgent attention by government and by all those with child care and child protection responsibilities. Some of the key recommendations were:

- The need to identify and keep track of vulnerable children.
- Improvements in identifying and recognizing child abuse.
- Services must be ethnically aware and sensitive to cultural issues.
- There must be greater consistency and clarity of response from agencies with protection responsibilities.
- Better information sharing and communication across different agencies.
- Need for common assessment frameworks across different agencies.
- Structural changes to the way child protection services are defined, organized, resourced and delivered.
- The need for new processes of inspection, monitoring and accountability.
- Need to improve the effectiveness of inter-agency working and training.
- The law on private fostering should be reviewed.
- Case Conferences should focus on establishing agreed plans to safeguard and promote the welfare of the child.
- The Child Protection Register should be replaced with a more effective system.
- There is a need for a Children's Commissioner for England (addressed in the Children Act, 2004).

The Laming Inquiry has created a point of reference in recent child protection history from which many subsequent changes and developments will be marked. It has influenced government thinking, for instance, with the publication of *Keeping Children Safe* – the government's response to The Victoria Climbié Inquiry report and Joint Chief Inspectors' report *Safeguarding Children* (Department for Education and Skills, 2003a) and the Green Paper, *Every Child Matters* (Department of Health, 2003a) which set out the government's far-reaching proposals for reforming the delivery of services for children, young people and families. The resulting Children Act was published in 2004. It provides the legal framework and, with the *National Service Framework for Children, Young People and Maternity Services*, also published in 2004, provides the strategic framework for re-shaping Children's Services in many fundamental ways including the introduction of Children's Trusts which bring together all child-focussed services under one umbrella organization. Congruent with this structural change is the shift of inspection of children's services to OFSTED. The latter have to report annually to government about the five outcomes for children's services, namely, children being healthy, staying safe, enjoying and achieving, making a positive contribution, and their economic well-being.

Recognizing the significance of these important changes and the need to focus on positive outcomes rather than internal structures and processes, the OFSTED Chief Inspector, David Bell, wrote:

'It's important to go beyond generalities of say, whether children are healthy as a whole, and to identify groups of vulnerable children and young people who have specific needs. We have to be careful that this not just Ofsted driving education inspection … this is about school, social care and education. I think that the danger is that everyone rushes around looking at structures and fails to remember that what matters are the outcomes.'

(Bell, 2004)

For more information concerning this aspect of the government's *National Child Care Strategy*, including *Quality Protects* and other related initiatives, and for details of the new children's legislation, the reader is recommended to visit the Department of Health and the Department for Education and Skills websites.

WHAT IS CHILD ABUSE?

What is child abuse? General definitions of child abuse (or child maltreatment) have been provided by the Department of Health (2003b) to promote shared understanding and agreement across different professional disciplines and agencies. These definitions refer to emotional abuse, child neglect, physical and sexual abuse. However, these categories represent a simplified labelling system for what is a very complex human and social problem. In reality, the abuse experienced by a child may fall under two or more categories at the same time, but there is still a tendency for agencies to select one dominant label category for linguistic convenience. Child Protection Registers do, however, tend to recognize this point and record abuse under combined headings, for example emotional and physical abuse or emotional and sexual abuse.

What is important from the child victim's point of view is that *abuse is abuse*, and the issue for them is their need for sensitive, effective and timely intervention that offers protection and freedom from further harm without destroying all the positive things the child values and needs to hang on to. This point was recognized by the Laming Inquiry into the death of Victoria Climbié (2003):

'Instead of responding creatively to the particular needs of the individual child in an effort to achieve agreed outcomes, professionals become preoccupied by the categorisation of children in light of eligibility criteria. This means that not only do fewer children receive help of an early, preventive nature, but that also the degree of danger is sometimes exaggerated in order to secure action.'
(The Laming Inquiry into the death of Victoria Climbié, 17–22 January 2003)

The notion of child abuse is also related to the legal concept of *significant harm*, a term employed by the Children Act 1989. The latter recognizes the important role of professional judgement in determining whether or not a particular set of circumstances for a child is harmful, and whether or not the actual or likely harm is *significant* within the context of child protection work and the law. The judgement is usually taken by professionals drawn from several different disciplines (e.g. social work, health, medicine and the police), who will assess and evaluate available evidence in order to ascertain whether the *threshold criteria* have or have not been met (see Simmonds, 1991).

Much of child protection work concerns abuse that has occurred *within* the family which we will discuss shortly. Occasionally though, abuse occurs *outside* the home, for example in a residential school, young offenders institution, in a children's home, at a youth club or camp or even within the context of church activities. The *National Service Framework for Children, Young People and Maternity Services* (DH/DfES, 2004) also highlights the vulnerability of children abused through prostitution and other forms of deliberate sexual exploitation. On some occasions, abuse has been skilfully organized by those responsible in such a way as to distract attention and divert suspicion away from their abusive, and unlawful, activities with children (Department of Health, 1995).

In some well-publicized cases, abuse has only come to light some considerable time after it occurred even though the abuse – whether physical, emotional and/or sexual – may have taken place over a period of many years. It is often difficult for those unfamiliar with the nature of abusive relationships to understand why the victims of such abuse had not spoken up earlier [see for example, Wilson and James (1995) for a discussion of this and other child abuse-related issues]. It reveals something of the way that power can be misused and physical and/or psychological control exerted in such a way that a perpetrator manages to maintain a hold over his or her victim, practically, emotionally and psychologically, to sustain the victim's silence for so long. According to the NSPCC, three-quarters of sexually abused children do not tell anyone at the time about their abuse, and many do not feel able to tell anyone about the experience later on (NSPCC, 2003).

The true extent of child abuse is difficult to quantify accurately, and reliance is usually placed on the data collected from child protection registers. According to the Department for Education and Skills (2003b), there were 26 600 children on child protection registers in England on 31 March 2003 (25 700 in March 2002). For Wales the figure was 2200, and for Northern Ireland it was 1608.

Figure 11.1 shows child protection registrations and re-registration over the past 10 years. Figure 11.2 shows rates of registration by age (DfES, 2003b). (For more detailed statistical information, the reader should consult the original documents.)

Also shown in Tables 11.1–11.3 are data for children on the child protection register according to age, gender and by category of abuse (DfES, 2003b).

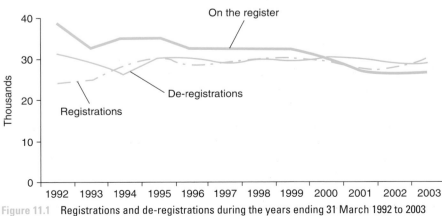

Figure 11.1 Registrations and de-registrations during the years ending 31 March 1992 to 2003 and the numbers on the register at 31 March each year. © Crown copyright 2004.

Table 11.1 **Registrations to and de-registrations from child protection registers during the years ending 31 March 1993–2003, and children on child protection registers at 31 March each year, by gender. © Crown copyright 2004**

Numbers, rates per 10 000 children aged under 18 years and percentages

England	Numbers[1]			Rates			Percentages[2]	
	All children[3]	Boys	Girls	All children[3]	Boys	Girls	Boys	Girls
On the register at 31 March								
1993	32 500	16 000	16 400	30	29	31	49	51
1994	34 900	17 400	17 400	32	31	32	50	50
1995	35 000	17 600	17 200	32	31	32	51	49
1996	32 400	16 200	16 000	29	29	29	50	50
1997	32 400	16 400	15 700	29	29	29	51	49
1998	31 600	16 000	15 500	28	28	28	51	49
1999	31 900	16 000	15 600	29	28	29	51	49
2000	30 300	15 400	14 600	27	27	27	51	49
2001	26 800	13 700	12 900	24	24	24	52	48
2002	25 700	13 300	12 200	23	23	22	52	48
2003	26 600	13 600	12 700	24	24	23	52	48
Registrations[4]								
1993	24 700	12 000	12 500	23	22	23	49	51
1994	28 500	14 100	14 200	26	25	26	50	50
1995	30 400	15 000	15 000	27	27	28	50	50
1996	28 300	13 900	13 900	25	24	25	50	50
1997	29 200	14 500	14 100	26	25	26	51	49
1998	30 000	14 800	14 600	27	26	27	50	50
1999	30 100	14 700	14 600	27	26	27	50	50
2000	29 300	14 500	13 900	26	25	26	51	49
2001	27 000	13 300	12 700	24	23	23	51	49
2002	27 800	14 000	12 800	25	25	24	52	48
2003	30 200	15 000	14 200	27	26	26	51	49
De-registrations[5]								
1993	29 400	14 300	15 000	27	26	28	49	51
1994	26 200	12 800	13 400	24	23	25	49	51
1995	30 200	15 000	15 200	27	27	28	50	50
1996	30 500	15 300	15 100	27	27	28	50	50
1997	28 900	14 400	14 500	26	25	26	50	50
1998	30 200	15 300	14 800	27	27	27	51	49
1999	29 400	14 800	14 600	26	26	27	51	49
2000	30 500	15 300	15 100	27	27	28	50	50
2001	30 200	15 400	14 700	27	27	27	51	49
2002	28 800	14 700	14 000	26	26	26	51	49
2003	29 200	15 100	14 000	26	27	26	52	48

1. Figures may not add up due to rounding.
2. Percentage calculations exclude unborn children.
3. The 'all children' figures include unborn children.
4. Where a child was registered more than once in the year within the same council, each registration has been counted.
5. Where a child was de-registered more than once in the year within the same council, each de-registration has been counted.

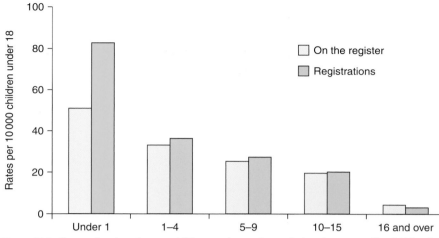

Figure 11.2 Rates of registrations to child protection registers during the year ending 31 March 2003, and rates on the register at that date, by age. © Crown copyright 2004.

Table 11.2 **Children and young people on child protection registers at 31 March 1993 to 2003, by age. © Crown copyright 2004**

		Numbers and percentages									
		Numbers[1]					Percentages[2]				
		Age at 31 March					Age at 31 March				
England	All ages[3]	Under 1	1–4	5–9	10–15	16 & over	Under 1	1–4	5–9	10–15	16 & over
1993	32 500	2300	9900	10 000	9100	1100	7	30	31	28	3
1994	34 900	2700	10 500	10 700	9700	1000	8	30	31	28	3
1995	35 000	2900	10 800	10 600	9600	900	8	31	30	27	3
1996	32 400	2600	9900	10 000	8800	890	8	31	31	27	3
1997	32 400	2800	9800	10 000	8700	810	9	30	31	27	2
1998	31 600	2800	9600	9800	8500	710	9	30	31	27	2
1999	31 900	3000	9700	9700	8600	650	9	30	30	27	2
2000	30 300	2800	9200	9100	8400	620	9	30	30	28	2
2001	26 800	2800	8000	8000	7400	560	10	30	30	27	2
2002	25 700	2600	7500	7600	7200	520	10	30	30	28	2
2003	26 600	2800	7600	7700	7600	510	11	29	29	29	2

1. Figures may not add up due to rounding.
2. Percentage calculations exclude unborn children.
3. The 'all children' figures include unborn children.

Another valuable source of information is the NSPCC, who maintain that each week at least one child dies as a result of physical abuse, and that this has been the case for the past 28 years (NSPCC, 2003). This is in spite of the significant investment of resources and all the work that has been undertaken to improve awareness and understanding of the problem, a huge investment in training and the development of

Table 11.3 Children and young people on child protection registers at 31 March 1999 to 2003, by category of abuse

England

Category of abuse	Numbers					Percentages				
	1999	2000	2001	2002	2003	1999	2000	2001	2002	2003
Neglect[2]	13 900	14 000	12 900	10 100	10 600	44	46	48	39	40
Physical abuse[2]	9100	8700	7300	4200	4300	29	29	27	16	16
Sexual abuse[3]	6600	5600	4500	2800	2700	21	18	17	11	10
Emotional abuse	5400	5500	4800	4500	5000	17	18	18	18	19
Categories not recommended by Working Together[3]	460	310	440	.	.	2	1	2	.	.
No category available (transfer pending conferencing)[3]	170	110	80	.	.	1	0	0	.	.
Mixed/not recommended by Working Together[4]	.	.	.	4100	4000	.	.	.	16	15

1. This table includes unborn children.
2. These three main categories also featured in the 'mixed' categories from 1998 to 2001 only. This table incorporates these 'mixed' categories into the main categories in order to show the total numbers of children for whom each category of abuse was cited on the register. The total of the percentages will exceed 100 for these years because children in the 'mixed' categories are counted more than once.
3. These categories were discontinued from 1 April 2001.
4. This category was introduced from 1 April 2001.

systems and services to protect children. The NSPCC research also indicates that most abuse is committed by someone whom the child knows and trusts, and that the abuse is often known about or suspected by another adult who could have done something to prevent it (NSPCC, 2003).

Each of the four categories of child abuse will now be discussed, together with examples to assist identification and recognition and a discussion of practice issues. The reader's attention is drawn to the helpful booklet provided free by the Department of Health (2003b), *What To Do If You're Worried A Child Is Being Abused,* which clearly sets out the steps that should be taken by different professionals who have serious concerns about the welfare of a child. The key child protection processes and the way that professionals and agencies should work together, and work in partnership with parents/ carers, are explained. Putting all these different elements together, one can obtain a better sense of there being a child protection system in operation, designed to protect and safeguard children. Getting the system to work effectively is but one of the many challenges facing child care and child protection workers.

CHILD NEGLECT

Child neglect has been defined as:

> '*The persistent failure to meet a child's basic physical and/or psychological needs, likely to result in the serious impairment of the child's health or development, such as failing to provide adequate food, shelter and clothing, or neglect of, or unresponsiveness to, a child's basic emotional needs.*'

(Department of Health, 2003b)

Examples of child neglect

The child may appear to be constantly hungry, fatigued, emaciated, inadequately and inappropriately dressed for the prevailing weather conditions, and have the appearance of being severely unkempt and uncared for. They may routinely be absent from nursery, playgroup or school without reasonable explanation. They may have a medical condition that remains untreated, be prone to regular, unexplained, accidents and may be left unsupervised and unattended in circumstances that are not appropriate for their age and capacity to cope. Such children may appear to be *failing to thrive* (for non-health-related reasons) and to all intents and purposes are not developing as one would expect given their age, circumstances and stage of development (Horwath, 2004).

The parent/carer's behaviour may reveal an indifference or lack of awareness of the care and safety of their child(ren). They may appear to be pre-occupied with their own needs and problems. In not being able to see further than their own emotional needs they may have little resources left over for their children's needs, emotionally, socially and practically. Many typical parenting tasks may simply not get done, or there may be no awareness that they should be done or done within a specific time frame. Parental behaviour may also resemble some of the features discussed under the heading of emotional abuse.

Child neglect is often confused with poverty. While the parents of some children are undoubtedly poor, they are clearly not all neglectful. Neglect may also be trivialized as referring to dirty children who are poor but happy. Affluence does not preclude parents from neglecting their children's safety and welfare. Material abundance does not equate with emotional warmth and meeting a child's social, emotional and developmental needs – but nor does it preclude it. These aspects may overlap with emotional abuse, and more especially with emotional neglect (Iwaniec, 1995).

Stevenson (1996) lends support to the therapeutic challenge for parents, carers and professionals to promote positive change in this context. She advocates the need for a clear framework and understanding of what it is that is being expected of the neglectful parent/carer and how change will be recognized and valued. It is clear that some parents have been aware of the criticisms made of them but were unclear as to what it was that the professionals wanted of them and what was realistic, given their particular life circumstances. Stevenson, however, is also clear about the need for professionals to recognize the dangers of collusion with struggling but seriously neglectful parents/carers and defining a point beyond which the removal of a child from the home may become a serious possibility.

Some attention has been paid to a consideration of the long-term harm caused by neglect (e.g. Rose, 1985) and also to the possibility that severe and prolonged neglect may lead to the death of a child (Moore, 1994). Moore writes that:

'Neglect is a serious form of child abuse (which) can have alarming consequences. Research shows that neglected children, living in poverty, have a higher death rate than children of other poor families.'

(Moore, 1994)

Notwithstanding this, it is often felt that this form of abuse is much less damaging than the other forms of abuse. There are several reasons for this – the effects of neglect are not usually sudden or dramatic, abuse is a longer-term process, professionals routinely work with families where there are elements of child neglect and become immune to it, many families who are poor and who live in poor circumstances are more susceptible to criticism of their life-style and more especially to their life chances. The parents/carers may have other serious personal and/or social difficulties that compound neglect of their children. For example, some parents may be severely depressed (Sheppard, 2001) or have other mental health difficulties that contribute to neglectful behaviour (Department of Health, 2001). There may be alcohol- or drug-related problems or domestic violence which exacerbates their child care and parenting capacity. Another reason may relate to the reluctance of professionals to be seen to impose their own personal values on another parent/carer, especially those who are clearly struggling to hold their head above water in difficult social circumstances. Lastly, there is contested debate around what constitutes *good enough parenting* in an increasingly affluent and materialistic society.

Stevenson (1996) has steered a pathway through the neglect debate in order to identify and separate out some of the key issues and implications for professionals working with neglectful parents/carers. She acknowledges the need to be realistic about what change and progress might be possible in particular family circumstances, and recognizes that there are constraints of time, resources and opportunities placed upon professional achievement. Furthermore, in some high-risk situations, where problems are multiple, complex and intractable, things may get to a point where there is an urgent need to take a difficult decision about whether the child should remain with his/her parents/carers or be removed.

While many professionals had argued that the problem of child neglect had itself been neglected (e.g. Moore, 1992), things are changing. As mentioned earlier, child neglect is currently the largest category recorded on child protection registers in England. Much is being done to work effectively with parents/carers who, for one reason or another, are neglecting their children (see for example Iwaniec, 2003). In many situations change and progress are being achieved, standards of parenting raised, and risks to children reduced. One approach is to draw up a contract with parents or carers which identifies the specific tasks, the changes that are required to raise standards and improve child care practices, a clear time frame to achieve it, and how they will be assisted with the process (Minty and Pattinson, 1994). Many professionals in health, social work and social care settings, in psychology and psychiatry, and trained volunteers, undertake a wide range of supportive and therapeutic work with parents and carers who have been neglecting their children and who set out to work together to achieve better and safer child care and parenting outcomes.

EMOTIONAL ABUSE

Emotional abuse has been defined as:

> '... the persistent emotional ill-treatment of a child such as to cause severe and persistent adverse effects on the child's emotional development. It may involve conveying to the child that they are worthless or unloved, inadequate or valued only in so far as they meet the needs of another person, age or developmentally inappropriate expectations being imposed on children, causing children frequently to feel frightened, or the exploitation or corruption of children.'

(Department of Health, 2003b)

Examples of emotional abuse

A child's observed behaviour, mood, deportment, language and development (physically, socially, cognitively, educationally and emotionally) may reveal delays and disturbances under one or more of the following headings, in severe measure: hypersensitivity and over-reaction, self-blaming and excessive self-criticism, acute fearfulness and weariness, persistently low self-esteem, solitary or isolating behaviour, emotional detachment, destructive behaviour to self or others and victimized behaviour.

The parents/carers may display a combination of the following behaviours, again in severe measure:

- rejection of the child as a person and all that he/she is and does;
- unable to see any intrinsic value in the child;
- denial of the child's right to exist as a separate person from their parent/carer;
- a child is only valued if they meet the needs/demands of parents/carers;
- hostility towards, or loathing of, the child;
- persistent hypercriticism of the child;
- emotional detachment and distancing from the child;
- constant ridiculing and belittling of the child;
- constant blaming or scapegoating of the child;
- parental behaviour that appears to be *low on warmth and high on criticism* (Department of Health, 1995).

Emotional abuse is not a single or fixed condition or state. Rather, it is more likely to have been caused by an ongoing abusive process lasting many months or years. The harm may not be immediately visible or obvious. Like other forms of child abuse it can be conceptualized along a continuum, ranging in nature and degree from very mild at one end to very severe and persistent at the other, with corresponding implications differentiated as to the impact upon the child, in both the short and long term. In effect, professionals will make a judgement about which point along the continuum a deteriorating situation has reached and decide if enough is enough.

Children who experience other forms of abuse, for example neglect, sexual abuse or physical abuse, are also likely to suffer from emotional abuse – an important factor that needs to be addressed equally as part of any Child Protection Plan and subsequent treatment intervention. This category, however, tends to reflect individual acts of abuse and fails to recognize collective forms of emotional harm caused to children by such acts as persistent bullying, racism, disablism, poverty, homelessness and 'bed and breakfast' living.

Professionals engaged in child care and child protection work frequently refer to the notion of emotional abuse as being rather a vague term, one that is difficult to determine and define. At the same time, they are likely to recognize that emotional abuse will be present in all the other categories of abuse, to a greater or lesser extent, as well as being present in its own right. O'Hagan (1993) has argued that emotional abuse can be identified if one only knows where to look, what to look out for and is clear about what questions should be asked. He subdivides emotional abuse into two categories – emotional abuse and psychological abuse. He defines these similarly as: parental/carers' behaviour that is sustained, repetitive and inappropriate to the child's expression of feelings, emotions and expressive behaviour (emotional abuse) and/or to the child's creative and developmental potential of crucially important mental faculties and mental processes, including the development of intelligence, language, perception, recognition, memory, attention and moral development (psychological abuse) (O'Hagan, 1993). He suggests that it is possible to identify a vulnerable child in an early years context (playgroup, child-minder, school, after-school club) and through careful monitoring and observation and with supporting evidence drawn from such media as: play, writing, drawing, mood, expression of feelings, demeanour and verbal and social interaction which, taken together with formal recording of behaviour and attainment, can reveal a great deal about the inner emotional and psychological state of the child and his/her feelings about his/her self, parents/carers and life generally. He argues a case for tracking and accurately recording a vulnerable child's observed behaviour, and his or her emotional state, over a period of time. This information could be added to that acquired by other professionals who may have different pieces of the jigsaw to fit together to build up a more comprehensive picture of the child's safety, health and well-being.

Another helpful conceptual and operational approach to the problem of emotional abuse has been provided by Iwaniec (1995) who draws a distinction between emotional abuse (an active process) and emotional neglect (a passive process). There are links here with O'Hagan's definitions, and, not surprisingly, with those provided by the Department of Health (2003b). Iwaniec's definition refers to:

'… the hostile or indifferent parental behaviour which damages the child's self esteem, degrades a sense of achievement, diminishes a sense of belonging, prevents healthy and vigorous development and takes away a child's sense of well-being.'

(Iwaniec, 1995, p. 25)

Iwaniec further describes emotional neglect in terms of the parent's/carer's inability to meet the child's emotional needs, providing little attention, stimulation or engagement, and failing to care, supervise, guide, teach and protect the child. She argues that parents and carers who have emotionally neglected their children often do so because of a combination of the following factors: ignorance, poor general awareness, depressive moods, mental illness, chaotic life-styles, poverty, lack of support and lack of good child-rearing modelling. Parents and carers who are just unable to give of themselves emotionally are often unable to give proper attention and respond to the demands of their own emotionally needy children. Child care and child protection workers are familiar with supporting very demanding and emotionally needy parents who often seem unable to look beyond their own needs and problems let alone address those of their needy children.

One such parent who could not bring herself to touch, cuddle or express emotional warmth in any way towards her own daughter, aged 7 years, sadly told the author about the way her own mother had emotionally 'starved' her (her word), emotionally retreating from her when she most wanted her and how she had been left with a powerful legacy of sad memories that have been hard to undo or disguise. She summarized her painful and damaging experiences in this way:

'The only times my mother ever touched me in the whole of my life was when I was born and when she used to hit me! She just couldn't bring herself to touch me in any other way. I just feel nothing at all for my own children now, even though I know it's wrong. I just have nothing inside me to give them.'

The young girl was subsequently registered on the child protection register under the category of emotional abuse and mother and child received a sustained period of therapeutic help to address the different social and emotional needs of each of them. Interestingly, the same mother felt able to touch, play and emotionally engage with her neighbour's children and those of her sister, but not with her own child.

The connection made by Iwaniec (1995) between neglect and emotional abuse seems especially helpful here in that it provides a conceptual bridge between the two child protection categories of neglect and emotional abuse as well as recognizing that these forms of abuse can be active or passive processes, or a combination of both. Parton (1996) also emphasizes the harm caused to a child by emotional neglect. Quoting from Messages from Research (Department of Health, 1995), he draws attention to the following important research finding:

'If (we) put to one side the most severe case, the most deleterious situations in terms of longer-term outcomes for children are those of emotional neglect, where the primary concern is the parenting style which fails to compensate for the inevitable deficiencies that become manifest in the course of the 20 years or so that it takes to bring up a child.'
(Parton, 1996, pp. 3–11)

What is clear is that emotional abuse is often present in the background of many children's lives, although its impact may be concealed, unrecognized or downplayed, because it lacks the drama, the suddenness and the visibility of other event-driven forms of abuse, such as sexual and physical abuse. Nonetheless, emotional abuse can leave a powerful legacy, the effects of which may continue for years unless something is actually done to help the child (and subsequently the young person and emerging adult). While there is a clear requirement to protect and safeguard the child, there is also a great need for imaginative and innovative therapeutic interventions for the needy and demanding parent/carer (e.g. Theme-Focused Family

Therapy, discussed by McCluskey, 2003). The demands placed upon the professional's time and resources may be substantial, and progress may be slow. The task is to work together to help improve the emotional climate of the family, address some of the many needs and issues of the parents/carers and to improve the health and well-being of the children. Many individual and group approaches to working with emotionally abusive parents/carers continue to be developed by statutory, voluntary and private care providers including those delivered by Family Centres, Community Resource Centres and through a variety of community-based projects.

SEXUAL ABUSE

Sexual abuse refers to:

'… *forcing or enticing a child or young person to take part in sexual activities, whether or not the child is aware of what is happening. The activities may involve physical contact including penetrative (e.g. rape or buggery) or non-penetrative acts. They may include involving children in looking at, or in the production of, pornographic material, or encouraging children to behave in sexually inappropriate ways.*'

(Department of Health, 2003b)

Examples of sexual abuse

A child may be overtly or covertly sexually abused. In the case of the latter, they may not even be aware that they have been sexually used by another person. Collecting evidence may therefore be more difficult than one might imagine, whatever form the abuse took. The child may feel able to speak of the abuse or describe uncomfortable and intrusive experiences or refer to unwelcome behaviour by an adult or young person within the home or outside it. There may be other clues available – physical, social, emotional, psychological and/or linguistic – about inappropriate sexual activities and sexual encounters that the child may have experienced. For example a child – male or female – may complain of physical pain, of soreness or even of bleeding or a rash, around their genital area, for non-medical reasons. Their social behaviour may gradually (or indeed suddenly) change and they may display anxiety about having to spend time alone with a particular individual. Their behaviour, play and language may appear overtly sexual and their interest in sexual play with other children may go well beyond what might be considered 'normal' sexual experimentation for their age. They may wish to copy adult sexual behaviour and insist on sexual play with other children, toys, pets, or they may display sexual knowledge beyond what is normal for their age or maturity level. For more information about the sexual abuse of boys, see Hunter (1991).

They may appear to be preoccupied with sexual thoughts and sexual fears, including flashbacks and past memories; they may be fearful about being touched, about undressing, and about their body generally. They may suddenly develop sleep disturbances, have nightmares or begin to wet the bed for no other obvious reason. Their mood and emotional state may change; their confidence may diminish and what was once a happy and outgoing child may gradually become withdrawn, solitary or avoid the company of others. For the most part, these factors would apply equally to boys and to girls. There are, however, clearly issues of context and of gender with sexual abuse; that is, the majority of perpetrators are likely to be male, but the mix of victims are both male and female (Department of Health, 2003b). Women, of course, do sexually abuse children, as Saradjian (1996) has discussed in her study of 50 women who were in treatment for sexual abuse.

Generally speaking, no single sign or symptom alone indicates sexual abuse (except possibly in the case of a small child having a sexually transmitted disease). Rather, one assesses the whole picture, weighing up all the evidence, seeking to understand the child's individual and family experiences, their explanations and circumstances, their state of mind and their feelings, in an holistic and comprehensive manner.

The parent's/carer's behaviour may provide few clues or indications that the child in their care is being sexually abused. Such abuse tends to be characterized by secrecy, and even when there are strong suspicions but little direct evidence, it may not be immediately obvious who is the perpetrator, what has taken place and over what period of time. Collecting independent and reliable evidence is notoriously difficult, a factor which seriously hampers the possibility of criminal prosecutions.

With child sexual abuse, it is important to ascertain what the family considers to be 'normal' sexual activity and also to discover what the child perceives to be 'normal' experimentation and developing curiosity. Smith and Grooke (1995) have pointed out that much of the UK literature has concentrated upon behaviour that is regarded as being sexually abnormal and 'deviant' rather than delineating what falls within the broad range of socially and culturally acceptable sexual experience and sexual development in contemporary society. The baseline, therefore, as to what is 'normal' sexual play and sexual experimentation varies for different children in the UK. It is not surprising therefore that judgements about what is 'normal', in a given cultural context, often seem debatable, value-laden and often rely on subjective opinion and experiences (Ghate and Spencer, 1995).

It is difficult therefore to avoid drawing upon one's personal moral values and social and cultural expectations in making professional judgements about child sexual abuse. It can also be very difficult to assess the true extent of significant harm in this context given the nature of sexual activities and the impact that it may, or may not, have upon a child, physically, socially, emotionally and psychologically, in the short term or over the longer term. The effects upon a child of sexual abuse will vary from child to child, depending upon several related factors, such as what was the relationship between the child and the abuser (the perpetrator), what sexual activity took place, over what period did it take place, where did it take place, how was the sexual activity 'experienced' by the child, what did it leave them feeling, was anyone else present, how often did this occur and so on.

It is important therefore for professionals, and for others, to ensure that they respond to the particular needs, risks and circumstances of each individual child in their own right rather than form a response to the label of sexual abuse (or more specifically, to the phrase, a 'case of sexual abuse') that has been placed on a child. This label is so powerful that it sometimes persists in the minds of the professionals long after the child concerned has socially and emotionally moved on. There may also be a tendency to continue attributing any subsequent problem and difficulties experienced by the child (and later on when they become a young person and an adult), to earlier sexual abuse, rather than to other 'normal' personal and social problems, life events and challenges. The stigma and power of the label of having been a victim of sexual abuse is also hard for survivors to shake off.

The effects upon the child (and subsequently upon a young person and emerging adult) of abusive sexual activities have been well documented. Some of these effects will now be discussed. According to Salter (1995), one common effect is post-traumatic stress disorder (PTSD) which is defined as:

'*A recurrent cycle of intrusive thoughts, images and feelings followed by periods of emotional denial and numbness. The intrusive phase may be marked by nightmares (which) sometimes shade into hypnagogic, i.e. imagery or flashbacks and survivors may waken from a nightmare only to see the perpetrator in the room.*'

(Salter, 1995, p. 185)

While many victims of sexual abuse confirm the presence of such symptoms, they also report additional consequences, especially where the abuse was not a sudden traumatic episode. This is not surprising, as PTSD was a term originally formed to describe the harmful effects of sudden events causing human tragedy such as accidents, earthquakes, explosions, plane crashes and ships sinking.

Finkelhor (1986) argued that, given the lengths that a perpetrator will go to prepare (groom) the victim for sexual activities, most child victims show few signs of PTSD because it (the abuse) is not seen to occur under conditions of danger or obvious threat. According to West (1991), the very idea of many paedophiles using force or threats to overcome a child's resistance to their advances would be seen as counter-productive and unsatisfying, and would risk denunciation, with all the dire consequences that would follow.

Salter (1995) has also provided a number of evidence-based descriptors of the short- and long-term effects of sexual abuse on children, building upon the work of Finkelhor (1986) and others in this area. In particular, she refers to anxiety and depression as two key consequences that occur most frequently as a result of sexual abuse. Over the longer term, Salter suggests that the anxiety and depression which adult survivors experience may be derived directly from affective flashbacks, secondary to cognitive distortions or current realities. The flashbacks may be triggered by such factors as the sudden memory of the smell of the abuser's body odour or aftershave, or close similarities of clothing, hair or beard style, the use of language, gestures or mannerisms of other people (Salter, 1995).

Other effects may include cognitive distortions in the victim's thinking – that is, the victim reconstructs the events in such a way that they may deny that anything took place. If they admit that something *did* take place, they may blame themselves and shift responsibility away from the perpetrator back onto themselves. The victim's faulty reasoning can lead them to believe that if it (i.e. the abuse) happened, then there must have been a reason for it and perhaps they were at fault or even deserved it in some way. Furthermore, the sense of violation, of being used, abused and exploited can also be turned inwards by the victim rather than outwards towards the perpetrator. In turning the anger inwards, many victims blame themselves for what happened to them and for not fighting back in some way. The anger, guilt, self-blame and low esteem felt against themselves can be something that is carried with them for many years, unless or until it is mediated by therapy, self-work or ameliorated by life events and experiences. Another effect might be *dissociation* – that is, creating mental and emotional separation in their mind between what happened to their mind and what happened, against their will, to their body. One can see how dissociation can be adopted as a strategy used to protect the mind from all the painful and angry feelings associated with the abusive experience.

Victims and survivors of sexual abuse also report fears and worries, over the longer term, around social and sexual intimacy. Their confidence and belief in themselves may have been so undermined that they wish to avoid situations in which close social contact is expected and sexual intimacy may occur. At the same time they may hanker for an intimate relationship with someone who will truly understand them and their experiences and help the healing process. However, intimacy may bring with it a risk of questions and the re-experience of past painful trauma, which for some people is the last thing that they wish to drag up again, having closed the door on it earlier in their life. On the other hand, the long-term damage caused by sexual abuse may manifest itself in reverse – in a desperate and compulsive desire for love, approval and acceptance by others, some victims indulge in excessive social and/or sexual intimacy. Some victims may be re-victimized as prostitutes or find themselves in relationships in which they are further sexually and/or physically exploited. Eating disorders are also common among survivors of sexual abuse, as are drug and alcohol addictions.

The experiences of a rape crisis centre in Washington, DC (2003) confirm the following consequences among women who had been victims of sexual abuse when they were children or young people:

- Orgasmic disorders – unable to have orgasms with partner, or extreme difficulty achieving orgasm.
- Masochistic practices – violent or humiliating practices necessary to obtain desire, arousal or orgasm.
- Desire disorders – general apathy towards sexual activity, spacing out during sex, little desire for sex, sex feels like an obligation.
- Having sex often and with many partners in the hopes of controlling one's sexuality.
- Experiencing negative feelings (guilt, fear, disgust, anger) while being touched or during intercourse.
- Compulsive masturbation.
- For women: vaginismus – collapsing of the vaginal wall, preventing penetration or causing vaginal pain.
- For men: erection problems or difficulty ejaculating (DC Rape Crisis Center, 2003).

For further up-to-date information about the effects of sexual abuse upon males, see Hopper (2003).

However, it is important to remember that not all survivors are affected in the same way, nor does each survivor experience all possible symptoms of abuse. The way a person experiences the effects of sexual abuse is influenced by his/her unique personality style, the particular circumstances of the abuse, the relationship to the person who abused them, and many other factors, as discussed above. Furthermore, it may take many months or years for a victim/survivor to feel able to articulate his/her thoughts and feelings about the experiences and the effects that it had upon him/her and his/her life. Sexual abuse has been termed the 'silent problem' because children often are either afraid to tell, having been threatened by the abuser to keep quiet, or are too young or too ashamed to put what has happened into words.

Healing may be a slow but effective process involving one of the 'talking therapies' such as individual counselling or group counselling to help the child (or young person or adult) address personal issues arising from the harm caused by the sexually abusive experience and from the aftermath upon his or herself, upon relationships and upon life in general.

PHYSICAL ABUSE

Physical abuse refers to:

> '*Hitting, shaking, throwing, poisoning, burning or scalding, drowning, suffocating or otherwise causing physical harm to a child, including by fabricating the symptoms of, or deliberately causing, ill health to a child.*'

(Department of Health, 2003b)

Examples of physical abuse

Children may appear with unexplained bruises, burns, bite marks or scald marks, or other physical injuries such as a black eye, cut lip or torn frenulum. Young children may have been severely shaken or attacked in such a way that there are no overt signs of external damage, but which may have caused serious internal injuries. They may hesitate to undress for fear of revealing their injuries, or they may have chunks of hair pulled out of their head. They may be afraid of returning home for fear of being hurt again by their parents or carers. Their behaviour, mood and general demeanour may also have suddenly changed for the worse and their performance at school or in nursery/playgroup may have deteriorated for no obvious reason. Such children may also have been a victim of physical bullying, racism or disablism.

The parents/carers may admit to hitting, punching, shaking or using a hard object or instrument upon their child. Conversely, they may deny all knowledge of the way that the injuries occurred, when given the location and nature of the injuries, and their circumstances, indicate that it is highly unrealistic and improbable that they could *not* know what had happened. The parents/carers may provide several different explanations to account for the injuries which conflict with each other and which lack plausibility or which are at odds with the evidence. They may have failed to have the child's physical injuries medically examined and treated, for no clear or valid reason. Sometimes, the parent or carer may be unaware of the extent of injuries caused to the child in their care or unconcerned and indifferent.

The idea that parents and carers who have a responsibility to care and protect children may actually harm them, has had a long and chequered history, which is described in standard texts on child abuse [see for example Parton (1985) or Corby (1993)]. As with other forms of child abuse, there is no scientific or watertight baseline for determining what constitutes physical abuse (let alone lawful chastisement). In contrast to Scandinavian countries and Austria, corporal punishment is unlawful and widely condemned, although that is not to suggest that physical abuse does not exist in those countries.

Much child abuse relates to the misuse of adult power and control, as is clearly the case with physical and sexual abuse (Smith *et al.*, 1995). Some awareness of the way in which parental control and power is exercised in families has been provided by Smith *et al.* (1995), who undertook an interesting study designed to examine control strategies in families. They found that variables such as poor marital relationships, family violence and serious aggression between siblings tend to correlate with high levels of physical punishment of the children, which was compounded in families that scored high on criticism and low on warmth scales.

With regard to some of the adverse consequences for the child of physical abuse, Corby (1993) has provided a summary of several research studies and reported experiences of the short- and long-term effects, from the perspective of the child's health and social, emotional and educational development (Corby, 1993). Moore *et al.* (1981) were first in the UK to report on the damaging long-term effects for a child of witnessing parental violence and of being caught up in the parents' lethal cycle of violence, reconciliation followed by violence and reconciliation, and so on.

There is no single explanation to account for physical abuse. Rather, a combination of adverse and potentially lethal factors may come together to create a situation of high risk and danger to a child:

■ *Cumulative factors*: a build-up of severe tension around conflictual and failing relationships coupled with a lack of a good social support network with no outlet to release cumulative stress and frustration.
■ *Situational factors*: acute stress associated with unsatisfactory housing, money worries, poverty, lack of positive outlets and social opportunities (life, work, relationships, etc.).
■ *Child-related factors*: the attitude and quality of attachment that the parent has to their child is important. The parent/carer may not want the child or have little if any positive feelings and attachment to the child. They may regard the child as being of the wrong sex, or see them as failing to live up to their unrealistic expectations. The child with a disability may come to be regarded as being 'responsible' for everything that has gone wrong in the parent/carers' life.
■ *Parental factors*: the parents/carers may have themselves been a victim of abuse, who have learned to turn to physical forms of control, and hit out when things are not done to order or on their terms. The parent/carer may have a serious mental health difficulty that adversely affects their capacity to understand, to cope and to care with challenging and demanding children. The parent/carer may be absorbed with their own problems or drug/alcohol habits. The parent's relationship may be failing, and conflict (and sometime violence) may be constantly present.
■ *Precipitating factors*: something unexpected that suddenly happens, an incident that marks 'the last straw', the unplanned and unforeseen event that pushed the parent/carer 'over the edge', and the child may bear the brunt of any violent consequences.

What is important here is that all but the last factor (the precipitating factor) is potentially knowable through undertaking a comprehensive assessment of a vulnerable child (i.e. a child in need) in his/her family context, and steps should be taken to reduce the identified risks to the child to safeguard him/her from further harm. The form of multi-agency assessment for vulnerable children (children in need) is well established (Department of Health, 2000; DH/DfES, 2004), and is a key tool used on a daily basis by child care and child protection professionals. The Framework for Assessment should also be undertaken with professionals who are conversant with the need to apply to their practice the findings from previous Child Abuse Inquiry Reports, such as the *Laming Inquiry Report* (Victoria Climbié Inquiry, 2003) and research-based publications, such as *Child Protection – Messages from Research* (Department of Health, 1995) and others such as Howitt (1992) and Reder *et al.* (1993).

MULTI-DISCIPLINARY CHILD PROTECTION WORK

The multi-disciplinary approach to protecting and safeguarding children from abuse is based on a number of premises. It recognizes that professional expertise comes from different areas, and that if professionals work together then the sum of the whole is greater than that of the individual parts. Furthermore, by being clear about their professional duties, tasks and responsibilities and by following the agreed, local child protection procedures, there is a better chance to protect and safeguard vulnerable children and to help them and their families. To be more effective, each professional needs a good understanding not only of their own procedures but also a good working knowledge and understanding of the procedures as they apply to the other professionals with whom they work to facilitate joined-up thinking and joined-up child protection practice.

The Department of Health (2003b) has clearly set out what it expects of each professional involved in protecting and safeguarding children, and how they should work together to form a child protection system. The child protection system therefore consists of people, resources, management processes, recording and report writing, training and shared learning and the application to practice of the law, policies, local procedures and the commitment to work together to protect and safeguard children from abuse. It is the operation of this system that is responsible for many of the subsequent decisions and processes that directly affect the welfare, care and protection of a child and which helps to form and consolidate an effective local practice culture. This inter-professional working is a key element of the Children Act 2004 and *The National Service Framework for Children, Young People and Maternity Services 2004*, and agencies are urged to have policies in place to assure robust cross-agency working practices, to audit the effectiveness of such practices, and to have governance arrangements in place to correct any deficits in practice that are identified.

Unfortunately, as the NSPCC reminds us, children do die each week (NSPCC, 2003) and the need to continue to improve training, shared understanding, communication and working together across organizational and professional boundaries is an ongoing challenge (Hallett and Birchell, 1995; DH/DfES, 2004). It is also a requirement of the Children Act 1989 and the Children Act 2004 that professionals seek to work in partnership with parents to provide a range of services that address complex issues facing children in need and help families who are facing serious difficulties in their lives.

We should remember that large numbers of children are protected and safeguarded every single day of the year, and their families supported and assisted by a range of child care and child protection professionals and services, working closely and effectively together.

Conclusion

This chapter set out to provide an introductory overview of the problem of child abuse, and the response to it through the operation of the child protection system. It raises many complex issues facing professionals and agencies with child care, child protection and safeguarding children responsibilities. Each of the four categories of abuse was considered in turn, and the point was made that, from the child's point of view, *abuse is abuse*, however the professional and agencies choose to categorize and classify it. Child protection is located in good child care practice. The child protection system is designed to provide a clear framework within which professionals and agencies should operate together to protect and safeguard children and to assist troubled parents and carers.

The expectations placed upon child care and child protection professionals and agencies is enormous, and working together is a positive strategy for combining the collective knowledge, experiences, skills and expertise of individuals who are confronted with this challenge on a daily basis. There is much to learn from Child Abuse Inquiries and from research and practice experience to apply to children in need. There is also a requirement to review critically the workings of the current child protection system as a whole and to recognize where structural, legal, policy and practice changes are needed in order to create a system that delivers better outcomes for children and their families.

Student activity

1. Using the National Service Framework (NSF) for Children, Young People and Maternity Services, Core Standard 5 (Safeguarding and Promoting the Welfare of Children and Young People) as a guide, identify the local policies and protocols in place in the locality where you are working as a student to protect children. Analyse these policies to see if they meet the requirements set out in the NSF.
2. Child protection register data 2003: What conclusions can you draw from the DfES child protection register data covering the past 10 years? What are these statistics unable to tell us about the true incidence and profiling of child abuse in England?
3. What implications do the statistics have for policy makers and professionals?

REFERENCES

Bell, D (2004): *For whom the Bell toils.* Interview with Health and Social Care, pp. 14–16, 13 April.

Corby, B (1993): *Child Abuse – Towards a Knowledge Base.* Buckingham: Open University Press.

Dale, P (1986): *Dangerous Families: Assessment and Treatment of Families.* London: Tavistock Publications.

DC Rape Crisis Center, Washington DC http://www.dcrcc.org/effects.htm Sourced: 10.5.2004.

Department for Education and Skills (2003a): *Keeping Children Safe. The Government's Response to The Victoria Climbié Inquiry Report and Joint Chief Inspectors' Report Safeguarding Children.*

Department for Education and Skills (2003b): *Statistics of Education: Referrals, Assessments and Children and Young People on Child Protection Registers: Year ending 31 March.*

Department of Health (1995): *Child Protection – Messages from Research.* London: HMSO.

Department of Health (2000): *Framework for the Assessment of Children in Need and their Families.* London: HMSO.

Department of Health (2001): *Child Psychiatry and Child Protection Litigation.* London: HMSO.

Department of Health (2003a): *Every Child Matters.* London: HMSO.

Department of Health (2003b): Home Office and Department for Education and Skills, *What To Do If You're Worried A Child Is Being Abused.* London: HMSO.

Department of Health/Department for Education and Skills (2004): *The National Service Framework for Children, Young People and Maternity Services.* London: DoH.

Department of Health, Home Office, Department for Education and Employment (1999): *Working Together to Safeguard Children: A Guide to Inter-agency Working to Safeguard and Promote the Welfare of Children.* London: HMSO.

Ghate, D and Spencer, I (1995): *The Prevalence of Child Sexual Abuse in Britain: A feasibility study for a large-scale notional survey of the general population.* London: HMSO.

Hallett, C and Birchell, E (1995): *Co-ordination and Child Protection: A Review of the Literature.* London: HMSO.

Hopper, J (2003): *Sexual Abuse of Males: Prevalence, Possible Lasting Effects and Resources.* http://www.jimhopper.com/male-ab Sourced: 9.5.2004.

Horwath, J (2004): Is this child neglect? The impact of difference in perceptions on social work practice. In Daniel, B and Taylor, J, *Neglect. Practice Issues for Health and Social Care.* London: Jessica Kingsley.

Howitt, D (1992): *Child Abuse Errors – When Good Intentions go Wrong.* Hemel Hempstead: Harvester Wheatsheaf.

Hunter, M (1991): *Abused Boys: The Neglected Victims of Sexual Abuse.* New York: Ballantine Books.

Iwaniec, D (1995): *The Emotionally Abused and Neglected Child.* Chichester: John Wiley & Sons.

Iwaniec, D (2003): Working with families who neglect their children. In Bell, M and Wilson, K (eds), *The Practitioner's Guide to Working with Families.* Basingstoke: Palgrave MacMillan.

McCluskey, U (2003): Theme focused family therapy: working with the dynamics of emotional abuse and neglect within an attachment and systems perspective. In Bell, M and Wilson, K (eds), *The Practitioner's Guide to Working with Families.* Basingstoke: Palgrave MacMillan.

Minty, B and Pattinson, G (1994): The nature of child neglect. *British Journal of Social Work,* **24**, 733–747.

Moore, J (1992): The neglect of the neglected child – child neglect. In Moore, J (ed.), *ABC of Child Protection.* Aldershot: Ashgate Publishing, pp. 80–94.

Moore, J (1994): Lethal weapon – neglect of children is a killer. *Community Care*, **1011**, 20.

Moore, J, Galcius, A and Pettican, K (1981): Emotional risk to children caught up in matrimonial conflict. *International Journal of Child Abuse and Neglect*, **9**, 225–235.

NSPCC (2003): *Facts and Figures about Child Abuse*. www.nspcc.org.uk

O'Hagan, K (1993): *Emotional and Psychological Abuse of Children*. Milton Keynes: Open University Press.

Parton, N (1985): *The Politics of Child Abuse*. Basingstoke: Macmillan.

Parton, N (1996): Child protection, family support and social work. *Child and Family Social Work*, **1**, 3–11.

Reder, P, Duncan, S and Gray, M (1993): *Beyond Blame – Child Abuse Tragedies Revisited*. London: Routledge.

Rose, S (1985): *Recognition of Child Abuse and Neglect*. Aldershot: Gower Medical Publishing.

Sedan, J, Hardiker, P and Barker, M (1996): Child protection revisited: balancing state intervention and family autonomy through social work processes. *Child and Family Social Work*, **1**, 57.

Salter, A (1995): *Transforming Trauma*. London: Sage Publications.

Saradjian, J (1996): *Women who Sexually Abuse Children*. Chichester: John Wiley & Sons.

Sheppard, M with Kelly, N (2001): Social work practice with depressed mothers in child and family care. Department of Health. London: HMSO.

Simmonds, J (1991): Making professional judgements of significant harm. In Adcock, M, White, R and Hollows, A (eds), *Significant Harm*. Croydon: Significant Publications.

Smith, M and Grooke, M (1995): *Normal Family Sexuality Knowledge in Children*. London: Royal College of Psychiatrists/Gorkill Press.

Smith, M, Bee, P and Nobes, G (1995): Parental control within the family: the nature and extent of parental violence to children. In *Messages from Research*. Department of Health. London: HMSO.

Stevenson, O (1996): Emotional abuse and neglect: a time for reappraisal. *Child and Family Social Work*, **1**, 13–18.

Thoburn, J, Lewis, A and Shemmings, D (1995): *Paternalism or Partnership? Family Involvement in the Child Protection Process*. Department of Health, London: HMSO.

Victoria Climbié Inquiry (2003): Report of an Inquiry by Lord Laming. Department of Health and the Home Office, London: HMSO.

West, DJ (1991): The effects of sex offences. In Hollin, C and Howells, K (eds), *Clinical Approaches to Sex Offenders and Victims*. Chichester: John Wiley & Sons, pp. 55–57.

Wilson, K and James, A (eds) (1995): *The Child Protection Handbook*. London: Bailliere Tindall.

12 YOUNG CHILDREN WITH DISABILITIES

Sue Hollinrake

This chapter aims to:

■ explore the experiences of disabled children and their families;

■ consider key changes in policy and practice developments in recent years in relation to disabled children and their families;

■ discuss some of the challenges currently presented to professionals working with disabled children and their families.

INTRODUCTION

It may now seem like stating the obvious that children with disabilities, whilst having additional specialist needs resulting from specific impairments, otherwise have the same needs as all children – a need for food and warmth, for love and affection, praise and recognition, stability, and stimulating activities and new experiences through play and education. However, it is not many decades ago that in this country a child's disability was often seen as the barrier to meeting many of these needs.

Institutionalization and exclusion from education provision meant that some children with disabilities often faced a bleak future (Oswin, 1971, 1978) or their parents battled for better provision and support in the face of many difficulties. Much has improved since the days when professionals might have encouraged parents to give up their profoundly disabled child to an institution but real inclusion in mainstream society for children with disabilities still entails the overcoming of significant barriers (Audit Commission, 2003a) and debates continue in education as to how best this can be achieved.

The *Family Resources Survey 2002–3* (Department for Work and Pensions, 2004) estimated that there are approximately 700 000 disabled children under the age of 16 in Great Britain. An estimated 1.2 million children have special educational needs (14% of all pupils) and 3 per cent of pupils have a statement of special educational needs (DH/DfES, 2004).

This chapter begins by identifying some of the key changes in policy and legislation which have affected the lives of young disabled children and their families in recent years, highlighting the shift in values underpinning these policies. The experiences of families are considered and challenges for practitioners working in this area are identified. In the ensuing discussion, disability is referred to in general terms as the scope of this chapter precludes discussion in any detailed way of issues concerning specific disabilities.

CHANGING VALUES: THE MOVE TOWARDS INCLUSION

Although this is a chapter focussing on young disabled children, a discussion on changing values also necessitates some consideration of disabled adults, since the pressure for change across all age groups has often come about as a result of actions taken in the realm of adulthood to secure the rights of disabled people to become full and active members of society. An understanding of the issues relating to the ideologies of disability which prevail in Western capitalist societies, and the various models which structure the provision of support services, is important (Finkelstein, 1991; Means and Smith, 1994; Oliver, 1983, 1990, 1994; Ryan and Thomas, 1980).

Through structural processes, people with disabilities have historically found themselves in powerless, subordinate positions and have consequently suffered discrimination, oppression and exclusion through a resulting lack of control over their lives (Ryan and Thomas, 1980), economic dependency and disadvantage (Sumpton 1988), stereotyping and labelling processes (Bond and Bond, 1994), and institutional policies and practices which reinforced these (Morris, 1969; Oswin, 1971, 1978).

An examination of social policy and legislation provides an appreciation of the crucial role of values, ideology and discourse in the field of disability generally, highlighting such issues as the allocation of value and worth, life chances and quality of life for disabled people. Maureen Oswin (1971) wrote a powerful account of the neglectful treatment of children with multiple disabilities living in long-stay hospitals which at that time offered a totally institutionalized way of living for them, excluded from the rest of society. Surprisingly, even shockingly, this research and her later publication *Children Living in Long-Stay Hospitals* (Oswin, 1978) based on further research received a hostile reception from some members of the medical and nursing professions, perhaps more worried about their jobs being under threat than about preventing the physical and emotional deprivation suffered by these children.

At that time, there were about 12 000 children living in long-stay hospitals in this country, many in children's wards attached to the large mental handicap hospitals, each housing about 20 or 30 children with severe physical and learning disabilities (Oswin, 2000).

Despite a movement away, in recent years, from the policies and practices of segregation towards inclusion, the 'out of sight, out of mind' approach has left a legacy of oppressive attitudes in the public mind with which disabled children and adults and their families still wrestle (Murray and Penman, 2000). There continues to be a struggle in confronting issues of human difference and a tendency to manage these issues in ways that have usually reinforced the differences negatively [from name-calling and bullying (Mencap, 1999) to negative media images] rather than valuing them or even perceiving them neutrally.

Concepts of normality often lie behind definitions of disability and these have been the subject of some debate. For physically disabled people, an inability to negotiate access to the physical environment such as buildings, transport and leisure activities has been viewed in terms of individual limitations rather than a collective lack of regard to their particular needs. In relation to learning disabilities, the medical profession has defined it in terms of a physical, organic abnormality, whilst educationalists have defined it as a statistical deviation from the norm, and psychologists as a deviation from socially acceptable behaviours. These concepts identify the individual as 'different' or 'abnormal', producing an individual 'personal tragedy' and 'deficit' model of disability, or 'medical model'. In contrast, the social model, with its emphasis on materially or socially constructed meanings, has developed more recently (Finklestein, 1980; Oliver, 1990).

The Disability and Advocacy Movements organized by people with both physical and learning disabilities have contributed significantly through their campaigning to a reclaiming of this territory and definition of the experience of people with disabilities. This has produced a climate of challenge to policy makers and a more enlightened professional approach. These activities have had a major influence on the development of the linked policies of de-institutionalization and care in the community for children and adults with disabilities, and have been a force for change in the organization and delivery of health and social services for people with disabilities throughout the 1980s and 1990s and into the twenty-first century. The idea of normalization (Wolfensberger, 1983) has permeated the philosophy behind community care and developed more generally into an approach to care and support that should empower recipients of services as active participants in the assessment of their needs and in the choice of interventions which is in marked contrast to the traditional medical model of the powerful expert professional and the passive patient.

Various pieces of legislation have contributed to the promotion of inclusion of disabled children and adults in society. The Disability Discrimination Act 1995 has brought measures to prevent discrimination against disabled people with regard to:

- employment;
- access to goods and services;
- land and property;
- education; and
- transport.

The Special Educational Needs and Disability Act 2001 [implemented in 2002 with its accompanying Code of Practice (Disability Rights Commission, 2002)] has since extended the scope of this earlier Act by imposing the mandate on schools (previously exempted) that they are not allowed to treat pupils with disabilities 'less favourably' than non-disabled pupils without being able to justify such treatment. They are also required to make reasonable adjustments so that pupils with disabilities are not substantially disadvantaged compared with non-disabled pupils, and plan strategically and make progress in increasing physical accessibility to schools and the curriculum. For parents of young disabled children seeking inclusive education provision, should local negotiations prove unhelpful, this Act may be used to challenge a school's inclusion practices if it is considered that reasonable steps have not been taken to ensure a child is properly included in mainstream activities.

The Carers and Disabled Children Act 2000 enables local authorities to provide services directly to the carer (or parent carer) in order to help support them in their caring role and to help maintain their health and well-being. The Act came into force in April 2001 and gave local authorities the power to supply certain services to carers and persons with parental responsibility for a disabled child following an assessment.

Parents and carers also have the right to ask for an assessment. The Act introduced direct payments for parents with a disabled child giving local authorities the power to make payments to them to directly secure the provision of services for their child, instead of services being provided under Section 17 of the Children Act 1989 for a child in need (see below), and to secure services to meet their own assessed needs (e.g. for a break from caring). This helps parents and their children to choose more inclusive provision and to tailor more flexible patterns of care to the child's individual needs.

The White Paper, Valuing People (DoH, 2001) has been an important milestone in the promotion of inclusion for people with learning difficulties and continues the drive towards more inclusive practice. It stresses the principles of rights, independence, choice and inclusion, and through person-centred planning and person-centred approaches (DoH, 2002), it emphasizes the necessity of ascertaining what individuals want and need, and the importance of working creatively towards achieving this.

There is an emphasis again on changing organizational culture and behaviour in order to achieve these goals (DoH, 2002). The Children's chapter in the White Paper (DoH, 2001) sets out the government's proposals for maximizing opportunities for disabled children. It focusses, in particular, on the learning needs of disabled children and their families, but does so within a framework which applies equally to all disabled children. It aims to improve, for example, partnership arrangements between the health service, education, leisure and social services departments. Its overarching objective for disabled children is:

'To ensure that disabled children gain maximum life chance benefits from educational opportunities, health care and social care, while living with their families or in other appropriate settings in the community where their assessed needs are adequately met and reviewed.'

(DoH, 2001)

In the field of child care, the Children Act 1989 was a major turning point in the inclusion of disabled children in mainstream child welfare legislation and service provision. It was the first piece of legislation in which disabled children were recognized as a group with special needs that had to be met by local authorities. It imposed a duty on local authorities to maintain a register of disabled children in their area and provided a definition of disability,

'A child is disabled if he is: deaf, blind or dumb or suffering from a mental disorder or is substantially and permanently handicapped by illness, injury, congenital or other disability.'

(Children Act 1989, Section 17, para. 11)

Unfortunately, the medical model of disability underpins this definition and the Act's approach to disabled children, who are constructed as a problem, with 'special needs' in contrast to the norm of able-bodied children. In this respect, the Children Act 1989 failed to take on board the gains of the Disability Movement in contesting definitions of disability. The Act also states that the aims of services for disabled children are:

'(a) to minimise the effect on disabled children within their area of their disabilities; and (b) to give such children the opportunity to lead lives which are as normal as possible.'

(Children Act 1989, Schedule 2, para. 6)

Again, the assumption of normality here, when linked to the concept of 'special needs', seems to avoid the debate about who should be 'normalized', and continues with the construction of disabled children as different and 'other' because they are not able-bodied.

The Children Act drew together and simplified the pre-existing legislative framework in relation to children and families and imposed new duties on local authorities such as the identification and assessment of 'children in need'. The local authority has a duty to respond to children in need in their area in a number of ways, through the provision of preventative services, aimed at preventing deterioration in family circumstances and at improving a child's health and development.

Children with disabilities are automatically regarded as 'children in need' within the terms of the Act. Aldgate and Tunstill (1995) found that in the years immediately following the implementation of the Act, services and budgets within local authorities for disabled children had expanded, with specialist teams of social workers and allied professionals being created to respond to need. However, local authorities can use the gate-keeping effect of definitions of thresholds of need and use severity of disability as a means of rationing services by targeting the more severely disabled children and leaving those with less severe or less definable disabilities to compete for priority within the non-specialist child support services.

Decisions about which services to provide should be based on an assessment of need. The concept of need and needs assessments have in recent years become central to health and social care professional practice as a result of both child care and community care legislation, guidance and policy. In relation to children, including children with disabilities, the Framework for the Assessment of Children in Need and their Families (DoH/DfEE/Home Office, 2000) and Standard 8 of the *National Service Framework for Children, Young People and Maternity Services* (DH/DfES, 2004) provide in-depth guidance and advice to professionals.

The progress made in this country in terms of service provision and its underlying principles, whilst still having some way to go (Audit Commission, 2003a), is sadly not reflected everywhere in the world (Jones, 2001). The needs and rights of disabled children are frequently overlooked because they experience the double invisibility of being a child and being disabled. Lack of awareness means that disabled children can become easily marginalized within the general children's agenda. The United Nations Convention on the Rights of the Child came into force in 1990 and was ratified by the British government in 1991. It proclaimed a number of rights for all children such as the right to life, to care and protection, to freedom of expression and thought. Article 23 also has specific things to say about disabled children as follows:

'… *that a mentally or physically disabled child should enjoy a full and decent life, in conditions which ensure dignity, promote self-reliance and facilitate the child's active participation in the community* …',

and also that disabled children have:

'… *the right to special care* …'

(United Nations, 1990)

The four guiding principles of the Convention as criteria of good practice are as follows:

- Non-discrimination.
- Survival and development.
- The best interests of the child.
- The child's right to have her/his opinion heard.

DIAGNOSIS AND DISCLOSURE

I have met many parents of children with disabilities over the past 30 years of working in this area, and very few have reported satisfaction with the way in which they learned the news of their son's or daughter's newly diagnosed disability. I have often been struck too by how readily parents will discuss their recollections in later years, which I have taken as an indicator of how alive the issues remain for them and how vivid their memories are of such a significant turning point in their lives. It can be a very traumatic time for parents and a period of great crisis (Audit Commission, 1994; Scope, 1994). Criticism of professional behaviour and support during this time is often very high.

In some ways this is not surprising, since 'the bearer of bad news' is rarely praised or appreciated for his or her efforts. However, in my experience, parents' vivid and clear memories of the way in which they were told often revealed insensitive and neglectful practice. Parents' complaints encompassed such approaches as one parent being told on their own and then left to share the news with the other parent; professionals avoiding or ignoring parents' anxieties about their child's development who were left feeling that they were over-anxious or 'fussy'; parents being given very bleak scenarios about their child's future in which negative projections about the impact of the disability on themselves as parents and on their child's future life chances were emphasized; parents being told in an abrupt and insensitive manner and then left to struggle on their own with the impact and to search by themselves for information and advice.

The tasks of diagnosing and then disclosing such information to parents often fall to medical professionals such as doctors and nurses. They are clearly difficult tasks, requiring skilled interventions. They are particularly difficult within a professional culture which still predominantly embraces a medical model, emphasising cure and treatment – approaches that may not have anything to offer to parents of disabled children. Additionally, wider cultural views that still marginalize disability and see disabled people as less valuable than non-disabled people can also have their influence on professional attitudes and approaches.

It is therefore vital that professionals undertaking these tasks are aware of their own values and beliefs about disability and have had the opportunity to examine, question and reflect on the discriminatory attitudes and stereotypes that will have been part of their own socialization. Valuing the child and respecting the parents are fundamental to good professional practice (Scope, 1994; DH/DfES, 2004).

Research studies that have focussed on the ways in which parents are told the news of their baby's or child's disability (Cunningham et al., 1984; Quine and Rutter, 1994) have demonstrated that where this is conveyed in an open, honest, direct and sensitive way, showing understanding for parental concerns and feelings, then there are significantly higher levels of satisfaction from parents about the professional support they have received. Additionally, in the longer term, there is a positive impact on parents' attitudes and their ability to adapt to parenting a disabled child.

In 1994, Scope published research that focussed on the experiences of parents at the time of diagnosis of disability or special needs called *Right From the Start* (Scope, 1994). The research highlighted good and bad practice in diagnosis and disclosure and promoted the notion of partnership with parents. A total of 103 parents of children with severe physical disabilities were interviewed, and only 37 per cent were satisfied with the professional management of the process. The research recommended that guidelines should be adopted by all health authorities and maternity hospitals and units, building on the good practice identified as already existing in some areas of the country. This work has been taken forward with the development of training materials and an ongoing Working Group to continue to press for change and to monitor progress. The need to get this right has been reinforced in the National Service Framework (DH/DfES, 2004).

Good practice demands that professionals working in this area have effective communication skills. They need to be able to impart information in non-specialist and non-jargonized language that can be understood and remembered by parents who are under stress. Sensitivity has to be used in gauging the amount of information a parent can digest at a particular time, along with their need for space and time to process information during a period of crisis and adjustment. Parents may need also to revisit issues at their own pace. For this reason, highly tuned interpersonal skills are needed not just in the initial phase of diagnosis and disclosure but in the weeks, months and even years which follow since future transitions may cause parents to re-examine their beliefs, views and attitudes about their son or daughter as they grow up and re-awaken earlier experiences. Other professionals who work with parents at later stages need to be aware of how the parents they are working with have managed their adjustment and be sensitive and responsive to their understanding of and adaptation to their child's disability with the passage of time. Working with parents from minority ethnic groups requires consideration of additional communication issues such as the use of interpreters and some knowledge of the family's culture, religion and beliefs, as misunderstandings and disagreements can arise more readily when language, culture values and understandings are different. Research has shown that service responses to parents of disabled children from minority ethnic communities are not always sensitive to their needs (Baxter *et al.*, 1990; Shah, 1992; Chamba *et al.*, 1999).

The psychological models that have been used to aid understanding of the impact on parents of having a disabled child derive from those concerning human reactions to bereavement and loss. The relevance of such models is based on the notion that parents are grieving the loss of the normal child they were expecting. Behind this lie culturally determined notions that disabled people are less valuable than non-disabled people. In these models, most notably described by Lindemann (1944), Kubler Ross (1969), Bowlby (1979) and Worden (1991), certain stages or phases of grief [including tasks which are to be completed in each stage (Worden, 1991)] are proposed, and though each of the above writers may vary in terms of the number and names of the phases, they broadly cover the following:

- shock and numbness;
- yearning and longing;
- denial;
- anger;
- bargaining;
- sadness and depression; and
- acceptance and re-organization.

These models have however been criticized for being prescriptive and fostering judgements about what is normal or abnormal, thus denying individual difference and diversity in the grieving process, and new models have emerged which refine the earlier models and emphasize the individual context of grief and social, behavioural and spiritual dimensions as well as the emotional and physical ones (Payne, 1999).

Olshansky (1962) developed the concept of 'chronic sorrow', later supported by the research of Wicker *et al.* (1981), which he applied to parents of disabled children, suggesting that the grieving process was ongoing and that later life cycle events and transitions often serve as a reminder of the original loss and re-awaken the process of grieving. This was not seen as an indication of poor adjustment to the loss but as a normal coping reaction.

Whilst in the context of a world which discriminates against and devalues disabled people, these models and stages may be useful in understanding the reactions of some parents of newly diagnosed children, there may be other emotional responses which should also not be overlooked such as relief that a diagnosis has been made after a long period of suspicion that the child was not developing as expected. Other parents may adopt a determination to overcome negative perceptions and view their child in a very positive and hopeful way. Parents will react in different ways and generalizations, and assumptions should not be made about how they are likely to think and feel.

Whilst there is a range of potential reactions and coping strategies for parents, some parents indicate understandably strong protective feelings towards their children and develop an intense bond, especially with those who remain highly dependent. This can have a stressful impact on the dynamics of the parental relationship (Heron, 1998) and can pose difficulties for siblings (Atkinson and Crawford, 1995). Early intervention and emotional support for parents is crucial to enable them to manage family relationships, balance different needs and enhance the amount of pleasurable interactions between the baby/young child and family members.

PRE-SCHOOL YEARS

Government policy in recent years has emphasized the need to improve the provision of both practical and emotional support for parents and their children in the early years following diagnosis. The Department for Education and Skills developed the Early Support Pilot Programme which is a pan-disability initiative to improve services for disabled children under 2 years old and their families, funded for four years between 2002 and 2006. It aims to develop more effective multi-agency family support, with the involvement of parents in the planning and delivery of services. Better information will be available for parents so that they are aware of the range of support services and their statutory entitlement. Better training to improve professional knowledge and skills is also being developed. The programme has produced practical guidance entitled *Together from the Start* (DfES, 2003) for professionals working with disabled children from birth to 2 years, aimed at achieving a family and child-centred response from professionals.

Linked with this is the development of care co-ordination through the role of key workers in a number of areas across the country. This initiative began in 1999 and seeks to minimize the difficulties parents can experience in having to negotiate a range of services to access support, often having to tell their story repeatedly to a trail of different professionals in order to get their needs met. The scheme responds to messages from research which have presented parents' views on this matter. Families who have someone who acts as a co-ordinator or 'key worker' tend to have better relationships with services, higher morale, fewer unmet needs, and are better informed (Glendinning, 1986; Beresford, 1995; Sloper and Turner, 1992).

In an attempt to promote social inclusion and raise standards in early years provision generally for children with disabilities as well as children and families with other social and educational needs, the Early Excellence Programmes were established by the government in 1997 following the White Paper *Excellence in Schools* (DfES, 1997) with the development of Early Excellence Centres (29 had been developed across the country by December 1999) to promote effective early identification and intervention for children with special educational needs, promoting where possible inclusion in mainstream provision and embracing other government initiatives and projects such as SureStart, Early Years Development and Education Action Zones. The aim is to provide good quality integrated early education and day care for children and their parents needing the support of centre-based provision. Another aim which is consistent with much other current social policy is to promote effective multi-agency co-operation between education, social services, health and other agencies. This theme of multi-agency and multi-professionals working together will be discussed later in the chapter.

All children need to play and have fun. However, there is a danger that when a child has additional needs due to a disability this important developmental experience can be lost due to a lack of opportunity. Play is essential to the development of communication, language and early numeracy and the acquisition of basic skills in these areas. Opportunities for inclusive play activities with non-disabled children are very important to the development of disabled children. The support of home learning specialists for pre-school children and their parents can also help with play and a range of other important developmental issues, offering stability, encouragement and support for parents in what can be an uncertain time for them.

EARLY SCHOOL YEARS

Children with disabilities currently access a range of educational provision across mainstream and special schools and units (i.e. just for children with statements of special educational needs) offering both separate and integrated opportunities. One in five children in England and Wales (1.9 million children) have special educational needs (which may be with or without a specific disability), and two-thirds of children with special educational needs attend mainstream schools (Audit Commission, 2003b).

The term 'special educational needs' was introduced in the 1981 Education Act and replaced the categories of handicap used in the 1944 Education Act. Inclusion in the education system is a fairly recent development for children with severe learning difficulties with the implementation in 1971 of the Education of Handicapped Children Act 1970. Prior to this, doctors had reserved for themselves the right to decide whether a child was 'educable' or 'ineducable'. Those who were deemed 'ineducable' were sent to Junior Training Centres run by local health authorities.

The 1993 and 1996 Education Acts continued to employ the term 'special educational needs', and a system of statutory assessment for children leading to provision has developed around this concept which is currently maintained through the Revised SEN Code of Practice (DfES, 2001). This is a guide for early education settings, state schools and local education authorities detailing the help they should give to children who have, or are thought to have, special educational needs. Schools and local education authorities must take account of the Code when they deal with a child with special educational needs. A Statement of Special Educational Needs resulting from an assessment is designed to ensure that the support needed by an individual child to progress educationally is available to him/her either in a mainstream or special school setting.

Formal assessment can provoke considerable concern for some parents who may be anxious about their child acquiring a label. The process can be very stressful and even intimidating for parents only just coming to terms with their child's disability.

On the other hand, for some parents it can come as a relief to have their child's needs assessed to provide a detailed picture of their needs and thereby help them to secure the right kind of educational support and provision for their child.

Statemented children can have a wide variety of needs related to a wide range of disabilities or difficulties from learning disability or physical disability, hearing or visual impairment to autism and Asperger's syndrome, and emotional and behavioural difficulties – or a combination of these, although the Code of Practice states that 'Statements will be rare for children under two…' (SEN Code of Practice 2001, Section 4.48).

For very young children who are screened and found to be deaf, then early intervention may be extremely important to facilitate communication between these children and their families and the development of linguistic skills, providing the parents have come to terms with the news of their child's deafness and are ready to make informed decisions. If the child has other disabilities in addition to deafness, such as visual impairment or physical disability, then it will be very important that a multi-professional assessment is undertaken as soon as possible to determine an appropriate support programme for the child.

The debate about integration versus segregation is a contentious one (Jerrom, 2002; Wilson, 2000; Gillen, 2002). The Audit Commission (2003b) found schools struggling to balance pressures to raise standards of attainment and become more inclusive. Opinions are still divided between those who promote inclusion for all pupils regardless of their disabilities and difficulties, and those who see a continuing role for special schools to cater for those with the most complex needs. Mainstream schools now take many children who would have previously been sent to special schools and the severity of disabilities and difficulties has thereby now increased in special schools – particularly as those children with profound and multiple disabilities are surviving much longer because of improvements in medical interventions.

Different models of inclusive practice have been developed across the country by individual schools and local education authorities responding to local needs, including special schools or units linking with mainstream schools and working together; generic special schools which range across, for example, MLD (moderate learning difficulties), SLD (severe learning difficulties) and autistic units all in the same building; regional centres for low-incidence disabilities such as visual or hearing impairments; the relocation of special schools and units on mainstream sites with dual registration for children in mainstream and special schools (for example with children with severe learning difficulties to help them to be a part of the school community and not an occasional addition). Resistance can be found in mainstream schools to inclusion, when it is seen as detrimental to other children and a change in attitude here through countering ignorance and fear is fundamental to pursuing this important shift in policy and practice. Scope has produced a very useful checklist and guide for parents to including children with cerebral palsy in mainstream primary and secondary schools (Brewis and James, undated). As Mittler (2000) points out, schools are society's agents for socializing children and young people and, as such, have a duty to promote inclusion effectively in order to challenge negative attitudes and promote by example the respect for, and valuing of, diversity and difference.

Many parents find the experience of the school years as positive and supportive. The school environment can act as a fairly easy contact point for other services, such as health and social care, where a multi-professional approach is fostered. Contact with other parents informally or through support groups contributes to a sense for parents of accessible sources of support, information and advice.

COMMUNICATION

For professionals working with young disabled children, ascertaining their wishes and feelings is an important aspect of any direct work with them. Some disabled children do not develop verbal communication, and familiarity with other communication systems such as Bliss, Makaton and British Sign Language will be extremely important for anyone interacting with these children.

For some children, the severity of their disability may appear to prevent them from communicating. There is an increased awareness of communication techniques in work with children and adults with severe learning difficulties (e.g. Caldwell, 1996; Porter *et al.*, 2001) where intellectual and communication difficulties limit the articulation of wishes, preferences and choices. Choice is a crucial aspect of growing personal autonomy and those who work directly with children with profound and complex learning difficulties know that, like everyone else, they make choices all the time – for example, gravitating repeatedly towards a particular individual or avoiding another. There is a need therefore to develop finely tuned communication skills such as listening and observation to pick up changes in expression or demeanour – what Beamer and Brookes (2001, p. 29) refer to as 'choice-making behaviour'. An internal dialogue and reflexive approach on the part of the professional worker are also necessary to ensure as accurate an interpretation of meaning as possible. Inclusion of the whole network of people who know the child well may be important as a means of accessing a detailed knowledge and understanding of the child's communication patterns and ways of expressing feelings and preferences.

DISABLED CHILDREN: VULNERABILITY AND PROTECTION

Child protection policy and practice are discussed in Chapter 11. Whilst it is not possible to explore this in any depth here, it is important briefly to outline issues about vulnerability and protection which are of particular significance for disabled children and their carers.

Disabled children are more vulnerable to neglect and abuse (physical, sexual and emotional) than non-disabled children (Westcott, 1991; Westcott and Cross, 1996; DH/DfES, 2004). There are a number of reasons for this. For many years the social context which made disabled children invisible led to professional inertia and indifference towards their vulnerability. The climate has changed, but prejudice, discrimination and oppression still remain factors to be challenged within organizations and within individual professional workers (Westcott and Cross, 1996; Colton, 2002). Disabled children often have a continuing physical and social dependency on carers as a result of their disability. There may also be multiple caregivers involved with a particular child's care due to respite care or residential schooling, which may expose that child to increased risk, particularly where distance from the family home makes regular contact difficult and parents are less able to monitor care and notice when it is inadequate or inappropriate. At home, pressure on families when a child has challenging behaviours or very demanding physical needs can also be a contributing factor to stress levels within a family, and in such instances regular support and breaks for parents are important in the protection of children through ensuring that parents are adequately supported themselves.

PARENTS' EXPERIENCES

There is a range of literature that has emerged during the past 20 years or so, highlighting the experiences of parents caring at home for a disabled child, and the difficulties commonly faced (e.g. Bayley, 1973; Kew, 1975; Gath, 1978; Wilkin, 1979; Worthington, 1982; Baldwin, 1985; Read, 1991; Shah, 1992; Dyson, 1993; Beresford, 1994; Burke and Cigno, 1996; Read, 2000; Redmond and Richardson, 2003; Evans, 2004).

Themes include the stresses which parents experience (Bayley, 1973; Glendinning, 1983; Quine and Pahl, 1986), though more recent research has highlighted the rewards of family caregiving (Clifford, 1990; Beresford, 1994). Other issues have been the struggles to secure the services they need (McCormack, 1978; Pahl and Quine, 1987), poor disclosure of the diagnosis (Cunningham and Davis, 1985), difficulties for siblings (Kew, 1975; Dyson, 1993; Atkinson and Crawford, 1995), and unhelpful professional attitudes and approaches (Beresford *et al.*, 1996; Hall, 1997).

Glendinning (1983) highlighted several important areas of support for families from social workers – someone to talk to, the provision of practical help, and sensitive responses to ambivalent feelings. Anderson (1982) also stressed the relevance of both emotional and practical support and the importance of focussing on both in order to achieve meaningful interventions.

The Audit Commission has produced an important report on services for disabled children (Audit Commission, 2003a). The researchers interviewed 240 disabled children, young people, and their families about their experiences. The study found that it is harder for disabled children and their families to contribute to everyday life in the way that others take for granted. At worst, this can result in the social exclusion of the whole family. Key issues for parents were barriers to economic participation, and concerns about housing, limited child care options and inaccessible benefits information. Play and leisure services were critical for children. Where there was flexibility and sensitivity to a child's needs, the opportunity to play with disabled and non-disabled peers was highly valued. Restricted access, service gaps or bullying cultures put pressure on the whole family. Parents and children said that their successful access to services, social activities, education and employment depended crucially on the accessibility of transport. The research confirmed that the so-called 'postcode lottery of care' was still very much in evidence. Much still depends on where families live and how hard parents are willing to push for services. They also found that often too little was being provided, too late, with long waits for information, equipment and treatment and that families have to negotiate a maze of services which is frustrating and confusing.

None of this is new, but pockets of good and innovative practice are developing through the initiatives outlined earlier and, as can be seen from the preceding discussion, change is accumulative and in the right direction. Parents and children are being listened to much more.

PARTNERSHIP

Working in partnership has become an important aspect of professional interaction with parents who use formal services. It has been part of a wider policy development towards more consumer power generally as the public sector became increasingly subjected to a market-style approach. The Children Act 1989 recognized the crucial role of families as the most appropriate place for children to be brought up. Supporting parents in doing this effectively, in partnership with professionals, is seen, in the majority of cases, as the most efficient use of public resources.

Research over the years has demonstrated that professional support for parents of disabled children is beneficial (Younghusband *et al.*, 1970; Hannam, 1975; Glendinning, 1983; Ayer and Alaszewski, 1984) and also that parents' unique knowledge and expertise about their child must be recognized (Beresford, 1995).

However, 'partnership' is not an easy concept in practice. Social work literature has paid much attention to trying to tease out its meaning and usefulness for practitioners. As Stevenson and Parsloe (1993) comment: 'Partnership is very vague since it suggests an equality which is rarely possible.' (Stevenson and Parsloe, 1993, p. 6).

Handy (1985) attempted to analyse the operation of power in organizations and described five aspects of 'social' power which could be used to exert influence over another person:

- physical power;
- resource power;
- position power;
- expert power;
- personal power.

Professionals can be seen to have resource power, position power (conferred via their perceived status and role) and expert power (knowledge gained through training that is ascribed to their particular role) and may be able to use personal power through the force of their own personality. Physical power in extreme cases may be wielded with the support of the organization by invoking state power through legislation to remove children from their families to prevent harm. Against this weighty armour parents and service users may have less overall power, though policy and practice in recent years has attempted to shift the balance towards them by ensuring consultation and consideration of their views, and making professional decision-making more transparent. Within the professional–parent relationship an explicit exploration of the expertise that each brings to the situation is a helpful way forward.

Solomon (1976), in relation to black service users or clients' interactions with formal welfare service provision, identified three potential sources of powerlessness which can be usefully generalized, covering negative self-images, negative experiences in engaging with external systems, and systems which consistently block and deny powerless groups the opportunity to take effective action. Solomon made a direct link between empowerment and the service delivery system: 'The success or failure of empowerment is directly related to the degree to which (the) service delivery system itself is an obstacle course or an opportunity system.' (Solomon, 1976, p. 29).

Interestingly, in the light of Solomon's comments, the National Report, Services for Disabled Children (Audit Commission, 2003a) found a jigsaw puzzle of services. Families still have to struggle through a maze of services to track down essential information. They then have to jump through a series of hoops to try and gain access to formal support. When they manage to be considered for help, families are asked to repeat their painful stories to a series of different staff. Services tend to work to their own priorities rather than plan jointly, so families fall through the gaps between services. It is hardly surprising that parents often feel that they are constantly fighting with support services to get the help they need.

Partnership between agencies has also been a policy aim of government for some time, both at strategic and operational levels, with limited success. Professional teams working in different organizations, with different management structures, different cultures, values, pressures and priorities can work against meeting the needs of children and families effectively and efficiently and in an holistic way. Developments within the Children Act (2004) seem to be emphasizing a need for a change in culture with greater emphasis on partnership and more joint working between agencies. Proposals include the development of a common assessment framework between agencies; more integrated services and organizational structures; improved information sharing; and more clearly defined accountability through the introduction of lead professionals where several different professionals are involved with a family. The lead professional will be responsible for ensuring a coherent and co-ordinated package of services for an individual child and family. There is a real need for what the National Service Framework (DH/DfES, 2004; p 24) calls 'seamless integrated working'.

Conclusion

Changes in culture can take time to manifest, but there are a number of government initiatives now working to improve services and to develop an integrated and inclusive approach for disabled children and their families through the Children's Trusts pilots; the Children's National Service Framework which has a working group specifically for disabled children and their families; the Quality Protects Programme in which disabled children have been a priority area and other programmes mentioned earlier such as early identification and intervention and care co-ordination schemes.

This chapter has looked very broadly at policy and practice issues and developments for disabled children and their families. Whilst progress remains patchy, with hard-pressed statutory agencies often struggling to provide an adequate service for an increasingly complex population of disabled children, it can be seen from the limited scope of this discussion that significant steps forward are being taken in the drive to provide a more inclusive experience for young disabled children and their families.

Student activity

Consider current barriers to inclusion for children with disabilities and their families (e.g. in pre-school facilities, schools, leisure and friendship) and strategies at individual and societal levels to overcome these. Discuss your considerations with a fellow student or colleague.

REFERENCES

Aldgate, J and Tunstill, J (1995): *Making Sense of Section 17. A Study for the Department of Health: Implementing Services for Children in Need within the 1989 Children Act.* London: HMSO.

Anderson, D (1982): *Social Work and Mental Handicap.* London: Macmillan.

Atkinson, N and Crawford, M (1995): *All in the Family: Siblings and Disability.* London: NCH Action for Children.

Audit Commission (1994): *Seen But Not Heard: Coordinating Community Child Health and Social Services for Children in Need.* London: HMSO.

Audit Commission (2003a): *National Report on Services for Disabled Children* (online) London: HMSO. http://www.audit-commission.gov.uk/reports (accessed 29.4.04).

Audit Commission (2003b): *National Report on Special Educational Needs* (online) London: HMSO. http://www.audit-commission.gov.uk/reports (accessed 29.4.04).

Ayer, S and Alaszewski, A (1984): *Community Care and the Mentally Handicapped: Services for mothers and their mentally handicapped children.* London: Croom Helm.

Baldwin, S (1985): *The Costs of Caring: Families with Disabled Children.* London: Routledge and Kegan Paul.

Bayley, M (1973): *Mental Handicap and Community Care.* London: Routledge and Kegan Paul.

Baxter, C, Kamaljit, P, Ward, L and Nadershaw, Z (1990): *Double Discrimination: Issues and Services for People with Learning Difficulties from Black and Ethnic Minority Communities.* London: King's Fund Centre.

Beamer, S and Brookes, M (2001): *Making Decisions. Best practice and new ideas for supporting people with high support needs to make decisions.* London: Values into Action.

Beresford, B (1994): *Positively Parents: Caring for a Severely Disabled Child.* London: HMSO.

Beresford, B (1995): *Expert Opinions: A survey of parents caring for a severely disabled child.* Bristol: Policy Press.

Beresford, B, Sloper, P, Baldwin, S and Newman, T (1996): *What Works in Services for Families with a Disabled Child?* Barkingside: Barnados.

Bond, J and Bond, S (1994): *Sociology and Health Care: An Introduction for Nurses and Other Health Care Professionals,* 2nd edn. London: Churchill Livingstone.

Bowlby, J (1979): *The Making and Breaking of Affectional Bonds.* London: Tavistock.

Brewis, L and James, J (undated): *A Guide to Including Children with Cerebral Palsy into Mainstream Primary and Secondary Schools.* London: Scope (online) http://www. scope.org.uk (accessed 12.4.04).

Burke, P and Cigno, K (1996): *Support for Families. Helping children with learning disabilities.* Aldershot: Avebury.

Caldwell, P (1996): *Getting in Touch.* Brighton: Pavilion.

Chamba, R, Ahmad, W, Hirst, M, Lawton, D and Beresford, B (1999): *On the Edge: Minority Ethnic Families Caring for a Severely Disabled Child.* Bristol: Policy Press.

Clifford, D (1990): *The Social Costs and Rewards of Care.* Aldershot: Avebury.

Colton, M (2002): Factors associated with abuse in residential child care institutions. *Children and Society,* **16**(1), 33–44.

Cunningham, C and Davis, H (1985): Early parent counselling. In Craft, M, Bicknell, J and Hollins, S (eds), *Mental Handicap. A Multi Disciplinary Approach.* Eastbourne: Bailliere Tindall.

Cunningham, C, Morgan, P and McGucken, R (1984): Down's syndrome: Is dissatisfaction with disclosure of diagnosis inevitable? *Developmental Medicine and Child Neurology*, **26**, 33–39.

Department for Education and Skills (1997): *White Paper, Excellence in Schools.* London: HMSO.

Department for Education and Skills (2001): *Revised Code of Practice for Special Educational Needs.* London: HMSO.

Department for Education and Skills/Department of Health (2003): *Together from the Start. Practical guidance for professionals working with disabled children (birth to third birthday) and their families.* London: HMSO.

Department for Work and Pensions (2004): *Family Resources Survey 2002–3.* www.dwp.gov.uk/asd/frs/

Department of Health (2001): *Valuing People. A New Strategy for Learning Disability for the 21st Century.* London: HMSO.

Department of Health (2002): *Planning with People. Towards Person Centred Approaches.* London: HMSO.

Department of Health, Department for Education and Employment and the Home Office (2000): *Framework for Assessing Children in Need and their Families.* London: The Stationery Office.

Department of Health and the Department for Education and Skills (2004): *The National Service Framework for Children, Young People and Maternity Services: Standard 8.* London: DH.

Disability Rights Commission (2002): *Code of Practice for Schools – Disability Discrimination Act 1995: Part 4.* London: TSO.

Dyson, LL (1993): Response to the presence of a child with disabilities: Parental stress and family functioning over time. *American Journal on Mental Retardation*, **98**, 207–218.

Evans, K (2004): One family's fight. *Community Care*, 1522, pp. 42–43, 13–19 May 2004.

Finkelstein, V (1980): *Attitudes and Disabled People: Issues for Discussion.* New York: World Rehabilitation Fund.

Finkelstein, V (1991): Disability: an administrative challenge? In Oliver, M (ed.), *Social Work, Disabled People and Disabling Environments.* London: Jessica Kingsley.

Gath, A (1978): *Down's Syndrome and the family – the early years.* London: Academic Press.

Gillen, S (2002): Can mainstream schools cope with children who have special needs? *Community Care*, 5 December.

Glendinning, C (1983): *Parents and their Disabled Children.* London: Routledge and Kegan Paul.

Glendinning, C (1986): *A Single Door: Social work with families of disabled children.* London: Allen and Unwin.

Hall, D (1997): Child development teams: are they fulfilling their purpose? *Child: Care, Health and Development*, **23**(1), 87–99.

Handy, C (1985): *Understanding Organisations.* Harmondsworth: Penguin.

Hannam, C (1975): *Parents and Mentally Handicapped Children.* Harmondsworth: Penguin.

Heron, C (1998): *Working with Carers.* London: Jessica Kingsley.

Jerrom, C (2002): Should special schools close? *Community Care*, 25 November.

Jones, H (2001): *Disabled Children's Rights: A Practical Guide.* International Save the Children Alliance. Sweden: Save the Children.

Kew, S (1975): *Handicap and Family Crisis. A Study of the Siblings of Handicapped Children.* London: Pitman.

Kubler Ross, E (1969): *On Death and Dying.* London: Tavistock/Routledge.

Lindemann, E (1944): The symptomatology and management of acute grief. *American Journal of Psychiatry*, **101**, 141.

McCormack, M (1978): *A Mentally Handicapped Child in the Family.* London: Constable.

Means, R and Smith, R (1994): *Community Care. Policy and Practice.* Basingstoke: Macmillan.

Mencap (1999): *Living in Fear.* London: Mencap.

Mittler, P (2000): *Working Towards Inclusive Education: Social Contexts.* London: Fulton.

Morris, P (1969): *Put Away: A Sociological Study of Institutions for the Mentally Retarded.* London Routledge and Kegan Paul.

Murray, P and Penman, J (eds) (2000): *Telling Our Own Stories. Reflections on family life in a disabling world.* Sheffield: Parents with Attitude.

Oliver, M (1983): *Social Work with Disabled People.* Basingstoke: Macmillan.

Oliver, M (1990): *The Politics of Disablement.* London: Macmillan.

Oliver, M (1994): Moving on: from welfare paternalism to welfare citizenship. *Journal of the Centre for Social Action*, **2** (1).

Olshansky, S (1962): Chronic sorrow, a response to having a mentally defective child. *Social Casework*, **43**, 190–193.

Oswin, M (1971): *The Empty Hours. A Study of the Weekend Life of Handicapped Children in Institutions.* Harmondsworth: Penguin.

Oswin, M (1978): *Children Living in Long-Stay Hospitals.* Spastics International Medical Publications Research Monograph No. 5. London: Heinemann Medical.

Oswin, M (2000): Revisiting the empty hours. In Brigham, L, Atkinson, D, Jackson, M, *et al.* (eds), *Crossing Boundaries. Change and Continuity in the History of Learning Disability.* Kidderminster: Bild.

Pahl, J and Quine, L (1987): Families with mentally handicapped children. In Orford, J (ed.), *Coping with Disorder in the Family.* London: Croom Helm.

Payne, S (1999): *Loss and Bereavement.* Buckingham: Open University Press.

Porter, J, Ouvry, C, Morgan, M and Downs, C (2001): Interpreting the communication of people with profound and multiple learning difficulties. *British Journal of Learning Disabilities*, **29**, 12–16.

Quine, L and Pahl, J (1986): Parents with severely mentally handicapped children: marriage and the stress of caring. In Chester, R and Divall, P (eds), *Mental Health, Illness and Handicap in Marriage.* Rugby: National Marriage Guidance Council.

Quine, L and Rutter, DR (1994): First diagnosis of severe mental and physical disability: a study of doctor–patient communication. *Journal of Child Psychology and Psychiatry*, **35**(7), 1273–1287.

Read, J (1991): There was never really any choice: the experience of mothers of disabled children in the United Kingdom. *Women's Studies International Forum*, **14**(6), 561–571.

Read, J (2000): *Disability, the Family and Society: Listening to Mothers.* Buckingham: Open University Press.

Redmond, B and Richardson, V (2003): Just getting on with it: exploring the service needs of mothers who care for young children with severe/profound and life-threatening intellectual disability. *Journal of Applied Research in Intellectual Disabilities*, **16**, 205–218.

Ryan, J and Thomas, F (1980): *The Politics of Mental Handicap.* Harmondsworth: Penguin.

Scope (1994): *Right from the Start.* London: Scope.

Shah, R (1992): *The Silent Minority. Asian Children with Disabilities.* London: National Children's Bureau.

Sloper, P and Turner, S (1992): Service needs of families of children with severe physical disability. *Child: Care, Health and Development*, **18**, 259–282.

Solomon, BB (1976): *Black Empowerment: Social Work in Oppressed Communities.* New York: Columbia University Press.

Stevenson, O and Parsloe, P (1993): *Community Care and Empowerment.* York: Joseph Rowntree Foundation.

Sumpton, R (1988): Poverty and mental handicap. In Becker, S and MacPherson, S (eds), *Public Issues, Private Pain: Social Work and Social Policy.* London: Social Services Insight.

United Nations Convention on the Rights of the Child (1990): New York: United Nations.

Westcott, HL (1991): The abuse of disabled children: a review of the literature. *Child: Care, Health and Development*, **17**(4), 243–258.

Westcott, HL and Cross, M (1996): *This Far and No Further: Towards Ending the Abuse of Disabled Children.* Birmingham: Venture Press.

Wickler, L, Wasow, M and Hatfield, E (1981): Chronic sorrow revisited: parents vs. professional depiction of the adjustment of parents of mentally retarded children. *American Journal of Orthopsychiatry*, **5**(1), 63–70.

Wilkin, D (1979): *Caring for the Mentally Handicapped Child.* London: Croom Helm.

Wilson, J (2000): Doing justice to inclusion. *European Journal of Special Needs Education*, **15**(3), 297–304

Wolfensberger, W (1983): Social role valorisation: a proposed new term for the principle of normalisation. *Mental Retardation*, **21**(6), 234–239.

Worden, JW (1991): *Grief Counselling and Grief Therapy*, 2nd edn. New York: Springer Publishing.

Worthington, A (1982): *Coming to Terms with Mental Handicap.* Huddersfield: Helena Press.

Younghusband, E, Birchall, D, Davie, R and Pringle, MLK (eds) (1970): *Living with Handicap.* London: National Children's Bureau.

CHILD HEALTH

Jayne Taylor and Val Thurtle

This chapter aims to:

- explore the origins of child health practice from an historical perspective;

- discuss the current situation within an holistic framework;

- examine the needs of children with ongoing health needs;

- examine personal and professional partnerships in relation to child health matters.

INTRODUCTION

Health is a very emotive subject. As we read in Chapter 2, one of the very first questions new parents ask after the birth of a baby relates to the *health* of the newborn infant. This concern with health continues throughout childhood and into adulthood. As a nation, we commonly greet each other with the question 'Hello – how are you'?, we write phrases such as 'hoping you are keeping well' in Christmas and birthday cards, and we lift our glasses to each other and say 'good health'.

The answers we give to questions such as 'how are you?' also frequently demonstrate our health-mindedness – 'I'm very well thank you', 'not too bad, although I've got a sore throat ... ', or 'I've had a terrible time of it recently with my back. I'm on four sorts of tablets, the doctor says ... '. One sometimes wonders if we would ever successfully start a conversation if we did not have health to talk about!

This concern extends beyond our own health to that of our children. Adults in general, and parents in particular, become very concerned when the health of a child or a group of children is threatened. The media frequently focusses upon such issues – the links between MMR and autism, the separation of conjoined twins, and so on. Our television screens show us 'fly-on-the wall' documentaries plotting the progress of children in hospital and stories relating to child health appear on an almost daily basis in our newspapers.

This chapter begins by looking at the origins of the current child health focus within our society, before moving on to examine the health of children today and its importance within our holistic philosophy. It then concludes by exploring professional and personal partnerships in relation to child health.

CHILD HEALTH: A NATIONAL CONCERN?

An historical concern?

Our nation's concern with child health is an interesting phenomenon, and it is useful to reflect for a moment upon the origin of this concern, so that we may be able to understand it more clearly and perhaps utilize it in a positive way. However, is this concern new? Certainly in the pre-Victorian era, and to some extent during the Victorian age, the value placed on the lives of children by the nation appeared to be less significant than it is today. That is not to say that parents did not love their children as much as we do now, but rather it reflects the treatment of children by society – particularly the children of the poor, and the orphaned. According to Cox (1983), many of these children grew up in the workhouses or, worse, ended up on the streets of the major cities. Kosky (1992), in an account of the founding of the Queen Elizabeth Hospital in Hackney Road, cites an account in the *Daily News* from 1870, which vividly describes the plight of such children:

> '*In this district of Bethnal Green, in the centre of which the new child's hospital stands, we know of hundreds of tiny breadwinners of two and a half years upwards. It is here that the trade of Lucifer boxes absorbs the energies of infants long before they can speak, and where street after street can be shown full of little workers who pass from infancy to childhood and from childhood to maturity without ever seeing a toy or gazing upon a green field.*'

Surprisingly, many attempts to help the plight of children met with marked opposition, mainly due to their ability to provide cheap labour for the powerful industrialists and at least some income (albeit meagre) for the family (Kosky, 1992). Whilst various Education Acts (e.g. those passed in 1887 and 1906) had introduced social reforms which made education both compulsory and free, and the Coal Mines Act (1845) and various pieces of legislation relating to factories, including the Ten Hours Act of 1847 and the Factory Act of 1901, had limited the legal number of working hours and improved the social conditions of children working in the factories, mines and mills, many children still worked long hours in appalling conditions, and had little or no schooling.

However, even during these seemingly 'dark ages' for children there were glimmers of the concerns with which we are familiar today. The public health movement of the mid-nineteenth century, for example, which developed following two cholera outbreaks in England, was a prime example of middle-class concern for the children of the poor (and marked the beginning of the health visiting service). Voluntary organizations such as Barnardos and the National Children's Home helped many, many homeless and orphaned children, and philanthropists such as Thomas Coram and Charles West campaigned tirelessly to open the Foundling Hospital in Coram Fields and the Hospital for Sick Children in London (more commonly known as Great Ormond Street Hospital), respectively.

Another development which influenced the nation's view of child health at the beginning of the last century resulted from the 1904 Interdepartmental Committee on Physical Deterioration. The knowledge that over half of the young men who had volunteered for the Boer War were unfit for service had prompted the instigation of the committee which recommended, among other reforms, the setting up of a school health service (Meredith Davies, 1975).

At this time there was also a growing interest in the infant welfare movement, which led to the establishment of the first milk depots, improved medical and nursing care, developments in pharmaceutics and better sanitation. These measures undoubtedly made a contribution to the fall in the infant mortality rate, which decreased from 163 per 1000 live births in 1899 to less than 100 per 1000 live births in 1915 (Clark, 1973).

Advances were also being made in our knowledge of epidemiology, and 'killer' diseases such as cholera and typhoid became more rare, although scarlet fever, tuberculosis, diphtheria and poliomyelitis were still prevalent (Department of Health and Social Security, 1976). In 1947, for example, 7984 cases of poliomyelitis were recorded, and almost 10 per cent of sufferers died. A second major epidemic between 1952 and 1954 saw 845 deaths in the UK (Department of Health and Social Security, 1976). The number of cases of tuberculosis gradually decreased with improved social conditions and diet, and with the introduction of mass screening and improved drugs, as well as the introduction of the BCG vaccination in the early 1950s. Diphtheria continued to kill 3000 children a year until the early 1940s, when mass immunization became available and both morbidity and mortality rates declined dramatically (Kosky and Lunnon, 1991).

Following the Second World War, and the decline of infectious and nutritional disorders, attention moved away from these childhood problems and tended to focus on children with chronic illness and disability (Hall, 1992). It was recognized that most childhood disability could be traced back to the perinatal period and that 'early intervention might lead to cure or at least substantial improvement' (Hall, 1992, p. 649). The conviction that if intervention occurred quickly enough disability would be minimized was a popular notion, and led to one of the most dramatic changes in the child health services during the twentieth century. No longer were health professionals to wait for parents to notice anomalies in their child's development and then to seek help. Instead, health professionals needed to go out and assess development in a proactive way so that intervention could be instigated as soon as possible. Nor, according to Hall (1992), was it thought sufficient only to focus upon those children who were thought to be at risk. All children should be brought into the assessment process, and routine developmental screening should be a universal activity.

As a result of these convictions our child health services developed along two almost mutually exclusive pathways during the last decades of the twentieth century. First, we had the preventative child health services – community-based health care professionals, including health visitors and school nurses, who spent significant amounts of their time undertaking mass screening of the childhood population. The preoccupation with screening was however, according to Hall and Elliman (2003), not only wasteful in terms of resource allocation, but also doubtful in terms of its efficacy, given that many of the screening tests being utilized were not based on sound evidence. The second pathway was the development of acute hospital services which have undergone radical change (Taylor *et al.*, 1999) over the period and will be subject to further change as a result of the implementation of the *National Service Framework (NSF) for Children, Young People and Maternity Services Part 1: standards for hospital services* (DH/DfES, 2004).

The problem for the child and the family is that the preventative and therapeutic services have tended to function in separate silos, with little common ground between the two. Add to this picture the input of social services who work in yet a third silo and we can start to see that it is possible for some families to be caught up in three bureaucratic systems. This is indeed the story we hear time and time again in our work with children – particularly those with ongoing health needs who have contact with all three services.

THE SITUATION TODAY

The situation at the beginning of the twenty-first century is one of variability. Changes are taking place in service delivery, but they are tending to be patchy. There are, for example, some excellent examples of good partnership working between community child health and social services, and between acute and community-based services. The key word though is 'patchy', and there is a definite commitment within central government to remove what is colloquially phrased the 'postcode lottery of care'. We explore more about this in Chapter 14. Things are, however, changing for the better, and we will explore some of these changes in the rest of this chapter. We start by looking at the preventative child health services and the growing emphasis on public health, followed by a brief look at other significant developments.

The view that routine broad-based screening will contribute to good child health has, to a large extent, remained consistent to the present day. Recently, however, the value of wide-ranging routine screening has been questioned in favour of a more limited core universal screening regime based on sound evidence of efficacy. Hall and Elliman (2003) argue that routine screening outside of a core programme makes little contribution to the detection of serious impairments which are more likely to be detected in the perinatal period through, for example, skilled neonatal examination, and by listening to parents' concerns. Consequently, in some areas of the country the practice of routine broad-based screening has virtually ceased. In any case, screening *per se* does not lead to good health but is a means of detecting difficulties – admittedly in many instances early detection may prevent the longer-term consequences of ill health. Hall and Elliman (2003) suggest that more emphasis should be placed on targeting resources to needy areas, utilizing processes that enable professionals to determine the needs of individual families, and meeting individual and community needs once they have been identified. *The National Service Framework for Children, Young People and Maternity Services* (DH/DfES, 2004) sets out a new Child Health Promotion framework which will be implemented over the next decade and will ensure a universal standard which includes some routine screening procedures, but also emphasizes the use of professional judgement to target resources effectively.

We must, however, recognize that not all illness and disability are by any means congenital and will not therefore be present during the perinatal period. The health of a child can be affected at any stage of development. Early years professionals working with children of all ages may be among the first to recognize changes in behaviour, physical or psychological symptoms, or other, sometimes subtle, changes which are indicative of health problems. This might be a health visitor or nursery nurse meeting a mother and child in a toddler group, a practice nurse giving a routine immunization, or a school nurse at school entry. Hall and Elliman (2003) recommend that pre-school records should be reviewed on school entry, height and weight should be measured at that point and child, parent(s) and school nurse should meet together to establish a relationship. Orthoptists should ideally screen all 4- to 5-year-olds and hearing tests are also carried out. Children with a known health problem or who have been identified as having difficulties will be seen more frequently but, as we have alluded to above, routine surveillance of all young children is not seen as necessary.

A second change which has occurred recently – and which is having an impact upon child health and the management of ill health – is the move away from hospital services towards a primary care-led National Health Service (see also Chapter 10). The government has placed responsibility for commissioning services within primary care, where some 90 per cent of care is actually delivered and the public health agenda has been given precedence in the development of services. Health in its widest sense is seen as central to child and human development. The promotion of health, taking account of physical, mental, emotional and social well-being, will ensure that young people can take advantage of their opportunities during their time of greatest growth and development, as well as reducing health problems in later life. To do this necessitates a wide or public health approach facilitating the well-being of children in the context of the family, school and community. This will require the assessment of health needs both on an individual and group basis. Such needs may be problem-orientated – looking at the causes of diseases or pathogenesis – but also highlight ways of promoting well-being or salutogenesis (Cowley, 2000). The philosophy of salutogenesis is concerned with identifying factors that create health and exploring factors that contribute to healing or a resistance to breakdown, physical or psychological. Activities and structures that build and create health should be developed by the children, parents and early years professionals concerned, so that all children develop to the highest possible level in terms of health and then, probably as a result, academic achievement.

Public health is a much-used term amongst community health professionals (Cowley, 2002), and is evident in government documents (DoH, 1999a, 2001a,b). There is much debate on the meaning of public health; the most frequently used starting point (Acheson, 1988) stresses the importance of 'the science and art of preventing disease, prolonging life and promoting health through the organised efforts of society'. In order to achieve maximum effectiveness health, education and social services departments will need to work together (this is discussed more fully later in this chapter). Examples of such a co-ordinated approach can be found in the evolution of Children's NHS Trusts, SureStart (see www.surestart.gov.uk), the Health Promoting Schools Programme (WHO, 1993) and, more recently, the National Healthy Schools Standard (Department for Education and Employment, 1999). In general terms, public health seeks to improve health and tackle inequalities by working with individuals, communities and government. In terms of young children, this might be realized through the design and implementation of programmes designed to encourage physical activity, promote a positive diet and reduce stress. It is not a case of health workers undertaking these programmes, rather an integrated approach with health, education, parents and children themselves as well as the local community addressing the issues together. Focussing on communities, Saving Lives (DoH, 1999a), for example, encourages all schools to become healthy schools, characterizing the principle that 'good health and social behaviour underpin effective learning and academic achievement which in turn promotes long term health gain' (p. 46).

Promoting public health has much to do with reducing inequalities and addressing poverty. The Acheson Report (Acheson, 1998) highlighted a multitude of health inequalities, many of which have been taken up as government initiatives, but specifically selects those that affect children and young people. Many derive directly from the impoverished circumstances in which some children are raised, while others relate to mental health issues and dental decay. The number of children in the UK living in a household which has an income below 50 per cent of the contemporaneous average after housing costs rose threefold between 1979 and 1999 (Bradshaw, 2002). The number of children still living in poverty within London (35 per cent of children compared with 30% nationally and 31% in the north) remains high. Links between poverty and child death are well established (Quiglars, 2001) and, while it is more difficult to demonstrate, there are indications that those living in poor socio-economic circumstances are more likely to have poorer health than their more affluent counterparts (Johnson, 2001). The very magnitude of the impact of inequalities is awesome. Those working with young children are likely to want to respond to the challenge by promoting healthier life-styles, for example encouraging cycling and walking, addressing nutrition and supporting children's emotional well-being by creating an accepting environment where they feel secure and can express their hopes, fears and concerns. The Acheson Report (Acheson, 1998) further advises the need to identify additional resources for children from less well-off groups, improving nutrition within schools, adding fluoride to water, and developing health-promoting schools.

Clearly, professionals working with children and families are ideally placed to participate in this somewhat challenging agenda. Talking specifically of school nurses, for example, *Making a Difference* (Department of Health, 1999b) points out they are '… playing a vital role in equipping young people with the knowledge to make healthy lifestyle choices' (p. 13). Such an outlook highlights the proactive nature of their work rather than merely responding to ill health and developmental difficulties. The document further advises that school nurses, by taking a public health role and leading teams of nurses and community and education workers, are expected to contribute to personal, health and social education and to citizenship training, work with parents to encourage positive parenting, promote positive mental health in young people as well as advise and co-ordinate health care to children with medical needs.

A third significant change which is gradually occurring at all levels within the health services relates to the relationship between professionals, children and their parents. 'Empowerment' of patients/clients and 'Patient and Public Involvement' are popular 'buzz words' to describe enabling of better decision-making through the acquisition of knowledge. The NHS performance assessment framework scores NHS organizations on the extent to which they respond to patient/client concerns and involve patients in the development and delivery of health services. Empowerment, it can be argued, has also been facilitated by the media and technological advancement in communication structures. As we mentioned at the beginning of this chapter, newspapers, the television and radio news liberally allocate their columns and time-slots to issues on child health and well-being. Usually, such news reports adversity, but it nevertheless serves an educative function and helps to empower through the acquisition of knowledge. Take a look also along the shelves in any large newsagent, and there will be a vast array of magazines devoted solely (or largely) to health. Many of these relate specifically to child health matters and play an important role in informing parents about current child health practices and child care issues, including prevention of ill health as well as health promotion. The internet too provides a multiplicity of sites and information about child health – it is possible to find information on almost any topic.

It is, however, important that we do not become complacent. Patterns of childhood morbidity and mortality indicate that there are both geographical and socio-economic variations, showing that there is still room for improvement. For example, data from the National Statistics Office show there are still a significant number of deaths attributed to '*signs and symptoms and ill-defined conditions*', which include sudden infant death syndrome as well as preventable deaths from other causes. The largest numbers of deaths, for example among boys aged 5 to 15 years are due to accidents, most attributable to transport; accidents are the second largest cause of death among girls of the same age, second only to cancer (National Statistics online, 2004).

Finally, we have seen over the past decade the emergence of new and different health issues affecting our children. Two examples are childhood obesity and sickle cell anaemia. The number of obese children in the UK has risen dramatically in recent years. The Health Survey for England (Joint Health Surveys Unit on behalf of the Department of Health, 2002) says that 8.5 per cent of 6-year-olds and 15 per cent of 15-year-olds were obese, with others also being overweight, if not obese. This seems to be more the case amongst those from an Asian background and those from less advantageous socio-economic backgrounds. It is a major issue in terms of their health in the future, with obesity contributing to the risk of heart disease and diabetes in later life, but also on their sense of well-being in the here and now, relevant to the issue of mental health mentioned above. The Health Development Agency (Mulvihill and Quigley, 2003) report there is evidence to support the use of multifaceted school-based interventions to reduce obesity and being overweight in school children. This might include nutrition teaching, physical activity promotion (government targets were established in 2004), more activity material to use in the curriculum and the modification of school meals and tuck shops. Such input would be to the benefit of children who are overweight and to those who may become so later in childhood.

Our second example of a new and emerging health issue challenging many health communities is sickle cell anaemia. Estimates are that 1 in 80 people of West African origin and 1 in 200 people of Jamaican origin have sickle cell anaemia. There are said to be over 9000 people in London with this condition, and they often feel poorly understood (Hall and Elliman, 2003). Sickle cell disease is a genetic condition. People with sickle cell anaemia have sickle haemoglobin (HbS), which is different from normal haemoglobin (HbA). If the gene giving the instruction to make HbS is inherited from one parent, the individual has sickle cell trait and can be a carrier of the condition. However, if the affected gene is inherited from both parents, they will only be able to make HbS. When HbS gives up its oxygen to the tissues, it sticks together to form long rods inside the red blood cells, making them rigid and sickle-shaped. The sickling causes pain which is often triggered by cold damp conditions, infections and dehydration. Those parents with such a child should know of the diagnosis and understand the limitations that sickle cell anaemia can impose on a child – the need for frequent drinks and easy access to lavatories and the triggering of pain by over-exertion or cold.

Obesity and sickle cell anaemia are by no means the only two issues that have emerged as significant problems over the past few years – there are clearly others such as HIV/AIDS, and a rise in autism-spectrum disorders, among others. A significant number of children are living with long-term (often complex) health needs, and it is on this group of children that we will now focus.

THE CHILD WITH ONGOING HEALTH NEEDS

The situation today is a complex one in terms of child health. We have hospital services for children which are generally for acute, short-term care, after which care tends to be transferred to community-based services. Far fewer children now die in early childhood as compared to 50 years ago (National Statistics online, 2004). Technology has led to more children who have experienced difficulties surviving through childhood and into adulthood, some with long-term health needs or disabilities. Hall and Elliman (2003) identify that some 3 per cent of all children have a disability of some sort, and about half of these disabilities are considered to be severe (see also Chapter 12). This means that there are increasing numbers of children within the community who are in some way 'ill' or who have additional needs, and who would traditionally have spent a longer period of time in hospital, or in some cases would have been

Table 13.1 Hypothetical example of professional involvement with one family

Professional	Input
Health visitor	Family health promotion and supportive relationship
Social worker (local authority)	Respite care, benefits, mobility issues
Social worker (SCOPE)	Respite care and specific advice
Community children's nurse	PEG feeding regime
Continence services nurse	Management of incontinence
Physiotherapist	Prevention of contractures and other therapy
School nurse	Management of health needs in the school setting and beyond
School teacher	Education
Classroom assistant	Educational support and general care
Speech and language therapist	Speech therapy
Occupational therapist	Support with home adaptations
Wheelchair services personnel	Provision of wheelchair
Hospital medical services	Regular review at out-patients
Community physician	Review of development
GP	Ongoing care as required
Practice nurse	Immunizations

permanently institutionalized. These children attend playgroups, nurseries and schools, and their care is shared by parents, educationalists and health and social care professionals within communities. Because many of these children have complex needs, it is unlikely that the 'sharing' of care will be with only one or even two professionals. A child with, for example, severe learning disabilities and physical disabilities might well be receiving aspects of their care from a dozen or more professional agencies. A hypothetical example is shown in Table 13.1 for a child aged 4 years with severe learning disabilities due to cerebral palsy who attends a special school.

This example is an extreme one, but for children with complex health needs and their families it is not an unusual one. In addition to the professionals involved in the care of such children (and we may not have thought of them all), there is likely to be a series of respite carers as well as other voluntary workers, family and friends.

Not all children with a disability will attend a special school, of course, or have such complex needs. The adoption of the principle of inclusion in education means that such children are increasingly attending mainstream schools. Excellence for all Children (DfEE, 1997) sets out stronger rights for the inclusion of children in mainstream education. If parents want a place for their child, the utmost must be done to facilitate this. This is fully supported in the Special Educational Needs Code of Practice (DfES, 2002). Not all children with special educational needs have a health problem, and not all those with a diagnosed health difficulty need support with their education, but there is a strong overlap in the two groups. Croll and Moses (2000) set out teachers' descriptions of children in Key Stage 2 (7- to 11-year-old) classes with special needs in a variety of classes and schools in 1998. In their classes, 26 per cent of children were seen as having special educational needs. Not surprisingly, learning was the most frequently mentioned nature of difficulty, with 23 per cent of children deemed to be in this category. Some 5 per cent of children were regarded as having an emotional and behavioural difficulty, and 4 per cent a health, sensory and physical difficulty. Clearly, these different groups of children overlap, with some children experiencing difficulties in all three areas. Sensory and physical difficulties may well be seen as a health concern and, within our holistic view (see the Introduction of this book), emotional and behavioural difficulties are also encompassed within health.

Croll and Moses' (2000) study confirmed earlier findings which noted that emotional and behavioural difficulties form the largest cause of difficulties among school children (British Paediatric Association, 1995). Awareness of this area of need has grown in the intervening years, with an increasing interest in the significance of mental health and behaviour difficulties amongst the school-age population. The Mental Health Foundation report (1999), *Bright Futures*, noted that one in five children are experiencing psychological problems including anxiety and depression as well as major developmental delays at any one time.

With the reduction of the number of places in special school and the commitment to the concept of inclusion there are more children with health needs in mainstream schools (Hall and Elliman, 2003). The majority cope well, gaining a full education and enriching the experience of their classmates. The practical healthcare of these children may be delegated to teachers, secretaries or classroom assistants, with support from community children's nurses or school nurses (DfEE, 1996). Whether the health need is epilepsy, eczema, asthma or some very rare condition, a care plan should be developed in partnership with educationalists, healthcare workers, support workers, parents and the child. This should ensure that care is co-ordinated, information is shared as necessary, medication or equipment is available, and intimate or invasive treatments can be given if required.

Children needing invasive treatment will remain the minority. Health in most schools for most children is concerned with promoting the best outcomes for all children. If this is done, the aims are for them to be happy and well in the here and now, to benefit from their education, and to develop into the healthy educated well-rounded adults of tomorrow.

At some time during their working lives most early years professionals will know or care for a child who is seriously ill, and who may ultimately die. For such children – who are often suddenly catapulted into the strange and sometimes frightening world of aggressive medical intervention – it is important that as many aspects of their life remain as stable as possible. They need the normality of familiar experiences, such as their regular school or nursery, to help them to cope with the unfamiliar experiences. Lavelle (1994) writes:

> '… *continuing formal education is important for two main reasons. First, it is the right of all children to have the opportunity to develop their potential abilities to the full and enjoy the enrichment which education brings to life, however long or short that life may be. Secondly, going back to school re-establishes the normal pattern of life for a child and reaffirms membership of the peer group. Being with your contemporaries locks you into life. Family life and relationships are easier to handle when the daily routine is a comfortable and familiar one.*'

(Lavelle, 1994, p. 87)

Clearly, these children present one of the greatest challenges for early years professionals, and sensitive and effective communication between parents and other agencies involved in the care of the child is of the utmost importance. When a child has been absent for a period of time because of serious illness, peers should be encouraged to make cards and pictures, etc., for their ill friend. Open and frank discussion with peers can smooth the way for the return of the child, who may be physically scarred or altered in some way. The return can be a daunting experience for the ill child, the healthy peers and the professional responsible for the group. We recommend an excellent text edited by Hill (1994) which gives sensible advice to professionals involved in the care of dying children and their families.

PARTNERSHIP WORKING

Health, social services and education have all been given prominence on recent governments' agendas, but they have been the remit of different services and implementation strategies, even though they are all concerned with the welfare of children (Mayall and Storey, 1998). The development of Children's NHS Trusts (DfES, 2003) – integrating education, social services and some health services – may take this further and lead to better integration of services and closer inter-disciplinary working, and ultimately to better services for children. This is important because of the impact that health and education particularly have on each other. For example, education influences a person's position in the work place, his or her academic achievements affecting the job that he or she will attain, which in turn influences his or her health outcomes. The Department of Education (1997) White Paper 'Excellence in Schools' refers to '… good education as a lifeline for children on the wrong side of the health divide' (p. 63). On the opposite side of the coin, the child who is wrestling with health difficulties and marked inequalities is unlikely to make the best use of his/her educational opportunities. Education may be seen as one of the main focusses of the school-aged child, but health and education are closely linked. These close links make it a nonsense to continue to segregate artificially the professionals who work in the respective services through, for example, the imposition of different terms and conditions of employment, professional affiliations and inspection regimes.

Our holistic philosophy advocates that all early years professionals have a responsibility towards the prevention of childhood mortality and morbidity and, as was discussed in this book's Introduction, whilst specialism (e.g. education, social work or health) is feasible within an holistic framework, intra/inter-agency collaboration and co-operation are vital for success. Each professional has a role to play which may be quite specific in terms of improving the health of the nation's children, health promotion, parental support and holistic assessment. Until such times as integrated children's services are the norm, professionals must recognize that there are many factors which influence a child's development, and make every effort to understand the roles of other professionals. We cannot assume that this will happen just because we all have the best interest of young children at heart. Each professional group requires an understanding of the others, which can best be achieved through shared learning, and the facilitation of skills such as advocacy, negotiation and communication, and ultimately through integrated early years services (see also the Introduction).

Conclusion

The health of children is an issue of national concern, and in this chapter we have discussed how the value placed upon children's health has developed over time and how children's health services have developed to respond to the needs of children and families. The health of children has to be the responsibility of all early years professionals who must take, and seek out, opportunities to promote the health of children and to prevent ill health. We cannot be complacent, however, as the way in which services have developed is not necessarily beneficial to children and their families – particularly those with complex needs. There is still a long way to go and still a need for greater integration of services. This can only be achieved through training and a enhanced understanding of inter-professional roles and responsibilities. Professional barriers must *never* be allowed to overshadow the need to provide excellent, integrated, child-focussed services.

Student activity

Identify a school-aged child with complex health needs. With the co-operation of the child and his or her parents, identify the different health, education and social care services with which the child/family has had contact, both currently and in the past. For each service identify the key aims of the services provided. Pay particular attention to any areas of overlap. Consider ways in which the number of contacts the child and family have with different services might be reduced.

REFERENCES

Acheson, D (1988): *Public Health in England: The Report of the Committee Inquiry into the Future Development of Public Health Function.* London: HMSO.

Acheson, D (1998): *Independent Inquiry into Inequalities in Health.* London: The Stationery Office.

Bradshaw, J (2002): Child poverty and child outcomes. *Children and Society*, **16**, 131–140.

British Paediatric Association (1995): *Health Needs of School Age Children* (Chair L. Polnay). London: British Paediatric Association.

Clark, J (1973): *A Family Visitor.* London: Royal College of Nursing.

Cowley, S (2000): *Situation and Process in Health Visiting in Appleton and Cowley. The Search for Health Needs.* London: Macmillan, pp. 25–46.

Cowley, S (ed.) (2002): *Public Health in Policy and Practice. A Sourcebook for Health Visitors and Community Nurses.* Edinburgh: Ballière Tindall.

Cox, C (1983): *Sociology: an Introduction for Nurses, Midwives and Health Visitors.* London: Butterworths.

Croll, P and Moses, D (2000): *Special Needs in the Primary School. One in Five?* London: Cassell.

Department of Education and Employment (1996): *Supporting Pupils with Medical Needs.* London: Stationery Office.

Department of Education and Employment (1997): *Excellence for all Children Meeting Special Educational Needs.* London: DfEE.

DFEE (1999): *National Healthy School Standard Guidance.* Nottingham: DfEE.

DfES (2002): *Special Educational Needs Code of Practice.* Nottingham: DfES.

DfES (2003): *Every Child Matters.* Nottingham: DfES.

Department of Health (1999a): *Saving Lives: Our Healthier Nation.* London: The Stationery Office.

Department of Health (1999b): *Making a Difference.* Leeds: Department of Health.

Department of Health (2001a): *Liberating the Talents.* London: Department of Health.

Department of Health (2001b): *Health Visitor Development Resource Pack.* London: The Stationery Office.

Department of Health/Department for Education and Skills (2004): *The National Service Framework for Children, Young People and Maternity Services.* London: Department of Health.

Department of Health and Social Security (1976): *Prevention and Health: Everybody's Business.* London: HMSO.

Hall, DMB (1992): Child Health Promotion, Screening and Surveillance. *Journal of Child Psychology and Psychiatry,* **34**, 649–658.

Hall, DMB and Elliman, D (eds) (2003): *Health for all Children,* 4th edn. Oxford: Oxford University Press.

Hill, L (ed.) (1994): *Caring for Dying Children and their Families.* London: Chapman & Hall.

Joint Health Surveys Unit on behalf of the Department of Health (2002): *Health Survey for England 2001.* London: Stationery Office.

Johnson, J (2001): Child morbidity. In Bradshaw, J (ed.), *Poverty: the outcomes for children.* London: Family Policy Studies Centre, pp. 40–55.

Kosky, J (ed.) (1992): *Queen Elizabeth Hospital for Sick Children: 125 Years of Achievement.* London: Queen Elizabeth Hospital.

Kosky, J and Lunnon, R (1991): *Great Ormond Street Hospital and the Story of Medicine.* London: Great Ormond Street Publications.

Lavelle, J (1994): Education and the sick child. In Hill, L (ed.), *Caring for Dying Children and their Families.* London: Chapman & Hall, pp. 87–105.

Mayall, B and Storey, S (1998): A school health service for children. *Children and Society,* **12**(2), 86–97.

Mental Health Foundation (1999): *Bright Futures.* London: Mental Health Foundation.

Meredith Davies, JB (1975): *Preventive Medicine, Community Health and Social Services,* 3rd edn. London: Ballière Tindall.

Mulvihill, C and Quigley, R (2003): *The Management of Obesity and Overweight: An Analysis of Reviews of Diet, Physical Activity and Behavioural Approaches. Evidence briefing.* London: Health Development Agency.

National Statistics online: Deaths by age, sex and underlying cause. www.statistics. gov.uk/STABASE/Expodata/spreadsheets/D8257.xls. Key demographic and health indicators. www.statistics.gov.uk/STABASE/Expodata/ spreadsheets/ D8378.xls

Quiglars, D (2001): Child mortality. In Bradshaw, J (ed.), *Poverty: The Outcomes for Children*. London: Family Policy Studies Centre, pp. 23–39.

Taylor, J, Muller D, Harris P and Wattley L (1999): *Nursing Children: Psychology, Research and Practice*, 2nd edn. London: Stanley Thornes.

World Health Organization (1993): *The European Network of Health-promoting Schools*. Copenhagen: WHO (Euro).

THE ILL CHILD

Val Thurtle and Jayne Taylor

This chapter aims to:

- identify the policy framework for ill children including the *National Service Framework for Children, Young People and Maternity Services*;

- explore Standard 6 and the impact this will have on service development for children who are ill;

- discuss ways of promoting empowerment of children with ill health and their families as a way of minimizing the impact of illness.

INTRODUCTION

As we have read throughout the earlier chapters in this book, there are many examples of health, social care and education services working together in a collaborative way to provide coherent services that have the child and his or her family at the centre.

This approach is even more important when the child is ill, whether the illness is an everyday self-limiting problem or a longer-term condition. It becomes paramount when the child's illness is life-threatening or life-limiting, or when the child has an illness which significantly disables his or her ability to carry out normal everyday activities (see Chapter 12). In this chapter we explore how professionals can work together to develop ideal child-centred pathways of care for ill children and their families. Our focus is mainly on community services, because this is where 90 per cent of the care of ill children takes place. We do refer briefly to hospital-based care, but only within the context of the care pathways discussed. We have however recommended some further reading at the end of this section for those readers who wish to explore hospital-based care in more detail.

THE POLICY FRAMEWORK

The development and delivery of services for children has moved at a rapid pace during the first few years of the new century, fuelled not least by the publication of the Kennedy Report into children's heart surgery at the Bristol Royal Infirmary (Kennedy, 2001) and the Laming Inquiry into the death of Victoria Climbié (Victoria Climbié Inquiry, 2003). The Laming report, in particular, highlighted that poor communication and a lack of partnership working between agencies played a significant part in the events that led to the death of Victoria. This accusation replayed similar accusations highlighted in almost every inquiry report into the death of a child at the hands of a carer over the preceding 30 years or so. It has become clear during the first five years of the new century that health, social care and education professionals must not work in isolation, must break out of their professional silos and engage in a programme of integrated working that will overcome the barriers to joint working we have all been talking about for too long, but doing little or nothing about.

In 2003, a Minister for Children, Young People and Families was appointed to drive forward this agenda for children. The purpose of the appointment was to ensure that all children have access to high-quality services and to safeguard against scandals such as Bristol and the death of Victoria Climbié ever occurring again. At around the same time, the publication of the Green Paper, *Every Child Matters* (DfES, 2003) asserted that we must give every child the best possible start in life, maximize their opportunities, and minimize risks to their health, safety and well-being. In March 2004 the publication of *Every Child Matters: Next Steps* (DfES, 2004) outlined how the proposals in the Green Paper would be realized. In the same year the Children Act (2004) was introduced, outlining a framework of accountability and partnership working through the establishment of Directors of Children's Services and Lead Members for children in each local authority, creating the new role of Children's Commissioner and setting up a new integrated inspection process. The Act also introduces measures to facilitate the sharing of information about children between different agencies through the establishment of protocols.

Alongside these policy initiatives the government is actively promoting the development of Children's Trusts to support the integration and co-ordination of service planning, commissioning and service delivery through the co-location of services, shared working and learning, and common assessment frameworks and information sharing (see also Chapter 10).

THE NATIONAL SERVICE FRAMEWORKS

These policy developments, among others, have been drawn together to provide a 10-year strategy for children with the publication of the *National Service Framework for Children, Young People and Maternity Services* (DH/DfES, 2004). The National Service Framework (NSF) programme was launched in April 1998 following the publication of two key documents (DoH, 1997, 1998). It was planned that one new framework would be introduced each year. The Children's NSF is clearly of great significance to all our readers, but is not the only NSF that has implications for children and their families, and it is worth mentioning briefly the NSF programme as it stands at the time of the publication of this book.

The NSFs were introduced to:

- Set national standards and identify key interventions for a defined service or care group.
- Put in place strategies to support implementation.
- Establish ways to ensure progress within an agreed time-scale.
- Form one of a range of measures to raise quality and decrease variations in service (other measures include the establishment of the National Institute for Clinical Excellence and national achievement targets).

The NSFs for mental health and coronary heart disease were the first to be produced, the comprehensive National Cancer Plan followed, and the NSFs for older people and for diabetes completed the first five priority areas – together the first five NSFs covered around half of total NHS expenditure. The NSF covering renal services was published in 2003 and 2005 (part two), and the NSF for long-term conditions was published in 2005. With the exception of the NSF for older people, the NSF programme has implications for the health and social care of children and their families affected by the relative conditions covered by the respective NSFs. Even the NSF for older people does have some relevance to children indirectly, in that it has paved the way for a common assessment framework allowing professionals from different agencies to share assessment material and information about their clients within agreed protocols.

In the NSF for children (DH/DfES, 2004), the National Clinical Director for Children wrote (p. 4):

'Children and young people are important. They are the living message we send to a time we will not see; nothing matters more to families than the health, welfare and future success of their children. They deserve the best care because they are the life-blood of the nation and are vital for our future economic survival and prosperity … The practical challenge is how to ensure that children's services locally are coherent in design and delivery, with good co-ordination, effective joint working between and across sectors and agencies, with smooth transitions and in partnership with children, young people and families.'

The first part of the NSF for children, young people and maternity services sets out five core standards for all children which aim to demonstrate how the practical challenges mentioned above can be realized. The first five standards are:

- Promoting health and well-being, identifying needs and intervening early.
- Supporting parenting.
- Child, young person and family-centred services.
- Growing up into adulthood.
- Safeguarding and promoting the welfare of children and young people.

These standards underpin the remaining standards within the NSF, which is further divided into two parts:

- Part two: which applies to children and young people in particular circumstances, such as those who have disabilities or mental health problems. Part two comprises five standards:
  - Children and young people who are ill.
  - Children in hospital.
  - Disabled children and young people and those with complex health needs (see Chapter 12).
  - The mental health and psychological well-being of children and young people.
  - Medicines management for children.
- Part three: which comprises the Standard for Maternity Services (see Chapter 2).

We will be utilizing Standard 6 of the National Service Framework to facilitate our exploration in this chapter about how we can best support children and their families during illness.

THE SHIFT FROM HOSPITAL SERVICES

Standard 6 of the NSF for children, young people and maternity services is concerned with children and young people who have an acute illness or injury and children who have (or are at risk of having) a long-term condition, which is not disabling. Standard 6 states that:

> *'All children and young people who are ill, or thought to be ill, or injured will have timely access to appropriate advice and to effective services which address their health, social, educational and emotional needs throughout the period of their illness.'*

When a child becomes ill – even if it is a relatively minor self-limiting illness – the equilibrium of normal family life becomes upset. The degree to which this happens will vary according to the nature of the illness and the context of the family. An illness that might seem devastating to one family might be played down or even ignored by another. A parent or carer may well adopt a 'wait and see' approach, use over-the-counter medication, and check their perception of the child's illness with significant others, such as grandparents or friends, in what is often termed the *lay referral system* (Freidson, 1970). What is evident in twenty-first-century healthcare for children is that health professionals do not have the monopoly in caring for, or making decisions about, the ill child. Parents are likely to be the most significant role players. When we consider everyday self-limiting illness they may well be the only health carers involved. In the NSF it is estimated that in 80 per cent of all childhood episodes of illness, parents do not involve the professional healthcare system at all (DH/DfES, 2004).

Although a significant amount of caring for ill children takes place within the family, children are actually avid users of the professional health services. A pre-school child will, in a typical year, see a general practitioner about six times, while a school-aged child will see the GP two to three times. Up to half of all children under 1 year old, and a quarter of older children, will visit an accident and emergency department, almost 10 per cent will attend hospital as an out-patient, and 7–10 per cent will be admitted to hospital. This latter statistic represents a marked reduction in hospital in-patient admissions over the latter half of the twentieth century. Consider for a moment the findings of the Platt Report from 1959 which highlighted that one-third of all children were admitted to hospital to have their tonsils removed, without counting admissions for other ailments. The Platt report, which paid deference to the work of psychologists such as Bowlby and Robertson (see Robertson and Robertson, 1989) who had vividly displayed on film the despair and misery that children experienced in hospital, was instrumental in bringing about the reduction in hospital admissions. The report recommended that children should only be admitted to hospital as a last resort and that care should be available to children in their own homes.

Keeping children out of hospital and providing community-based services to support children who are ill and their families is an admirable aspiration but does nevertheless bring with it a different set of issues that need to be addressed. Not least is the very *ad hoc* way that the shift from hospital- to community-based child care has taken place. The lack of trained community-based children's nurses, for example, has placed the burden of professional care with health visitors, general practitioners, practice nurses, parents and generic district nurses, many of whom will have had little or no training in the specific needs of ill children and their families. Where community children's nursing services exist they often comprise a single nurse who cannot provide continuous cover to support families. What seems to be evident is that care has shifted from hospitals to communities in some areas, regardless of whether tangible support services exist or not. This was highlighted by the Audit Commission in 1993 and again in the NSF for children (DH/DfES, 2004). The NSF outlines a training strategy so that practitioners without child-specific qualifications but who are working with ill children can gain the skills and knowledge they need to work effectively and safely. They do not suggest that service delivery stops, but that service developers view the next few years as a transitional period during which time sufficient numbers of qualified children's practitioners should be fully trained, whilst in the interim general practitioners receive training in certain core aspects of working with children.

The provision of qualified children's practitioners is not going to be a case of replacing generic workers with children's workers. What is evident is that the number of ill children in the community is ever-increasing for a number of reasons and that this will lead to a demand for more and more workers competent in the care of ill children. First, improved surgical and anaesthetic procedures allow children to be discharged more quickly from hospital; indeed, in some cases they no longer need to spend the night as an increasing number of procedures are carried out on a day-case basis. This will increase even more over the next decade as new, locally based treatment centres are developed. Second, the number of very premature babies who now survive has increased, and some of these tiny infants who would previously have spent many months in hospital are discharged into the community so that separation of the family is minimized. A number of these babies do however come home with significant health needs, with some requiring 24-hour care. Third, there are those children with a long-term illness such as cystic fibrosis, diabetes, cerebral palsy, epilepsy or leukaemia, which may previously have necessitated frequent admissions to hospital for pharmaceutical and other interventions. These children are more usually being cared for in the community because frequent admissions have been shown to have adverse effects on the child's well-being (Taylor *et al.*, 1999).

DEVELOPING LOCAL CHILDREN'S CLINICAL NETWORKS

When children and their families do come into contact with the professional health services it is often a traumatic time. Children tend to become ill very quickly, and it is often difficult to separate what might be a relatively trivial ailment from a more serious condition that may require the child to be admitted to hospital. It is important therefore that children and their families have access to healthcare systems that are designed to maximize timely assessment and diagnosis so that they receive appropriate care in the appropriate setting.

The NSF supports the development of local children's clinical networks, which provide an integrated, safe and comprehensive service to support children and their families during illness. The components of a local children's clinical network are (DH/DfES, 2004):

- NHS Direct.
- The ambulance service.
- Primary care provision; for example, GP, out-of-hours provision, walk-in centres.

- Community pharmacy.
- Accident and Emergency/Minor Injuries Units.
- In-patient provision.
- Community children's nursing services.
- Children's community teams providing health and social care and family support.
- Specialist clinical networks to provide expert advice 24 hours a day at a local level.
- Other local health services.
- Administrative support.
- Formal links with education and social services.

The local children's clinical network should operate effectively at all points in the child's illness experience. The idea is that everyone within the network – and particularly the child and the family – are aware of where and to whom they should go for support in the event of a specific need arising. There should be clear clinical and managerial leadership and accountability for the clinical network, common and agreed protocols for careful management of resources, trust and collaboration between the respective parts of the network and robust audit and governance arrangements (DH/DfES, 2004). The NSF includes a number of exemplars of how a clinical network should operate, more of which will be developed over time. One exemplar already published is for asthma, which demonstrates how the network will work in an acute episode of asthma. When the child or family notices the onset of an acute exacerbation and the child fails to respond to self-care, the child will be assessed and treated at a point of first contact, which might be the GP, a professional at a walk-in centre, NHS Direct, or an Accident and Emergency department. If necessary, the child may be referred to the paediatric team or treated at the point of first contact if it is possible to manage the asthma, thus allowing the child and family to return to self-care. Either option may lead to a review of the child's asthma, which may result in identification of a need to develop the child and/or parent's skill and knowledge in self-care. Links to the school health service may be appropriate, and so on. The aim is to develop pathways of care through the system, with easy and known access to services that are required at a particular point in time.

The other important aspect of the clinical network is that there is a robust system to support children, not only when needs arise due to acute episodes of illness but also when the needs of a child with a specific long-term illness such as Type 1 diabetes change over time. Parts of the clinical network that are in place to support the child at the beginning of the illness and around the time of diagnosis such as the specialist paediatric team and NHS Direct become less important and significant to the child and family over time, when other parts of the network take over. It is possible to plan this to some extent. For example, we know that starting school can be a particularly traumatic time for children and parents, and a different part of the network such as the school nursing service will have an important role during this time.

EMPOWERING CHILDREN AND FAMILIES AND DEVELOPING FAMILY-CENTRED CARE

Developing a local children's clinical network relies heavily on parents being empowered to make decisions and knowing who they need to contact in any given situation, mainly because they are the family and the constant in the child's life. As noted above, while various parts of the network play differing parts in the child's care pathway, the family will be there at all times. The literature is full of references to *empowerment of the family* and *family-centred care* but Campbell and Summersgill (1993), in commenting on family-centred care, note that it is often unexplained, and that there have been few attempts to define exactly what this means. If care workers have this problem, it is difficult to see how parents coping with an ill child can understand it.

In order to empower parents and promote and support family-centred care, parents need to be fully informed about the child's illness, the choices available to them, sources of support and intervention, and any other information that will help the parents to become 'expert' in their understanding of their child's illness. In many instances parents will become more knowledgeable about a particular illness than the professionals involved (remember that the parent is learning about one illness trajectory whereas most professionals have to be knowledgeable about many), and some professionals find this unsettling. In one study of Canadian families whose children had persistent otitis media with effusion (Wuest and Stern, 1990), great efforts were made by the families to obtain knowledge and skills that would allow them to participate fully in the management of their children's condition. However, the families became disenchanted because they believed that the professionals involved were not taking notice of their opinions and feelings. Wuest and Stern concluded that there is a real need for professionals and parents to work together. True partnership (in this case the parent–professional partnership) is about sharing, and this must be a two-way process. Remember that the aim is to empower parents so if they know a lot more than you do, you have achieved your aim! Parents and children – if and when they are able – should be encouraged to become 'expert patients' through the expert patient programme which is run through Primary Care Trusts (PCTs). Enabling children to participate in the Expert Patient Programmes may mean assisting them to develop self-confidence and self-management skills. PCTs should encourage parents and children to participate in the development of services that are designed for them.

Not every parent will be willing or able to spend hours scouring the internet or searching for information in library, nor will they wish to become 'expert patients'. Many will rely on the relevant professionals to help them gain knowledge. Unbiased and complete information should be shared with parents, and pathways of care should be developed that meet the family's needs, socially, emotionally and financially. They need to be fully informed, and the information must be provided in an appropriate way that is sensitive to developmental, cultural, social and language differences. This includes copies of relevant reports, letters and other communications about the child, which should be shared with the family according to current government policy (see www.dh.gov.uk/policyandguidance/organisationpolicy/publicand-patientinvolvement/copyingletterstopatients/fs/en).

Early years workers should be aware that information needs will vary between families and at various times during the child's illness. For example, at the time of diagnosis parents will need a great deal of information, but this should be given at a pace determined by the parents. Some will want to know everything there is to know, whereas others will need time to assimilate the diagnosis and will want information in more of a 'drip-feed' fashion. Professionals should be aware too that information imparted at the time of diagnosis is not sufficient, and their responsibility does not end at that point. When new information is discovered (e.g. through research), it is helpful if the professional can explain what this means rather than leaving it to parents to guess when they hear a news story on the radio or read it in the newspaper.

The overall aim is to empower parents so that they are better able to cope with their child's illness. This is not a hollow aspiration but one which is based on sound evidence that coping behaviour will influence positively or negatively the outcomes of the illness for the child and for the family (Boekaerts and Roder, 1999) particularly when the child has a long-term illness. Effective coping results in relevant adaptation to the child's illness, whereas ineffective coping can have harmful consequences and lead to mal-adaptation. One of the purposes of professional intervention must therefore be to maximize and facilitate coping skills which, according to Eiser (1990), will lead to greater independence and competence.

The child too, if he or she is able, should be empowered so that he or she can exercise the right to be included in decision-making processes. For many children – and particularly those with long-term conditions – their role includes taking on significant aspects of self-care as they move towards adulthood. This may mean taking on responsibility for self-medication, exercise regimes, avoidance of certain activities that will exacerbate a particular condition, or undertaking other therapeutic interventions that might once have been performed only by health professionals but which mean a greater degree of independence if the child can carry out the intervention alone.

Professionals need to be aware that where a child has a long-term illness (and this may be right at the start, depending on the age and stage of development of the child), they will become increasingly autonomous and parental advocacy will usually diminish. This requires professionals to make judgements about when it is appropriate rhetorically to put the child in the 'driving seat' and allow them to make judgements about what information is given to the parents. For example, an adolescent may no longer wish parents to be involved in routine physical examinations, and may wish to be given information without parents being present. Professionals need to be cautious to maintain the patient's confidentiality (in this case the child) whilst balancing the parents' need for information (DH/DfES, 2004). It can sometimes be a tricky job to balance the demands and needs of the child and parents.

MINIMIZING THE IMPACT OF ILLNESS

We have discussed above the need to empower parents and children through information and encouraging them to become experts in their illness trajectories. Illness – particularly if it is long-term – can however have a devastating effect on all aspects of the child and family's life and early years workers will need to work with families to minimize the impact of illness to allow the child to lead as normal a life as possible. This applies to children with non-life-threatening illness as well as to those who may eventually die as a result of their illness.

One of the most tangible difficulties is the impact of illness on educational opportunities. Episodes in hospital for example can mean children missing vital time at school, and it also impacts on normal friendships and other extra-curricular activities. Guidelines have been published to guide organizations to provide staff, facilities and equipment for education to continue when a child is in hospital (DoH/DfEE, 1996). Hospital staff will need to develop good communication channels with the child's school to help the child develop and achieve full educational potential. The NSF discusses the need for health and education services to develop joint protocols to ensure the smooth transition from school to hospital and hospital back to school, where an admission is planned (DH/DfES, 2004). The named teacher and named health contact in consultation with the child and family should develop, monitor and review healthcare plans which detail respective support requirements. When a child's needs change – for example, if medication or treatment is revised – the care plans should be altered accordingly and all parties informed.

It is not only hospital admissions that can have an adverse impact on education. Children who need frequently to attend out-patient departments or assessment centres can be helped by sensitive scheduling of appointments; for example, at the start or end of the list so that they spend a minimum time away from school. Schools should also encourage children and parents to attend school for part-days if, for example, the child is unwell in the morning but feels better later in the day. For example, some parents – if a child has a fit first thing in the morning – will keep them away from school for the whole day, yet the child may be feeling fine within an hour or two and be quite well enough to attend.

Encouraging children to participate in other normal childhood activities and in friendship groups is also an important way of minimizing the impact of illness. Parents may be reluctant for their children to participate in activities that cannot be overseen by themselves or a trusted teacher, and they can develop an over-protective attitude to the ill child (Hurst, 1996). Other parents and friends may likewise have fears about a child with a particular health need being entrusted to them. Helping parents and children to find a healthy balance that enables the ill child to participate in activities safely can be achieved through simple suggestions. Examples include encouraging a friend and parent to visit the ill child at home first and giving a range of emergency contact numbers. Likewise, encouraging the parent of the ill child to write down a few facts about the illness or provide leaflets about an illness can all be useful.

Conclusion

In this chapter we have looked at children with ill health and how, as early years workers, we should be working towards reducing the impact of illness on the child and family through empowerment and effective working practices across agencies. The approach needs to be individualized to the context of the family, and includes ensuring that families have information designed to meet their needs in every way.

The *National Service Framework for Children, Young People and Maternity Services* (DH/DfES, 2004) provides a 10-year strategy for the development of child-centred services, and alongside other policy initiatives – notably Standard 6 – advocates the setting up of local children's clinical networks, which will provide joined-up services with clear pathways through the healthcare system.

Liaison and partnership working between agencies and in collaboration with children and their families is a vital component of minimizing the impact of ill health on a child's longer-term social and emotional outcomes.

> We finished by looking at the vision of the team that developed Standard 6 of the National Service Framework. They want to see:
>
> ■ Children and young people who are ill receiving timely, high-quality and effective care as close to home as possible.
> ■ Children and young people who are ill and their families being cared for within a local system which co-ordinates health, social care and education in a way that meets their individual needs (DH/DfES, 2004, p. 4).

Student activity

Look at the *NSF for Children, Young People and Maternity Services* and find the two published exemplars on asthma and autism, which have been produced to support the implementation of the framework.

Identify a child you know or with whom you are working, and develop a map similar to those in the exemplars for the child's condition which highlights possible routes through the healthcare system and links to other agencies.

REFERENCES

Boekaerts, M and Roder, T (1999): Stress, coping, and adjustment in children with a chronic disease: a review of the literature. *Disability and Rehabilitation*, **21**(7), 311–337.

Campbell, S and Summersgill, P (1993): Keeping it in the family: defining and developing family-centred care. *Child Health*, **1**, 17–20.

DfES (2003): *Every Child Matters*. London: The Stationery Office.

DfES (2004): *Every Child Matters: Next Steps*. London: The Stationery Office.

Department of Health (1997): *The New NHS: Modern, Dependable*. London: DoH.

Department of Health (1998): *A First Class Service: Quality in the NHS*. London: DoH.

Department of Health/Department for Education and Employment (1996): *Supporting Pupils with Medical Needs*. London: DfEE.

Department of Health/Department for Education and Skills (2004): *National Service Framework for Children, Young People and Maternity Services*. London: DoH.

Eiser, C (1990): Psychological effects of chronic disease. *Journal of Child Psychology and Psychiatry*, **31**(1), 85–98.

Freidson, E (1970): *Profession of Medicine*. New York: Dodd, Mead and Company.

Hurst, R (1996): A disabled person's viewpoint. In Kurtz, Z and Hopkins A (eds), *Services for Young People with Chronic Disorders: In their Transition from Childhood to Adult Life*. London: Royal College of Physicians.

Kennedy, I (2001): *The Report of the Public Health Inquiry into Children's Heart Surgery at the Bristol Royal Infirmary 1984–1995.* London: The Stationery Office.

Platt, H (1959): *The Welfare of Children in Hospital: Report of the Committee on Child Health Services.* London: HMSO.

Robertson, J and Robertson, J (1989): *Separation and the Very Young.* London: Free Association Press.

Taylor, J, Muller, D, Harris, P and Wattley, L (1999): *Nursing Children: Psychology, Research and Practice*, 3rd edn. London: Nelson Thornes.

Victoria Climbié Inquiry (2003): Report of an Inquiry by Lord Laming, Department of Health and Home Office. London: HMSO.

Wuest, J and Stern, P (1990): The impact of fluctuating relationships with the Canadian health care system on family management of otitis media with effusion. *Journal of Advanced Nursing*, **15**, 556–563.

FURTHER READING

DH/DfES (2004): *National Service Framework for Children, Young People and Maternity Services: Standard 7.* London: DoH.

Taylor, J, Muller, D, Harris, P and Wattley, L (1999): *Nursing Children: Psychology, Research and Practice*, 3rd edn. London: Nelson Thornes.

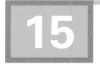

CHILDREN OF THE WORLD

Jayne Taylor

This chapter aims to:

- explore the experiences of children in developing countries using the Human Development Index and the Convention on the Rights of the Child as a framework;

- focus on the holistic needs of children in developing countries, with particular emphasis on life expectancy and health, education and wealth;

- examine ways in which international aid is focussed on the developing world.

INTRODUCTION

'*All children have rights: the right to protection, to education, to food and medical care, and to much more. Every child, no matter where he or she lives, has the right to grow up feeling safe and cared for: a simple thought, which few would openly challenge. But, sadly, the reality is quite different.*'

(Audrey Hepburn, in: United Nations International Children's Emergency Fund, 1989)

The inclusion of this chapter on the lives of children of the world is justified on two grounds. First, it adds a truly international perspective to the study of early childhood, and enables the reader to gain some insights into the everyday existence of those children who live in less-developed parts of the world. Second, it perhaps allows the reader to reflect on the reality of disadvantage which has been referred to throughout the rest of the book. This does not mean to say that we in any way condone the despair, neglect and poverty in which some children exist in this country. Rather, we wish to put this existence into a context. Those of us who are concerned with and have an interest in children during their early years are moved by the plight of disadvantaged children, wherever they live, regardless of their religious affiliation, ethnicity, culture or creed. We recognize that children have rights such as those outlined in the Convention on the Rights of the Child, and we recognize that children are special.

This chapter explores the lives of children in the less-developed world from an holistic perspective, with the ultimate aim of enabling the reader to develop a broader view of those early years.

Definitions

It is important that we begin by clarifying what we mean by the developing countries, before we can explore more fully the lives of children who live there. At one time, the term *Third World* was used synonymously with the developing world, with countries being classified according to their economic or 'civilized' level as being first, second, third or fourth. Countries such as the UK, most of Europe, the USA and Australia were included in the First World category, the former Eastern Bloc countries were defined within the Second World category, the Third World category included countries within Southern Asia, South America and Africa, and the Fourth World category included specific tribal peoples such as the African Bushmen, the Australian Aborigines and the South American Indians.

Clearly, however, there were problems in utilizing such broad categories. In the first place, the terms first, second, third and fourth imply some hierarchical classification, suggesting that first is 'better' than second, second is 'better' than third, and so on. Second, critics also argued that the terminology was essentially ethnocentric, and did not acknowledge that because something is inherently different this does not make it better or worse.

The International Bank for Reconstruction and Development (known as the World Bank) chooses to classify countries according to the gross national income (GNI) per capita – previously referred to as the gross national product (GNP). Based on the GNI per capita, each country is classified as low income, middle income (sub-divided into lower middle and upper middle), or high income. The World Bank looks at indicators such as debt and measures the ratio of debt and income. In addition, the World Bank compiles data about development organized into six sections: World View, People, Environment, Economy, States and Markets, and Global Links (World Bank, 2004). However, there are also weaknesses within this system. For example, the GNI is not a sensitive measure in cultures where goods and services are exchanged without financial accreditation, and does not account for how a country chooses to spend its wealth.

The term *developing countries* is therefore the preferable terminology created by the United Nations, particularly when considered alongside the United Nations development measure known as the Human Development Index (HDI) which accounts for life expectancy, educational attainment and adjusted real income (wealth). Developed countries are all nations in Europe, including the countries that were part of the former Soviet Union, as well as North America, Japan, Australia and New Zealand. All other nations of the world are considered to be developing countries. However, the words *developing* and *developed* also suggest a hierarchy and imply that something is not yet fully formed and will eventually develop. Inadvertently it also suggests that being fully developed is a wholly desirable attribute, and yet we are aware from the readings throughout this text that not all children who live in the developed world experience the ideal. Poverty, ill health and cruelty exist for children in the UK and other Western 'developed' countries, and their lives are far from ideal. It is also true to say that some children residing in developing countries have lives that are enriched by cultures and pleasures which children in the developed world will never be fortunate enough to experience.

As we have mentioned above, we prefer the term 'developing countries' when considered along with the HDI. The framework for the discussion within this chapter is based on the HDI and related articles within the Convention on the Rights of the Child. However, we acknowledge that this is not an ideal classification system, which universally reflects the reality of growing up and living in different parts of the world.

The rights of the child

In 1989, a single legal instrument entitled the Convention on the Rights of the Child was approved by the international community and brought together the rights that every child is entitled to, regardless of sex, social origin or religion. The key word here is *every* – whilst some of the articles contained within the Convention may seem far removed from the children we are used to working with, there are children within all societies that face disadvantage, poverty, homelessness, violence and other adversity. Children in developing countries may face extreme forms of disadvantage and the Convention applies equally to them – they have the same rights as children living in more wealthy parts of the world.

The Convention on the Rights of the Child was predicated by a series of Declarations of the Rights of the Child. The League of Nations endorsed the first Declaration in 1924, and a second Declaration was endorsed in 1948 by the United Nations General Assembly. Work began almost immediately on a more detailed Declaration, which was endorsed in 1959. This set out 10 principles.

The principles set out in the Declaration of the Rights of the Child were statements of moral and ethical intent and were not legally binding. In order to carry the weight of international law, a convention or covenant was required and, spurred on by the United Nations-sponsored International Year of the Child, a working party was formed to develop the Convention on the Rights of the Child. The Declaration of Human Rights, the International Covenant on Civil and Political Rights and the International Covenant on Economic, Social and Cultural Rights heavily influenced its work in the formation of the 41 substantive articles that make up the Convention, which was unanimously adopted in 1989 by the United Nations General Assembly and came into force in 1990.

By 1995, a total of 185 states had ratified the Convention, making it the most widely and rapidly ratified human rights treaty in history (UNICEF, 2004), and by 2003 a total of 192 countries had formally ratified it. In 2002, two additional protocols were adopted on the involvement of children in armed conflict, and on the sale of children, child prostitution and child pornography, in order to strengthen the provision of the Convention in these areas.

THE HEALTH OF CHILDREN

The Rights of the Child – Article 24(1)

'*State parties recognize the right of the child to the enjoyment of the highest attainable standard of health and to facilities for the treatment of illness and rehabilitation of health. State parties shall strive to ensure that no child is deprived of his or her rights of access to such health services.*'

Throughout this text we have discussed the need to take an holistic perspective when considering children during the early years. This approach is also adopted by the United Nations in its HDI in recognition that it is the tripartite combination of life expectancy, education and wealth that contributes to our experiences of life. In many respects these three components are interwoven, and certainly each will influence the other two. However, for the purpose of clarity we shall discuss each in turn before considering the overall picture at the end of the chapter. We shall therefore commence our discussion by looking at life expectancy and health in relation to children in developing countries.

It is interesting to reflect for a moment on the major causes of death among populations within the developed world, and to make comparisons with the developing world – although a note of caution should be added here about a shortage of comparable specific data on health, particularly from developing countries (Wagstaff, 2000: Haggett, 2000). In developed countries the major causes of death are circulatory and degenerative diseases, followed by cancers. Many of these causes are attributable either directly or indirectly to life-style (e.g. diet, smoking, lack of exercise, alcohol). In the developing world the picture has historically been very different, with the major causes of death being infectious and parasitic diseases (Meade and Earickson, 2000) and HIV/AIDS (WHO, 2000a). Indeed, it is a similar scenario to that which existed in the UK during the last century, although the causal organisms are different (see also Chapter 13). However, there are evident changes in terms of mortality in developing countries, with HIV- and AIDS-related deaths affecting both the child and adult populations of many countries, particularly in Africa. The World Health Organization (WHO) estimates that the widespread use of antiretroviral therapy (ART) would reduce HIV/AIDS-related deaths considerably and have introduced an initiative called '3 by 5' – aiming to treat 3 million people living with HIV/AIDS in the developing world with ART by 2005. Smoking-related deaths are also likely to increase over the next few decades due to a rise in tobacco use.

In terms of child mortality, approximately 10.5 million children under the age of 5 died in 1999. Of these children, 3.8 million were from Africa, 2.5 million were from India, and 750 000 were from China (WHO, 2000a). This was 2.2 million fewer deaths than in 1990. The causes of death in developing countries are attributable to the effects of measles, pertussis, tetanus, tuberculosis and malaria, diarrhoea and starvation (approximately 8 million children die each year from these last two causes). These and other diseases led to marked differences between developed and developing countries in terms of life expectancy at birth and infant and child mortality rates (the numbers of deaths in the first year of life per 1000 live births and the likelihood of a child dying before his or her fifth birthday, respectively). The reduction in deaths over the decade were mainly attributable to a reduction in death from diarrhoea due to widespread use of oral rehydration therapy (estimated to have reduced deaths from diarrhoea from 3.3 million to 1.5 million) and to mass measles immunization campaigns. However, there is no room for complacency, and certainly no evidence that the death rates will continue to spiral downwards. WHO data show that in seven countries, five of which are in Africa, child mortality actually rose.

Life expectancy

The Rights of the Child – Article 6

'1. *State Parties recognize that every child has the inherent right to life.*
2. *State Parties shall ensure to the maximum extent possible the survival and development of the child.*'

Life expectancy is a useful indicator, although the lack of data generated within some countries in relation to death registrations does lead to some doubt as to its usefulness as an entirely reliable indicator. What is evident from basic indicators is that a child born in 1999 in Japan, which currently leads the world league tables, has a healthy life expectancy of 74.5 years, which is almost triple that of a child born in Sierra Leone (a healthy life expectancy of 26 years, the world's lowest) (WHO, 2000b). However, there are a number of factors which may influence healthy life expectancy at birth which will be discussed later in this chapter. For example, war, drought and crop failure can have a marked impact on statistics such as those mentioned above.

Infant mortality

The infant mortality rate (IMR) is one of the most reliable indicators of the health of a country because it is relatively easy to measure, even in countries without sophisticated registration systems, by asking appropriate samples of the adult population about the numbers of children born live who have subsequently died. There is also a positive correlation between infant mortality, child and adult mortality. What the infant mortality rate for a country cannot do is give an indication about variations within countries at a given point in time – it will only allow for comparisons to be made between countries and within countries *over* time. However, these are both useful comparisons, particularly the latter, which is a good indicator of progression. Looking at the IMR between the various regions of the world, Angola has the highest IMR of 261.5. This can be compared with the highest IMRs in each of the other regions which are Haiti (IMR 88.9), Afghanistan (176.2), Azerbaijan (78.3), Myanmar (111.5) and Cambodia (137.2). To put this into context, the IMR for the UK is 5.8 (WHO, 2000c). Looking over time, the probability of a child dying before his or her first birthday in 2000 globally was 7 per cent, compared with 10 per cent in 1990, 12 per cent in 1980, and 25 per cent in 1950. Progress is due to better nutrition, better sanitation, water and housing, access to electricity and access to medical care and education (WHO, 2000c).

Infant mortality rates are attributable to similar causes to those mentioned above in relation to child mortality. However, there are other factors which lead to early childhood deaths which are less significant during later childhood. These factors are generally associated with the perinatal period. For example, it is estimated that moderate to severe birth asphyxia will affect 3 per cent of the 120 million babies born in developing counties each year, and 900 000 babies will die as a result (WHO, 1998). The reasons for birth asphyxia are many, and include factors associated with maternal health prior to birth, such as having many children, heavy work and poor maternal nutrition, intrapartum factors such as maternal haemorrhage and cord prolapse, and post-natal factors such as hypothermia which, even in hot climates, is exacerbated by washing but not drying babies after birth. Sadly, many of these deaths could be prevented if mothers and their babies in developing countries had access to trained personnel and incubators, and if some traditional practices, such as rubbing babies with mustard oil and not breast-feeding for the first three days of life, were avoided. However, effectively conveying such messages to relatively isolated people is extremely difficult, particularly in countries where illiteracy is common among women. Traditional practices frequently have cultural or religious significance, and prevention of such practices requires a consistent and innovative approach to health promotion. The difficulties are compounded by the fact that many mothers may be unable to access medical services, or deliberately choose not to access such services because of a misconception that medicine and hospitals are for the ill. They are therefore not an entirely accessible population. Given all of these difficulties, there *are* examples of cases where whole communities have taken account of such issues. The large-scale introduction of barefoot doctors in rural China has resulted in a marked drop in maternal mortality rates (Koblinsky *et al.*, 1999), for example, and Quezon City, in the Philippines, campaigned to become the 'first mother–baby-friendly city', and mobilized the entire community – government, health professionals, women and men – towards positive partnerships in child bearing. Since that first initiative, WHO have called for all women to have access to a trained birth attendant (WHO, 2002a) and the baby-friendly hospital initiative strategy has been initiated jointly by WHO and UNICEF, aiming to create healthcare environments where breastfeeding is the norm.

A further issue which is also of great importance in relation to infant mortality is son preference. The extent to which this contributes to infant mortality is unknown, as governments are clearly unwilling (or unable) to publicize selective abortion rates for female fetuses, or the extent to which female infanticide is practised. In 1995 and 1996 the broadcasting on television of *The Dying Rooms* documentaries brought this hidden problem vividly to the forefront of UK society by focussing on the abandonment and killing of female children in China, as a result of the 'one-child-only policy', combined with the traditional view of a patriarchal society which values male children more highly than female children. Many female children are apparently placed in understaffed orphanages where they spend their short lives physically restrained, without affection, play or education. This clearly contravenes the convention on the Rights of the Child. According to Hussain *et al.* (2000), son preference exists in other cultures such as Bangladesh and India – girl children have a higher child mortality rate due to discrimination against them in terms of food allocation and access to healthcare.

The Rights of the Child – Article 19(1)

> 'State Parties shall take all appropriate legislative, administrative, social and educational measures to protect children from all forms of physical or mental violence, injury or abuse, neglect or negligent treatment, maltreatment or exploitation, including sexual abuse, while in the care of parents(s), legal guardian(s) or any other person who has care of the child.'

Child morbidity

Where child mortality is attributed to particular causes, it is usually the case that child morbidity can be attributed in a similar way. For example, diarrhoea and malnourishment are significant causes of illness among children, as well as being major causes of mortality. It is estimated that diarrhoea in children under the age of 5 years accounts for 1.8 billion episodes and claims the lives of 3 million children each year (Haggett, 2000). Large-scale education about the benefits of oral rehydration (which re-establishes the body's fluid and electrolyte balance) has taken place in the developing world, and such treatment is both cheap and easy to administer. However, many children continue either to die or to be severely affected by diarrhoea, often because of the underlying disease, or because they do not receive adequate help.

Another cheap and easily administered measure which can prevent acute enteritis and other childhood mortality and morbidity is to discourage bottle-feeding in favour of breastfeeding. In 2002, the Fifty-fifth World Assembly reported that 55 per cent of infant deaths from diarrhoea and respiratory infection were due to inappropriate feeding. An estimated 57 000 children aged from 6 to 59 months die annually in nine West African countries alone due to vitamin A deficiency, which also causes blindness and increases the risk of other infections (WHO, 2001). Many of these deaths would be preventable if babies were exclusively and uninterruptedly breast-fed during the first 6 months of life – which forms part of the Global Strategy on Infant and Young Child Feeding (WHO, 2002b). However, the bottle-feeding industry is large and commercially lucrative, and Palmer (1999) and Baby Milk Action (2000) suggest that the baby milk industry continues to discourage breastfeeding through the advertising (both covert and overt) of their products. World-wide, less than 35 per cent of infants are breast-fed exclusively for the first 4 months.

HIV- and AIDS-related illnesses also affect many millions of children in the developing, as well as the developed, world. First, there are the children who are HIV-positive, who have had the virus transmitted to them either vertically (from mother to baby *in utero* or during birth), from contaminated blood products, from infected needles, through sexual contact, or via breast milk. Diarrhoea is a predominant symptom and death occurs rapidly, often because of prevailing social conditions. Second, children are affected when their parents or carers are HIV-positive or become ill with or die of AIDS-related disease. The stigma associated with HIV and AIDS is as apparent in the developing world as it is in the developed world, and many children suffer because they are associated with the disease – even though they themselves may not be HIV-positive. Third, the HIV/AIDS issue has had a further 'knock-on' effect which is affecting children in developing countries, as scarce research funding into killer diseases such as malaria has been diverted to AIDS prevention.

Other significant causes of child morbidity can be attributed to perinatal factors. We mentioned in the previous section that almost a million children die of birth asphyxia each year. There are also over 3 million children who survive but are disabled by epilepsy, cerebral palsy and learning difficulties. As the lifespan of such children increases due to better medical care, they are increasingly outliving their primary carers (WHO, 2003). These children clearly require special healthcare and education as set out in the Convention on the Rights of the Child.

The Rights of the Child – Article 23(1)

'*State Parties recognize that a mentally or physically disabled child should enjoy a full and decent life, in conditions which ensure dignity, promote self-reliance and facilitate the child's active participation in the community.*'

Traditionally, however, children with such disabilities have been placed in large institutions in urban areas (WHO, 2003), which are a consequence of colonial influence, with the British system of providing care for these children being transposed to different areas of the world, regardless of their relevance to local culture. Such institutions served only to isolate these children from their families and their culture, and whilst their health and development may have been optimized, it was virtually impossible for them ever to be integrated back into their own societies in later years. The current view is that children should be provided with home-based care by utilizing a system of people who can provide intervention. If possible, there should be a family member who, with professional support, education and back-up, can provide therapy. Some developing countries have introduced a tier of workers (front-line workers) who operate between the professionals and the family. Other countries aim to provide day care with specialist input, with the children being enabled to remain with their families for the rest of the time. The WHO (2003) is trying to work with countries to implement rehabilitation services that best match the social and economic situations that persist to address all issues related to the full participation of people with disabilities. A key aim is to develop an early detection and intervention tool for children from birth to 3 years so that they can derive maximum benefit from community rehabilitation. This philosophy is in line with the Convention on the Rights of the Child.

The Rights of the Child – Articles 23(2) and (3)

(2) 'State Parties recognize the right of the disabled child to special care and shall encourage and ensure the extension, subject to available resources, to the eligible child and those responsible for his or her care, of assistance for which application is made and which is appropriate to the child's condition and to the circumstances of the parents or others caring for the child.'

(3) 'Recognizing the special needs of the disabled child, assistance extended in accordance with paragraph 2 of the present article shall be provided free of charge, whenever possible, taking into account the financial resources of the parents or others caring for the child and shall be designed to ensure that the disabled child has effective access to and receives education, training, health care services, rehabilitation services, preparation for employment and recreation opportunities in a manner conducive to the child's achieving the fullest possible social integration and individual development, including his or her cultural and spiritual development.'

Even diseases which are relatively minor in developed countries, or which have been eradicated, carry high mortality and morbidity rates in developing countries. One example of such a disease is measles, which it should theoretically be possible to eradicate, or at least effectively to control, if total immunization could be achieved. In countries such as Namibia, a mass campaign from 1997 reduced the cases of measles from 4000 to less than 100 per year. Unfortunately, despite these large-scale vaccination programmes, we are a long way from achieving global eradication. Child morbidity in developing countries, including measles, is heavily influenced by a number of factors which, if overcome, could have a significant impact upon the health of children. These include:

- poor sanitation and water supply;
- lack of education about control and spread of disease;
- overcrowded housing/large families;
- deficient healthcare systems;
- environmental conditions;
- lack of immunization policies;
- poverty;
- war;
- national debt;
- bottle-feeding (rather than breastfeeding);
- malnutrition.

Improving, maintaining and promoting the health of children in the developing world is a complex and difficult problem which is hampered by many factors. However, improvements have been and continue to be made. Methods of health intervention and promotion are at last being adapted that are suitable and appropriate for the cultures which they aim to support. This has happened because objective systems of evaluation have been set up, which are the key to success. We can only hope that the days of building large urban institutions for children with severe learning disabilities, or of imposing Westernized, didactic health promotion campaigns, or of donating incubators for babies which are unsuitable for the climate and cannot be mended when they break down, are over.

THE EDUCATION OF CHILDREN

The Rights of the Child – Article 28(1a and b)

(1) 'State Parties recognize the right of the child to education and with a view to achieving the right progressively and on the basis of equal opportunity, they shall, in particular:

– Make primary education compulsory and available free to all;
– Encourage the development of different forms of secondary education including general and vocational education, make them available and accessible to every child, and take appropriate measures such as the introduction of free education and offering financial assistance in case of need.'

The World Declaration on Education for All was issued in 1990 by the United Nations International Children's Emergency Fund (UNICEF), and adopted by the World Conference on Education for All in Jomtien, Thailand. It reiterates Article 28 of the Convention on the Rights of the Child. Further to this adoption, The Dakar Framework for Action – Education for All: Meeting Our Collective Commitments was adopted by the World Education Forum in 2000. As was mentioned earlier, it is extremely difficult to separate life expectancy, education and wealth, because each of these factors is dependent upon and influences the others. For example, with regard to health and life expectancy we have considered how a lack of education, particularly literacy, can affect health promotion. We have also discussed how children with severe learning disabilities were effectively removed from their own cultures and placed in urban institutions, thus depriving them of education which would promote their 'general culture'. Life expectancy, health and education are also influenced by the wealth of a country, or by the unequal distribution of wealth within a country, just as the wealth of a country will influence healthcare and education systems.

Education in the developing world aims to achieve similar outcomes to education in the developed world. Children require educational opportunities that will enable them to acquire the skills of literacy, numeracy, oral expression and problem-solving, as well as to develop skills, knowledge, values and attitudes appropriate to their culture. The education of children is also important for the future economy of developing countries and the United Nations in its Millenium Development Goals has set a target to secure access to education for all children by 2015. The ability to train professionals such as doctors, nurses, engineers and teachers enables a country to decrease its dependence on the developed world and can help to increase the quality of life of individuals and families.

However, there are still many children in the developing world who are deprived of education, or who receive only a limited education for a short period of time. UNESCO reported that in sub-Saharan Africa, four out of every 10 children do not attend primary school, and even where primary enrolment rates are increasing, such as in Latin America, the drop-out rates are high (NetAid, 2004). There is also a marked gender difference in illiteracy rates, with 66 per cent of illiterate people being female (UNESCO, 2001). Whilst looking at literacy rates does give a 'snapshot' view of a particular country, it does not provide detailed information about the education systems within countries, or about the levels of education within those systems. Literacy, whilst clearly being very important, is only one outcome measure, and there are many more. It is also possible that many children who *do* receive education remain illiterate because the quality of education is so poor. Other children remain illiterate because they *do not* receive education in any form.

The United Nations Education, Scientific and Cultural Organisation (UNESCO) was set up with the aim of restoring education systems following the Second World War. It now operates in partnership with governments to enable them to put educational policies into practice, including the provision of education for adults as well as for children. A great deal of progress has been made where governments are committed to education in terms of providing primary education (NetAid, 2004). However, in very poor countries this may mean very large classes of children and severely restricted learning and teaching resources, making teaching very difficult. In many countries there are gender differences in the extent to which education is received. There is a clear need for parents and local communities to be involved in decision-making about their children's education, so that they may feel an increased sense of commitment to education.

In other countries where the government is not committed to education, or where there is war, education provision can be non-existent for some children.

In some countries the education provision varies considerably, with certain children being excluded from the education system altogether. For example, there are millions of children worldwide, colloquially known as 'street children', who have been forced to live and work on the streets of large cities for a number of reasons. In Bangladesh alone there are an estimated 3 million street children (Bokolamulla, 2003). This growing urban tragedy is more prevalent in, but not solely confined to, the poorest developing countries. For example, in parts of South America, such as Brazil, Mexico and Colombia, the number of children who roam the streets of large cities is an ever-present problem, with very young children being forced to work to live – some shining shoes or washing cars, whilst others turn to prostitution as a means of earning money. In some places these children are seen as being no more valuable than vermin, and are hunted down and murdered by adults wishing to clear them from the streets. They receive no formal education, and have often been 'written off' by the societies in which they live. In a study by Rizzini and Mandel Butler (2003), children living on the streets of Rio de Janeiro spoke of their fears of the military police, the municipal guards and private security guards who the children greatly fear and consider to be their main enemies rather than people with whom they feel safe. The children spoke of guards who had threatened death and physical violence:

> *There are many wrongs on the street, the guards chasing you, taking our things away, hitting us, aggression. When V. is on duty he disses us. He is a guard that we have here, he works with a gun. He said I would turn into compost the next time he catches me here so late. That is, that I am going to die, right?'*

Clearly the experiences of these children are dire, and the increase in the numbers of such children is an embarrassment to many governments worldwide, particularly in the developed world. The fact that very young children should be forced to call the streets their home and work from a very early age is an appalling situation which is totally in conflict with the Convention on the Rights of the Child.

The Rights of the Child – Article 27(1)

> *'State Parties recognize the right of every child to a standard of living adequate for the child's physical, mental, spiritual, moral and social development.'*

The Rights of the Child – Article 32(1)

'State Parties recognize the right of the child to be protected from economic exploitation and from performing any work that is likely to be hazardous or to interfere with the child's education, or to be harmful to the child's health or physical, mental, spiritual, moral or social development.'

However, the situation is not entirely negative for street children and other children in developing countries. A variety of projects worldwide are improving education for children – some under the auspices of UNESCO and others independent of them. One example of such a project is the Catholic Action for Street Children operating in Ghana which aims to contact street children and gradually to build relationships with them. They provide a day centre and programmes including literacy and skills training to help older children learn a trade (see www.hrw.org). A further project, Casa Alianza, operates similar programmes in Guatemala, where over 700 children and young people on the streets are murdered each year. Their aims are to provide safety, sanctuary, advocacy, a regular structure, choice and where possible reunification with families.

WEALTH

The final measure accounted for by the HDI, referred to at the beginning of this chapter, is adjusted real income or wealth. We mentioned previously some of the difficulties in considering wealth, in that measures such as the GNI do not account for how a country spends its wealth, or indeed the extent to which countries are using, selling or destroying their natural resources. However, there are very great differences in the living standards of people, including children, in different countries, and large-scale poverty is evident in the developing world, associated with hunger and mass misery.

In 1997, the United Nations launched its 'Agenda for Development' (UN, 1997), recognizing many of these issues and urging unified action for change. The report made recommendations to improve poverty within the developing world, including:

- Sustainable economic growth and social development of all countries to improve standards of living through the eradication of poverty, hunger, disease and illiteracy.
- The provision of adequate shelter and secure employment for all.
- The preservation of the environment.
- Democracy, respect for all human rights and fundamental freedoms.
- The empowerment of women and their full participation on a basis of equality in all spheres of society.

One of the key areas addressed within the Agenda is the promotion of a non-discriminatory, transparent and predictable multilateral trading system and promotion of investment and transfer of knowledge and technology, as well as the need for a strategy to find durable solutions to the debt problem (discussed later). However, before we move on to discuss debt we need first to acknowledge some other variables that affect sustainable growth, namely the difficulties experienced within the poorer countries that are compounded by political instability and war, and land which is unsuitable for growing essential crops, resulting in hunger and starvation.

Political instability and war

Political instability and war have many effects on civilians, including children. Not only does the infrastructure of a country stagnate, but it is also often destroyed. For example, the war in Somalia caused mass starvation, large cities such as Mogadishu were reduced to rubble, and for months on end electricity and water supplies were non-existent. Many children died of starvation or were injured or killed during the fighting. Others died because of disease associated with poor sanitation, and many more were orphaned and left Somalia as refugees. The problem with this and other conflicts, including more recently those in Rwanda, Serbia and Croatia, where large-scale 'ethnic cleansing' took place, is that when peace is restored, the difficulties of reuniting the many children who have been separated from their families are immense and often insurmountable. In many cases children are denied not only a nationality of their own but also even a name of their own, and are subject to racial discrimination. This contravenes the Convention on the Rights of the Child.

The Rights of the Child – Article 7

'*The child shall be registered immediately after birth and shall have the right from birth to a name, the right to acquire a nationality and, as far as possible, the right to know and be cared for by his or her parents.*'

The Rights of the Child – Article 2(1)

'*State Parties shall respect and ensure the rights set forth in the present convention for each child within their jurisdiction without discrimination of any kind, irrespective of the child's or his or her parent's or legal guardian's race, colour, sex, language, religion, political or other opinion, national, ethnic or social origin, property, disability, birth or other status.*'

War also brings less obvious challenges. Whilst children are frequently denied education during times of war, the existing professionals within a country are also denied education. For example, Swinburne (1994) described the situation of health professionals in Sarajevo during the conflict there, and discussed the academic stagnation and difficulty in keeping up to date with developments.

The lack of advancement as a result of war has many detrimental effects on children (and adults), and whilst we have seen many examples of how developed countries have come to the aid of individual children in order to overcome the deficits of, for instance, medical technology as a result of war, there are many, many more children who do not receive such aid. There are also longer-term effects on children. For example, the WHO (1997) has reported on the mass rape of women in situations of armed conflict and displacement. In the Rwanda conflict, many women were infected with HIV as a result of rape, with the subsequent effects on their children discussed earlier.

Developed countries, usually in collaboration with UNICEF and international charities such as the Red Cross, aim to provide assistance to civilians caught up in war. However, the problems faced by foreign workers in developing countries during times of war are enormous. For example, the equipment they are used to dealing with in the developed world, which might be available in the field, is difficult to operate within war zones where electricity supplies may be unreliable or lacking. The types of wounds which health professionals encounter may also be unlike any they have experienced before (Esser, 2002).

Food and hunger

Developing countries are often not self-sufficient in terms of their food production for several reasons. First, they may be politically unstable, with unstructured agricultural policies. Second, the populations of some countries tend to exceed the capacity of farmers to grow sufficient crops. Third, the land is frequently poor and only amenable to the growth of limited crops. Fourth, the international commodities markets are often working against the individual farmer in developing countries. Finally, ecological changes within the world are resulting in seemingly natural disasters and crop failures which can in part be attributed to environmental damage caused within the country or as a consequence of practices in other countries.

At present only 11 per cent of the world's surface is farmed for crops, while a further 20 per cent is apparently cultivable. The development of new, high-yielding strains of wheat, corn and rice, and the development of fertilizers, herbicides, pesticides and irrigation techniques have contributed to what is known in the developed world as the *Green Revolution* – and bumper harvests have been the result. However, current methods of modern farming are not without problems. The chemicals needed to produce high-yield crops are derived from fossil fuels, mechanized farming also depletes energy resources, and the spraying of crops with pesticides can pollute both the atmosphere and the water supply.

There are differences in the types of crops which can be successfully grown in different parts of the world. In many parts of the developing world, environmental variation is such that there tends to be an over-reliance on single crops. If the main crop fails, the results are catastrophic in terms of human life and the country's economic infrastructure. A further problem arises when a country relies on a single crop and overproduces it, which forces down the price of the commodity on the world market.

The distribution of the world's food supply has given rise to some speculation in recent years. If the global harvest were to be shared out, there would easily be enough food to feed everyone. Famines are the result of complexities relating to politics, economics, war and problems of storage and distribution. One short-term response to starvation in the developing world is to transport stockpiled surplus food to the places where it is needed most. In the long term, however, this does nothing to help farming in developing countries. Pouring surplus cheap and free food into developing countries lowers food prices, and can lead to less food being grown locally as it becomes financially non-viable to continue to farm. Except in emergency situations, the general view is that the most successful strategy involves enabling the development of appropriate technology, transportation systems, education programmes and administration systems.

The problems of mass starvation were vividly brought to the attention of the developed world in the 1980s by the first Band Aid and the work of Bob Geldof, who was moved to action after seeing a news report about starvation in Ethiopia in 1984. Geldof visited Ethiopia and, on his return, organized Band Aid – a massive musical extravaganza and other projects which raised millions of pounds for Africa. The importance of the aid to Africa was that it was channelled into projects which aimed to solve the longer-term problems of feeding vast populations, rather than just dumping excess food from the developed world.

Following Geldof's success, the General Agreement on Tariffs and Trade (GATT) drew up Article XXXVI, which attempted to discriminate positively in favour of developing countries in terms of export, access to world markets, financial support, and the elimination of barriers and custom duties, as well as introducing measures to stabilize world markets (General Agreement on Tariffs and Trade, 1986). This preferential treatment was reaffirmed by the World Trade Organisation in 1999 (WTO, 1999). These longer-term policies can only benefit those in developing countries, but the compounding factors mentioned above will probably always mean that organizations such as UNICEF will need to provide emergency food aid to the developing world.

Debt

Many developing countries struggle continually under huge foreign debt. They are forced to take drastic measures to repay both the debt and the resulting interest which accumulates on it, and consequently less money is available to solve the current problems within these countries, including education and child health.

There is international recognition of the fact that the cycle of debt in which some countries have found themselves must be broken, whether by the cancellation of a debt or its re-scheduling. There was indeed commitment to the cancellation of much debt in countries classified as the most Heavily Indebted Poor Countries (HIPC) in an initiative launched by the World Bank and the International Monetary Fund (IMF) in 1996. Forty-two countries (most from sub-Saharan Africa) are eligible for classification as HIPCs. There is however no easy answer to the debt problem in the developing world. The HIPC Initiative had only limited success, and in response to massive popular campaigning by the International Jubilee 2000 coalition, creditor countries agreed in 1999 to enhance the HIPC initiative to provide greater levels of cancellation of debts. However, Beattie (2004) reports that the process has been further delayed because of disputes among rich nations on how much relief to grant.

There is evidence that where debt is cancelled, the effects on development are staggering. In Tanzania, for example, the debt cancellation has enabled the implementation of a five-year education development plan which has seen the abolition of school fees, marked success in the attainment of gender parity in the education system, a 50 per cent increase in enrolments in primary schools, the building of 31 825 classrooms, the recruitment of over 17 000 new teachers, and much more beside (letter from the President of Tanzania to Jubilee Research, 2004). The removal of debt has, in effect, had a positive impact on education targets and employment, and in the longer term will no doubt impact on health – an example of how our three interrelated themes really do interact in practice.

Conclusion

This chapter has focussed upon three key elements of childhood experience, although there are clearly many others that are vitally important. Many children growing up in the developing world suffer disadvantage in the form of poverty, poor health and limited educational opportunities, and many never reach adulthood.

However, there is hope for children in the developing world, and it does give us at least some satisfaction to know that there is international recognition that investment in today's children will bring benefits to tomorrow's societies. Policies aimed at helping children in the developing world must however be culturally sensitive and appropriate, consistently carried out, child-friendly and, above all, they must be evaluated fully in order to provide evidence of their efficacy.

The Convention on the Rights of the Child outlines the principles which should be afforded to *all* children. We have referred to some of the 41 articles throughout this chapter, but as a final note we would urge the reader to read the full convention.

REFERENCES

Baby Milk Action (2000): *UNICEF Statement to the European Parliament Development and Cooperation Committee – Special Meeting on Standard Setting by European Enterprises In Developing Countries.* Baby Milk Action Press Release, 23 November.

Beattie, A (2004): Debt relief initiative for poor countries held up. *Financial Times*, 12 February.

Bokolamulla, D (2003): Interaction with developing countries – education for street children in Bangladesh. *E-journal of the WSC-SD.*

Esser, JA (2002): Post traumatic stress disorder and reaction. In Zubenko, WN and Capozzoli, J (eds), *Children and Disasters: A Practical Guide to Healing and Recovery.* Oxford: Oxford University Press.

General Agreement on Tariffs and Trade (GATT) (1986): *Trade and Development Article XXXVI.* Geneva: GATT.

Haggett, P (2000): *The Geographical Structure of Epidemics.* Oxford: Clarendon Press.

Hussain, R, Fikree, FF and Berendes, HW (2000): The role of son preference in reproductive behaviour in Pakistan. *Bulletin of the World Health Organization*, **78**(3), 379–385.

Koblinsky, MA, Campbell, O and Heichelheim, J (1999): Organizing delivery care: what works for safe motherhood. *Bulletin of the World Health Organization*, **77**(5), 399–406.

Meade, MS and Earickson, RJ (2000): *Medical Geography*, 2nd edn. New York: Guildford Press.

NetAid (2004): *Why Education?* Retrieved from www.netaid.org/learn/Index_htm.

Palmer, G (1999): *Politics of Breast-feeding*, 2nd edn. London: Independent Publisher Group.

President of Tanzania (2004): Letter sent to Ms Ann Pettifor, Director of Jubilee Research. Retrieved from www.jubilee2000uk.org/latest/tanzania04304.htm.

Rizzini, I and Mandel Butler, U (2003): Life trajectories of children and adolescents living on the streets of Rio de Janeiro. *Children, Youth and Environments*, **13**(1). Spring. Retrieved from http://cye.colorado.edu.

Swinburne, C (1994): War babies. *Nursing Times*, **90**, 23.

UNESCO (2001): *United Nations General Assembly Resolution.* Retrieved from www.unesco.org/education/efa/ed_for_all/background/un_resolution_1997.shtml.

United Nations (1997): *Agenda for Development.* New York: UN.

United Nations International Children's Emergency Fund (2004): *The Convention on the Rights of the Child*. Retrieved from www.unicef.org/crc/convention.htm.

Wagstaff, A (2000): Socio-economic inequalities in child mortality: comparisons across nine developing countries. *Bulletin of the World Health Organization*, **78**(1), 19–29.

World Bank (2004): *World Development Indicators*. Geneva: World Bank.

World Health Organization (1997): *Violence Against Women: In Situations of Armed Conflict and Displacement*. Geneva: WHO.

World Health Organization (1998): *Basic Newborn Resuscitation*. Geneva: WHO.

World Health Organization (2000a): *Drop In World Child Mortality reaches Target, New Study Shows But Many Countries Lagging*. WHO Press Release WHO/67, 12 October.

World Health Organization (2000b): *WHO Issue New Health Life Expectancy Rankings*. WHO Press Release, 4 June.

World Health Organization (2000c): *Infant and Child Mortality Rates*. Retrieved from www.who.Int/child-adolescent-health/overview/CHILD_HEALTH/mortality_rates_00.pdf.

World Health Organization (2001): 51st Session of the WHO regional committee for Africa. Retrieved from www.afro.who.Int/press/2001/regionalcommittee/re51005.html.

World Health Organization (2002a): *Global Action for Skilled Attendants for Pregnant Women*. Retrieved from www.who.Int/reproductive-health/mpr/mpr_global_action.pdf.

World Health Organization (2002b): *Global Strategy on Infant and Young Child Feeding*. Geneva: WHO.

World Health Organization (2003): *Future Trends and Challenges In Rehabilitation*. Retrieved from www.who.Int/ncd/disability/trends.htm.

World Trade Organization (1999): *Preferential Tariff Treatment for Least Developed Countries*. WT/L/304 Report.

WEBSITES

For a full copy of the Convention on the Rights of the Child – www.unicef.org/crc/convention.htm.

For information about projects concerning Street Child – www.hrw.org.

PERSPECTIVES ON EARLY CHILDHOOD RESEARCH

Jayne Taylor

This chapter aims to:

■ explore the value of research to the early years professional;

■ discuss methodological issues in early years research;

■ examine ethical considerations involved in undertaking research using child subjects.

INTRODUCTION

Imagine two staff nurses watching two women enter a children's ward. Both women are of a similar age and appearance. One is dressed in casual attire, whilst the other is wearing a smart business suit. Each woman holds a suitcase and the hand of a small boy. Both boys are about to be admitted to hospital. One of them, when passing the open door of the playroom, looks up at his mother, and on receiving her assent he runs to join the children who are playing there. His mother smiles and continues to walk towards the nurses. The other boy clutches his mother's hand very tightly and starts to cry softly.

One of the nurses turns to the other:

Nurse 1: I wonder why two seemingly similar children in a similar situation react so differently.
Nurse 2: There could be a hundred and one reasons.
Nurse 1: Yes, but if we could find out why, we could help little chaps like this one – he's so frightened. Imagine the ward full of happy, playing kids!
Nurse 2: Bliss!

Similar scenes are undoubtedly played out in nurseries, playgroups, schools, hospitals and crèches each time a group of new children arrives on the scene. The individual differences as well as the similarities which exist between children have both puzzled and fascinated professionals, and given them the motivation and material to enable them to delve into the complex world of the child through research. Many answers to countless questions have been discovered through investigation, but many questions remain unanswered, and indeed always will. Children change as society progresses, and they need to develop new behaviours in order to adapt to a complex and demanding world. There will always be questions which can be addressed through research, and as answers to existing questions are found, new and different questions will emerge.

We have included this chapter within the book for two main reasons. First, we wish to present a text that will support the training of early years professionals, and research awareness, at the very least, is an expectation of most if not all training programmes. Second, we have included this chapter because, as a writing team, we are firmly committed to the notion of research as a valuable asset in the advancement of practice. Early years professionals should be able to use other people's research intelligently by developing their own critical reading skills and, where necessary, to undertake research themselves. They should work from an established knowledge base which they understand, and seek to advance knowledge and theory through research.

The chapter begins by exploring the value of research to practice, and then moves on to examine different approaches and methodologies which have specific relevance to the study of children. We shall also focus on the ethical implications of undertaking research which involves children, with particular reference to early years professionals working within health settings. However, we must emphasize that we cannot cover all aspects of research methodology within the scope of one chapter. There are many excellent books which do this, and we have included a selection in the further reading section at the end of the chapter.

THE VALUE OF RESEARCH IN THE EARLY YEARS

In the Introduction, we discussed why the study of early childhood is important, with reference to its value as an emerging discipline in its own right, and also to the need for professionals to be able to map the childhood/adulthood continuum and explore the influence of childhood experience on adult behaviour.

Throughout the other chapters in this volume we have referred to the work of researchers who have undertaken studies for both purposes, although clearly there are fewer works which follow the progress of children into adulthood, because of the methodological challenges such an approach entails. It is because of the contributions of all of these researchers that we have the body of knowledge relating to the early years which exists today.

Drawing upon previous research serves a number of purposes. It can, for example, enable the investigation of a particular problem through the study of literature and lead to greater understanding of a certain phenomenon, which can in turn lead to changes in and advancement of practice. It can also predicate further empirical study of an area by informing the future researcher of existing work, tried and tested methodologies, and the problems, pitfalls and potential limitations of a specific approach. Existing research can enable researchers to approach topics in a similar or different setting, but it can also inform them so that they do not unnecessarily undertake work which has already been done. Studying previous research is almost always a prerequisite of future research-based activity. We shall explore this in more detail.

Using existing knowledge to inform practice

Look again at the vignette presented at the beginning of this chapter. The first nurse is making an assumption that the two children are *similar*. They may indeed be of a similar age and be similar in their looks. What the nurse does not know, however, at this stage is that the 'happy' child has been into hospital before, although never to this particular ward. His mother has spent a great deal of time preparing him for this admission, including borrowing books about hospitals from the library and engaging the help of the child's nursery-school teacher. At nursery all of the children in the little boy's class have been investigating hospitals and have built a small toy ward. They have a nurse's uniform and a doctor's coat. The little boy's experience of being a patient has been utilized to the full, and he has been able to impress friends with his superior knowledge! His mother also brought him to the 'Saturday Club' held at the hospital the previous week. This club is for all pending admissions, so that the children and parents have the opportunity to become familiar with the environment and some of the equipment. The little boy had taken a ride on a trolley which was made to look like Thomas the Tank Engine, and had listened to his own heartbeat via a stethoscope. The other little boy had done none of these things, and was only told he was to be admitted to hospital the day before.

The nurse is also making assumptions about the mothers of these two children. The mother of the happy child feels comfortable in the hospital setting. She is familiar with the environment, hospital routines and procedures. The suitcase she carries contains her belongings as well as those of her child because she will be staying in hospital with her son throughout his admission. The case also contains what she describes as her 'hospital survival kit', consisting of magazines, a good book, some ear-plugs, chocolate, orange juice, coffee and a comfortable tracksuit.

The mother of the unhappy child, by contrast, feels very uncomfortable. Her only experience of hospital, other than when she gave birth to her son, was as a small child. Her memories are unhappy – separation from her parents, pain, being in a ward with very elderly ladies, smells, unpleasant noises, and someone dying. Her childhood ordeal has given her a persistent fear of hospitals, and she has avoided telling her son about his admission for as long as possible because she knows she cannot cope with his questions. She is not going to stay overnight with him, although she knows she ought to do so. The guilt that she feels about this is making her even more tense. All she wants to do is hand her son over to the nurse as quickly as possible and leave.

The second nurse was right – there are potentially a 'hundred and one' reasons why these children behave differently. However, by talking to both mothers and visiting the library, the nurses will identify the most likely reasons for the differences in behaviour. They can narrow down the reasons for the differences by studying and understanding previous research. They may, for example, find the following.

- Mothers who have had negative experiences of hospital as children are less likely to visit or stay with their children than non-fearful mothers. The fear of mothers is more likely to lead to stressful reactions in the child (see Taylor *et al.*, 1999). The fearful mothers tend to be reluctant to have contact with hospital staff.
- Encouraging a mother (or parent) to stay with a child during hospitalization reduces the social discontinuity between hospital and home which can distress young children (Miron, 1990).
- Preparation for the experiences of hospital can help young children to cope and reduce stress (Murphy-Taylor, 1999). Preparation should involve parents (Kristensson-Hallstrom *et al.*, 1997) and nurseries and playgroups, etc. The use of leaflets and books is an excellent way of introducing children to hospitals in a non-threatening manner (Stone and Glasper, 1997).

- Pre-admission visits to the hospital can also reduce anxiety in children during hospitalization (Marriner, 1988; Kiely, 1989). Using play as a way of introducing some of the equipment that children will encounter can be extremely beneficial (Haiat *et al.,* 2003).

As a result of reading about previous research in this area, it may be possible to change practice so that mothers such as the mother of the unhappy child can be helped in positive ways to cope with their fears.

Using research to inform practice is the first (and an essential) step towards making progress, and as professionals we should strive to ensure that each and every part of our practice is informed by research. In the scenario described above, the nurses would have been able to find, through thorough and systematic searching of the literature, that there are research findings which can inform practice in this particular field.

Developing critical reading skills

The use of literature to inform practice is not entirely straightforward. Undertaking a literature review in itself can be complex, and involves library skills which take time to develop. Most of us only use libraries in a very superficial way, and it is only when we become familiar with a library that we can begin to use it to its full potential. In addition, the increasing use of databases, CD-ROMs and the internet have revolutionized our ability to access material quickly.

However, when material has been identified it may, in some fields, reveal conflicting views about certain topics. This is particularly so when the area being researched is new. You may recall, for example, the contrasting information which emerged during the early 1980s about the transmission of human immunodeficiency virus (HIV), which led to a certain amount of panic. It was only as more research was undertaken and reliable data emerged about the virus that some of the previous literature was shown to be incorrect.

It is important that early years professionals are able to make informed decisions about when research is reliable and valid, so that they do not make changes to practice on the basis of 'bad' research. There are clearly a number of ways of learning critical reading skills, and there are many good books which can help (see the further reading section at the end of this chapter). There are also many professional training programmes which require students to undertake supervised research themselves and, whilst the value of this has been questioned, it is a good way of learning to understand the somewhat mystical language of research and developing skills which will help with critical reading. It is to research activity that we shall now turn.

UNDERTAKING RESEARCH WITH CHILDREN

We have stated previously that this chapter is not intended to give a step-by-step guide to undertaking research – that would be neither possible nor appropriate. The main intention is to focus upon aspects of research involving children which are *different* to those which involve adults, so that the early years professional undertaking research may more ably transfer knowledge designed to apply to adult subjects to children in early years settings. Those areas of research methodology where there seem to be a few tangible differences (e.g. identification of problems, question formation) are not discussed. However, we shall commence with a few very broad principles which apply when undertaking research with children.

Overarching principles

As you have read throughout this book, children are not small adults. They perceive events differently to adults, their understanding of experience is different to that of adults, and the social contexts within which they exist are different to those of adults. Children are very special and deserve special consideration. They are also fascinating because of the way in which they rapidly develop physically, socially, psychologically and emotionally, and because of their ways of knowing and understanding.

The researcher who wishes to study children, particularly during the early years, is faced with a wealth of potential, as well as a few methodological 'headaches'! For example, traditional methods of collecting data may be inappropriate or even impossible because of the child's stage of development. Imagine the stupidity of asking a group of 2-year-olds to complete a questionnaire!

The early years researcher must possess those vital qualities which are essential to early years workers in all settings, namely well-developed skills of observation (see Chapter 1, pp. 6–19), knowledge of child development, a liking for children, patience and an ability to communicate through a variety of media. In many ways young children themselves can provide the researcher with an apt role model! From the first days of life children set out on a voyage of discovery. They explore, investigate, examine, categorize experiences, draw conclusions and seek to extend the boundaries of their knowledge. A very early text (Murray and Brown Smith, 1922) discusses the philosophy of Froebel (see also the Introduction), which summarizes this point admirably. He wrote that:

> 'Like things must be ranged together, unlike things separated. ... The child loves all things that enter his small horizon and extend his little world. To him the least thing is a new discovery, but it must not come dead into the little world, nor lie dead therein, lest it obscure the small horizon and crush the little world. Therefore the child would know why he loves this thing, he would know all its properties. For this reason he examines the object on all sides; for this reason he tears and breaks it; for this reason he puts it in his mouth and bites it. We reprove the child for naughtiness and foolishness; and yet he is wiser than we who reprove him.'
>
> (Murray and Brown Smith, 1922, p. 47)

The thorough way in which children investigate new experiences or seek to find solutions, the way in which they systematically approach problems and extend the boundaries of their knowledge – these are the principles of undertaking research with young children.

Methodological differences

When engaging upon early years research, the researcher needs to employ all of the skills and knowledge referred to above in order to ensure that the research yields results which are both reliable and valid. Three of the main problems, which are interrelated, are sampling, data collection and ethical implications (which will be discussed separately in the next section of this chapter).

Samples are the foundation of research and provide the researcher with the medium to answer research questions through data collection. A sample is anything which is smaller than a full population, and samples are used because it is rarely possible to study an entire population, although this does happen sometimes (e.g. the United Kingdom 10-yearly Population Census, or Graham and Rutter's Isle of Wight Study – you will find reviews of this famous study in most British texts on child psychology). The basis of sampling involves two general laws: the first is that a relatively large, randomly selected sample will represent the characteristics of the sample population; the second is that larger groups of data are more highly stable than smaller groups of data.

The importance of sampling during early childhood relates to the homogeneity of groups of children. You will recall the discussions in various chapters so far in this book about children's development, particularly in terms of their cognition and their social development. It is extremely difficult to identify an homogeneous group of children because age is a relatively poor predictor of cognitive and social development. Therefore, bias in sampling is a problem faced by many early years researchers. There are ways of overcoming bias, but the researcher must be aware that a group of intellectually intact pre-school children (spanning a five-year period from 0 to 5 years) is likely to be a far less homogeneous group than a group of intellectually intact adults (spanning, for example, a five-year period from 34 to 39 years).

However, many early years researchers are not concerned with being able to generalize their results across populations, but *are* concerned with their own practice in their own familiar settings. Samples which are 'convenient' may be biased and non-random and, regardless of the size of the sample, bias will remain in evidence. This presents no difficulty as long as it is recognized and acknowledged that the results cannot be generalized beyond the sample.

The second main problem relating to undertaking research during the early years concerns *data collection*. We have already mentioned the difficulty of using questionnaires among groups of young children. Similar difficulties are equally evident when using other self-report methods, such as rating scales. However, as with other data collection methods, modification can enable their use. For example, collecting data about postoperative pain using a numerical rating scale with young children may prove very unsuccessful, but by adapting the scale and using pictures of 'smiley' faces (see Whaley and Wong, 1991), or photographs as in the 'Oucher Scale' (Beyer and Aradine, 1987), success can be achieved. These tools have been shown to be reliable in measuring pain (Keck *et al.*, 1996). Using colour to symbolize levels of response is also a useful means of collecting data from children (see, for example, Sandberg *et al.*, 1993, who used colour-coded post-boxes). Similarly, a questionnaire designed to elicit information from hospitalized patients about food was modified by the author for use on the children's wards to include a 4-point scale which included the headings 'yuk', 'a bit yuk', 'OK' and 'yummy', instead of the adult version of 'not very good', 'all right', 'good' and 'very good'.

Observation is one of the most important data-collection methods for the early years researcher, and indeed it is one of the most important skills of the early years professional, as was discussed in Chapter 1. One particular observation technique derived from ethology, which involves the observation of children in their natural settings, is particularly useful. Observer effects (i.e. changes in behaviour caused by the intrusiveness of the observer within the situation) are problematic, but young children tend to adapt relatively quickly to the presence of, for example, a new adult within their nursery class. Observer effects can be minimized, therefore, by allowing the children being studied to adapt to the presence of the researcher [see for example Hawthorn's (1975) classic study of children in hospital], or by the researcher blending into the natural setting of the child.

Researchers using observation as a data-collection tool frequently need to adapt their methods to suit the cognitive level of the child. Whereas researchers using adult subjects may be able to ask their subject to use complex skills, early years researchers will use observation of the medium of play and toys in order to collect data (see for example, Smallwood, 1988; Cummings and El-Sheikh, 1991; Egeland and Kreutzer, 1991; Pellegrini, 2001; Susuki and Kato, 2003).

Interviews involving young children can also be problematic for the early years researcher, particularly in terms of the reliability of data. We have stressed many times that children and adults perceive experiences in different ways (Bower, 1977), and the reporting of interview data may lead to inaccuracies because of the *interpretation* of a child's language by the researcher. Children may, in fact, use quite complex language, but have limited understanding of the meaning of their words (see Luria and Yudovich, 1959, for a fascinating and detailed record of children's conversation), and they may be paraphrasing words that they have heard adults using, or they may understand but not have the language acquisition to be able to verbalize adequately. Others may pronounce words in strange ways, or use 'pet' words which stand for something completely different! However, it is important to stress that it is valuable to seek information directly from children, rather than relying on data from adults *about* children. Compas and Phares (1991) explore this issue and suggest that wide variations may exist between the reportings of teachers, parents and the children themselves in relation to specific data, which is something to consider when undertaking research and when reading other people's research. This is perhaps not quite so simple, however, when considering research with children who are, for example, ill. A sensible compromise advocated by Dimond (1996) is that such research should only involve children where it is absolutely essential and the information required cannot be obtained by using adult subjects.

The need for small-scale studies

Well-designed research on a small scale, using small convenient samples and data-collection methods which are appropriate to the child's level of understanding, provides the building blocks of professional knowledge because such research contributes to the generation of theory and, ultimately, to the advancement of practice. Much of the existing knowledge we work with today was originally derived from small beginnings. Axline's (1964) study of Dibs provided the basis for further study in the field of play therapy, and even Piaget himself formulated many of his early working hypotheses through close observation of his own three children! However, whether the research is on a small or large scale, whether it uses observation, questionnaires, interviews or other forms of data collection, it is always necessary to give due consideration to the ethical implications of undertaking research. It is to this important area that we shall now turn.

ETHICAL IMPLICATIONS OF RESEARCH INVOLVING CHILDREN

All researchers have a responsibility to analyse the ethical implications of their work, whether they work in the health services, the educational sector, social services or elsewhere. However, this responsibility is greatly amplified when the research being undertaken can be linked to the health or illness of children. Such research comes under the auspices of the Department of Health's Research Governance Framework (2001, p. 3), which covers:

'All research which relates to the responsibilities of the Secretary of State for Health – that is research concerned with the protection and promotion of public health, research undertaken in or by the Department of Health, its non-departmental public bodies and the NHS, and research undertaken by or within social care services that might have an impact on the quality of those services. This includes clinical and non-clinical research, research undertaken by NHS staff using NHS resources, and research undertaken by industry, the charities, the research councils and universities within the health and social care systems.'

There are, however, clearly some types of research which will carry stronger ethical implications than others and, as a starting point, researchers should always define very clearly what the child will be asked to do in order to participate in the research. If the research is *invasive*, either physiologically, psychologically or socially, then its moral acceptability should be questioned. This applies not only to healthcare workers but to *all* researchers using child subjects, because of the potential detrimental effects on the child. Brykczynska (1989) clarifies this point further:

'Invasiveness is not only about a concept of physiological invasiveness; children sharing ideas about life at home, for the benefit of the researcher, can become just as upset at the insistent questions of researchers, as children having blood taken.'

(Brykczynska, 1989, p. 121)

Brykczynska (1989) goes on to discuss how both of these examples involve invading the private world of the child and, because children do not perceive events in the same way as adults, seemingly *harmless* experiences can be potentially *harmful* to the child. This poses difficulties for the researcher, parents and others (e.g. members of ethical committees, research supervisors, managers who control access to physical environments) who have to make an informed judgement about the potential effects of involving a child or group of children. This problem has long been recognized, but there is no easy answer, although we shall explore further criteria which can be utilized. However, it is useful to remember the words used in the Platt Report:

'It is never safe to assume that a child will be afraid of an experience that an adult regards as frightening, or conversely that an experience which has no terrors for an adult will have none for a child.'

(Platt, 1959, p. 28)

One of the main criteria which should be applied relates to whether the research is *therapeutic* or *non-therapeutic*. Dimond (1996) defines therapeutic research as that which takes place when '… the subject stands to receive direct benefit from the research which is undertaken as part of his or her treatment' (p. 123). Non-therapeutic research is defined as research conducted without '… any direct or indirect benefit to the data subject' (p. 123).

Therapeutic research is evidently less contentious than non-therapeutic research which, when it involves children, is only acceptable as long as ethical principles and ethical codes are adhered to, and if there will be direct benefit to other children, and provided that the research has obtained the assent of children and the consent of parents (Brykczynska, 1989). It is perhaps prudent always to ask whether it is absolutely necessary to use children at all, or if it is possible to obtain the information required from adult subjects (Dimond, 1996), although it is worth mentioning that the level of agreement between parents and children concerning their individual interpretation of experiences is not always high (Sandberg *et al.*, 1993). However, if children must be used, then the researcher must ensure that the correct procedures and protocols are followed to protect the rights of the child.

Post-war codes of ethics

Following the Second World War and the War Crimes Trial in Nuremberg, and as a direct result of the atrocities which were carried out during the war under the guise of 'research', the Nuremberg code was declared in 1946 as a set of guidelines which should govern the behaviour of those undertaking research on human subjects. This code, and others which have since been developed, have application to working with child subjects, particularly as many of the atrocities which made the design of such codes necessary involved child subjects. Doctor Josef Mengele, Chief Medical Officer of Auschwitz-Birkenau Concentration Camp, involved many children, usually twins, in inhumane research in an attempt to discover the secret of multiple births so that the Aryan *Ubermensch* (super-race) could be multiplied at a faster rate than normal and world power achieved (Vigorito, 1992). Segal (1992) documents that this research included cruel, scientifically senseless and sometimes lethal methods carried out in atrocious conditions, resulting in needless suffering and the early death of innocent children.

The War Crimes Trial, and particularly what became known as the 'medical case', brought to light many issues surrounding experimentation on human subjects, and the need to ensure that the 'safety rails' such as the Hippocratic Oath, which should protect human subjects, cannot be removed again (Neuhaus, 1992). The Nuremberg code (Nuremberg Military Tribunals, 1949), the Universal Declaration of Human Rights (United Nations, 1948), the Declaration of Helsinki (World Medical Association, 1964, amended in 1975, 1983, 1989, 1996 and 2000), the European Commission Directive 91/507/EEC (European Commission, 1991) and other profession-specific codes such as the British Psychological Society's Code (BPS, 2000) and British Sociological Association's statement of ethical practice (BSA, 2002) have all been developed because of the recognition of the vulnerability of human beings and the need to preserve and protect human rights. Derived from, and incorporated within, the various codes mentioned above are the basic ethical principles upon which all research should be based (after Beauchamp and Childress, 2001):

- respect for persons and their autonomy;
- justice and fair treatment;
- beneficence;
- non-maleficence.

Whilst it is not possible to explore these principles further, there are many excellent texts which do so and which are cited in the further reading section at the end of this chapter.

Consent issues

It has already been mentioned above that the assent of children involved in research (if they are able to give such assent) and the consent of those with parental responsibility should be sought prior to their involvement in the research (Brkzynska, 1989). This is particularly important in that the Children Act (1989) (Department of Health,

1989) purports that there should be participation on the part of children in making decisions in cases where they have sufficient intelligence and maturity (although deciding upon what constitutes *sufficient* is open to interpretation). Dimond (1996) suggests that mentally competent 16- and 17-year-olds should give informed consent to their own involvement in research. Children below the age of 16 years should be asked to consent if they have sufficient understanding to do so. However, Dimond advises that the consent of parents should also be sought, particularly if the risks involved are considered to be significant.

Conclusion

This chapter has focussed on two main areas. First, it is important to emphasize that research is of great value to all of us who work with children. It is research which has enabled us to develop those theories which underpin our practice, and it is important that we are able both to access previous research and to develop skills so that we may critically read and intelligently use previous research. It also enables us to undertake further research and to build upon the existing body of knowledge so that the boundaries of practice can be extended.

However, it is important to recognize that undertaking early years research is not straightforward, and we may need to adapt and modify methodologies so that the design of the research is appropriate to the age and cognitive and social development of the child. Undertaking research with child subjects also involves additional ethical considerations which were discussed in the last section of this chapter.

Research involving children can be problematic, but the rewards of systematic study in the complex world of the child make the efforts of the researcher very worthwhile.

Student activity

Find a research article that has directly used children as research subjects (it can be about anything and can be a classic article or one from a recent journal).

- Read the article carefully.
- Identify any possible ethical implications, particularly any risks or harm to the child. What steps (if any) did the researchers take to ensure that their research met ethical standards?

REFERENCES

Axline, V (1964): *Dibs in Search of Self*. Harmondsworth: Penguin.

Beauchamp, TL and Childress, JF (2001): *Principles of Biomedical Ethics*, 5th edn. New York: Oxford University Press.

Beyer, J and Aradine, CR (1987): Patterns of pediatric pain intensity: a methodological investigation of a self-report scale. *Clinical Journal of Pain*, **3**, 130–141.

British Psychological Society (2000): *Code of Ethics*. Leicester: BPS.

British Sociological Association (2002): *Statement of Ethical Practice*. Durham: BSA.

Bower, T (1977): *The Perceptual World of the Child*. London: Fontana/Open Books.

Bryczynska, GM (1989): Ethical considerations in paediatric nursing research. In *Ethics in Paediatric Nursing*. London: Chapman & Hall, pp. 119–141.

Compas, BE and Phares, V (1991) Stress during childhood and adolescence: sources of risk and vulnerability. In Cummings, EM, Greene, AL and Karraker, KH (eds), *Life-Span Developmental Psychology: Perspectives on Stress and Coping*. Hillsdale, NJ: Lawrence Erlbaum Associates, pp. 111–130.

Cummings, EM and El-Sheikh, M (1991): Children's coping with angry environments: a process-oriented approach. In Cummings, EM, Greene, AL and Karraker, KH (eds), *Life-Span Developmental Psychology: Perspectives on Stress and Coping*. Hillsdale, NJ: Lawrence Erlbaum Associates, pp. 131–150.

Department of Health (1989): *The Children Act*. London: HMSO.

Department of Health (2001): *Research Governance Framework for Health and Social Care*. London: DoH.

Dimond, B (1996): Legal issues. In De Raeve, L (ed.), *Nursing Research: and Ethical and Legal Appraisal*. London: Ballière Tindall, pp. 118–137.

Egeland, B and Kreutzer, T (1991): A longitudinal study of the effects of maternal stress and protective factors on the development of high-risk children. In Cummings, EM, Greene, AL and Karraker, KH (eds), *Life-Span Developmental Psychology: Perspectives on Stress and Coping*. Hillsdale, NJ: Lawrence Erlbaum Associates, pp. 61–84.

European Commission (1991): European Commission Directive 91/507/EEC. Brussels: European Commission.

Haiat, H, Bar-Mor, G and Shochat, M (2003) The world of the child: a world of play even in hospital. *Journal of Pediatric Nursing*, **18**(3), 209–214.

Hawthorn, P (1975): *Nurse I want my Mummy!* London: Royal College of Nursing.

Keck, JF, Gerkensmeyer, JE, Joyce, BA and Schade, JG (1996): Reliability and validity of the faces and word descriptor scales to measure procedural pain. *Journal of Pediatric Nursing*, **11**(6), 368–374.

Kiely, T (1989): Preparing children for admission to hospital. *Nursing Series*, **3**, 42–44.

Kristensson-Hallstrom, I, Elander, G and Malmfors, G (1997): Increased parental participation in a paediatric day care unit. *Journal of Clinical Nursing*, **6**(4), 297–302.

Luria, AR and Yudovich, F (1959): *Speech and the Development of Mental Processes in the Child*. Harmondsworth: Penguin.

Marriner, J (1988): A children's tour. *Nursing Times*, **84**, 39–40.

Miron, J (1990): What children think about hospitals. *The Canadian Nurse*, **86**, 23–25.

Murphy-Taylor, C (1999): The benefits of preparing children and parents for day surgery. *British Journal of Nursing*, **8**(12), 801–804.

Murray, ER and Brown Smith, H (1922): *The Child Under Eight*. London: Edward Arnold.

Neuhaus, RJ (1992): The way they were, the way we are. In Caplan, AL (ed.), *When Medicine went Mad: Bioethics and the Holocaust*. Totowa, NJ: Humana Press, pp. 211–232.

Nuremberg Military Tribunals (1949): Nuremberg Code. Washington, DC: US Government Printing Office.

Pellegrini, AD (2001): Practitioner review: the role of direct observation in the assessment of young children. *Journal of Child Psychology and Psychiatry*, **42**(7), 861–869.

Platt, H (1959): *The Welfare of Children in Hospital: Report of the Committee on Child Health Services*. London: HMSO.

Sandberg, S, Rutter, M, Giles, S, *et al.* (1993): Assessment of psychosocial experiences in childhood: methodological issues and illustrative findings. *Journal of Child Psychology and Psychiatry*, **34**, 879–897.

Segal, NL (1992): Twin research at Auschwitz-Birkenau: implications for the use of Nazi data today. In Caplan, AL (ed.), *When Medicine went Mad: Bioethics and the Holocaust*. Totowa, NJ: Humana Press, pp. 281–300.

Smallwood, S (1988): Preparing children for surgery. *Association of Operating Room Nursing Journal*, **47**, 177–185.

Stone, KJ and Glasper, EA (1997): Can leaflets assist parents in preparing children for hospital? *British Journal of Nursing*, **6**(18), 1054–1058.

Susuki, LK and Kato, PM (2003): Psychosocial support for patients in pediatric oncology: the influences of parents, school, peers and technology. *Journal of Pediatric Oncology and Nursing*, **20**(4), 159–174.

Taylor, J, Muller, D, Wattley, L and Harris, P (1999): *Nursing Children: Psychology, Research and Practice*, 3rd edn. London: Stanley Thornes.

Vigorito, SS (1992): A profile of Nazi medicine: the Nazi doctor – his methods and goals. In Caplan, AL (ed.), *When Medicine went Mad: Bioethics and the Holocaust*. Totowa, NJ: Humana Press, pp. 9–14.

Whaley, LF and Wong, DL (1991): *Nursing Care of Infants and Children*, 4th edn. St Louis, MO: Mosby.

World Medical Association (1964) (amended in 1975, 1983 and 1989): *Declaration of Helsinki. World Medical Assembly*. Helsinki: World Medical Association.

United Nations (1948): *Universal Declaration of Human Rights*. New York: United Nations.

FURTHER READING

Beauchamp, TL and Childress, JF (2001): *Principles of Biomedical Ethics*, 5th edn. New York. Oxford University Press.

Christensen, P and James, A (eds) (2000): *Research with Children: Perspectives and Practices*. London: Falmer.

Cohen, L and Manion, L (2000): *Research Methods in Education*, 5th edn. London: Routledge.

Curtin, C (2001): Eliciting children's voices in qualitative research. *American Journal of Occupational Therapy*, **55**(3), 295–302.

Greig, A and Taylor, J (1999): *Doing Research with Children*. London: Sage.

Lewis, A and Lindsay, GE (eds) (2000): *Researching Children's Perspectives*. Buckingham. Open University Press.

Oppenheim, AN (1992): *Questionnaire Design and Attitude Measurement*, new edn. London: Pinter.

Polit, DF, Beck, CT and Hungler, BP (2001): *Essentials of Nursing Research*, 5th edn. Philadelphia, PA: Lippincott.

Yin, RK (2004): *Applications of Case Study Research*, 2nd edn. Newbury Park, CA: Sage.

WORKING WITH YOUNG CHILDREN AND THEIR FAMILIES

Jayne Taylor

INTRODUCTION

We come to the study of early childhood with a personal set of experiences of our own childhood, of our education, of our professional practice (or intended practice), of other people's children and, perhaps, experiences of our own children. We also bring to our studies a perspective, and we will each have an agenda or a personal set of aims which will relate to our personal reasons for choosing to study early childhood. For example, a student may ultimately wish to qualify as an early years teacher and will therefore focus his or her study upon education, or a student may wish to work as a children's nurse, in which case a health bias through the study of early childhood will be preferable. Other students may already have professional qualifications but wish to enhance their practice through further study.

What soon becomes apparent when studying early childhood is that the 'subject' chosen for study (that is, children and childhood) is vast, complex and strangely addictive. As mentioned above, we will have a personal agenda and may come to our studies wishing to focus specifically upon one aspect of childhood, such as health or education or social policy. What we soon realize is that it is almost impossible to study discrete areas of early childhood without gaining a fundamental knowledge of other areas – which brings us back to our holistic perspective. In our introductory chapter we emphasized the importance of holism, which does not attempt to separate these areas, recognizing instead that for the child and the family these aspects of childhood are inextricably interwoven. Separation of these aspects of childhood does not reflect the real essence of childhood and family life, and it soon becomes apparent that there are a common set of skills and a baseline of knowledge which all early years workers require, as well as the necessity to understand the context of childhood and family life.

Whether you have read this book from cover to cover or only delved into certain chapters, you will have noticed that the chapters fall generally into four types. There are those that examine the skills of the competent early years professional, such as Chapter 1 (Early Childhood Studies: first principles) and Chapter 16 (Perspectives on early childhood research). These chapters highlight the essential skills which are common across specialisms, in particular the scientific study of early childhood and the importance of competences such as observation.

Then there are those chapters which explore developmental aspects of childhood, including Chapter 2 (New beginnings: factors affecting health and well-being in the Infant), Chapter 3 (Physical growth and development), Chapter 4 (Personal, social and affective development), Chapter 5 (Children's relationships) and Chapter 6 (Play, language and learning). These chapters explore developmental processes and, because these are common to all children, we consider that knowledge relating to them is essential for all early years practitioners, regardless of specialism. Knowledge of play, for example, is pivotal to our understanding of childhood, our ability to communicate with children, and a child's ability to communicate with us. Observing children at play can, if we have the requisite knowledge, tell us about the ways in which children perceive their worlds, about the nature of childhood itself, and about the child's stage of development. Knowledge, coupled with a well-developed ability to observe and assess, will allow the practitioner to see beyond the outer child and will enable understanding of the complex set of experiences which make up the life of the child. As Froebel says, 'play at first is just natural life'.

Then there are those chapters which examine issues relating to the context of child and family life, policy and provision, including Chapter 7 (Early childhood education and care), Chapter 8 (The early school pathway), Chapter 9 (The child in society), Chapter 10 (Social policy: the state, the family and young children), Chapter 13 (Child health) and Chapter 15 (Children of the world). With the exception of the last of these, all explore the development of factors and systems that influence the lives of children and their families. Chapter 15, which explores the lives of children in developing countries, takes an even broader view, examining issues relating to policy, education, health and healthcare provision.

Chapter 11 (Child protection, welfare and the law), Chapter 12 (Young children with disabilities) and Chapter 14 (The Ill Child) discuss issues which face children, families and early years practitioners during adversity. Whilst there are clearly many more issues that we could have included which focus on children who experience life events which lead to difficulties, we felt that these three areas are those which the early years practitioners are most likely to encounter during their everyday working lives. For these children, in particular, the holistic framework which has been a recurring theme throughout the book is of the utmost importance. The children who are the focus of these three chapters will have contact with a range of early years professionals, and communication and collaboration are essential for the provision of competent care.

This final chapter aims to look at these issues in the context of working with children and their families, by drawing together the themes which permeate the book. These themes are communication and collaboration, developmental issues, the family in context, and finally we shall return to our principle theme, which is holism.

Before we look at each of these themes, however, we would like to just reflect for a minute, particularly for those who have read and used the first edition of this book, on what has been a remarkable shift in the way in which children and families have moved towards the centre of many of the policy and other initiatives we have discussed throughout the text. Whilst current practice may not always place children and families centre-stage, there is a real and tangible commitment to ensure that they are empowered to influence their relationships with professionals and the services that are delivered on their behalf. We applaud this shift, and urge practitioners to ensure that their individual and collective practice conforms with the aspirations of policy makers to put children and families at the heart of decision-making.

COMMUNICATION AND COLLABORATION

As we mentioned above, the early years practitioner is unlikely to work in total isolation, regardless of his or her chosen specialism. Team-work is the norm when working with children and their families, whether it involves working with fellow professionals or across professional boundaries. When I first began working as a health visitor, a discerning manager gave me an excellent piece of advice which was that, every day, before leaving work, I should ensure that a colleague would be able to take over my case-load without any difficulty – in case I was run over by a tram. Whilst it was unlikely that a tram would run me over (we had no trams in Great Yarmouth!), the advice was sound and taught me an important lesson. Working with children and families was the pleasant part of my work, and the aspect which had attracted me to health visiting in the first place. The record-keeping, communication of problems to the manager and referral to other agencies were the infrastructure of my practice and, whilst these were also the mundane and sometimes tedious aspects of the job, they were absolutely fundamental to my professional practice. This principle is as true today as it was then, even though the methods may have changed with parent-held records, databases and electronic communication systems.

However, communicating with colleagues and other professionals is not always easy. There are many actual and potential barriers to communication, and in professional practice these barriers operate at different levels. There may be barriers between the early years practitioner and the child and family, between colleagues working within the same sphere of practice, or between different professional groups.

Barriers which exist between the early years practitioner and the child and family may arise for a number of reasons. First, the practitioner may not be aware of the cognitive abilities of the child (or indeed of the family), and communication may be at an inappropriate level. This was discussed more fully in Chapter 6. Second, the ethnocentrism of the practitioner may mean that communication is inappropriate in terms of its content or delivery. Practitioners should take care not to impose values from their own class, religion or culture upon families. Finally, there may be reasons why even seemingly appropriate communication is ineffective, for example because the child and family are in a state of denial. This is a relatively normal stage for families to pass through when they have to face bad news about the health and well-being of a child (although in Chapter 12 we discuss how in many instances 'bad news' is given in an inappropriate way). It can also be apparent, however, when a parent is told about the deviant behaviour of a beloved (and normally good) child by a teacher, for example. Some parents will not seem to believe what is being said about the child because it is outside their own experience of him or her and cannot be aligned with their previous understanding and knowledge of that child's behaviour.

Barriers that exist between early years practitioners from within the same specialism can also be particularly awkward. These barriers tend to be of a personal nature, and should never be allowed to affect the care of children or families. However, there are occasions when a lack of communication about very simple matters will have detrimental effects. For example, if one practitioner gives a mother advice about how to wean her baby and a second practitioner (maybe inadvertently) contradicts this advice, the mother may become very confused, and in the end follows the advice of neither professional. The development of clear protocols and standards, based on the best possible available evidence, within organizations about what constitutes appropriate advice in a given situation can be extremely useful and beneficial to both the practitioner who gives the advice and the parent who receives it.

Barriers to communication that exist between professional groups can be very difficult to break down, and can also be potentially harmful to the child and family. For example, we have been given anecdotal evidence about children and families who have 'fallen through the net' and not received appropriate care in terms of family support, benefits and other tangible forms of care, because each professional group has assumed that the others have taken responsibility for care. There is also case-study evidence from some of the major child abuse inquiries which indicates that this does indeed happen, with devastating consequences. Corby writes:

> 'Almost all the inquiries published since 1973 have highlighted failures of systems to act in a co-ordinated way and failures of individuals to co-operate and communicate effectively in events leading up to children's deaths.'

(Corby, 1995, p. 211)

Non-effective communication and collaboration are not always connected to a reticence on the part of professional groups to break down barriers, nor do they always result in no one group taking responsibility for care. In some instances the problems stem from too many groups wishing to take responsibility and ownership for care, which results in the child and family becoming 'swamped' by well-meaning practitioners. Take the example of a child who, after a long struggle against cancer, faces the final hours of life at home with her family. The child has known many professionals over a number of years who have been responsible for various aspects of her care. At this very private and special time for the family, their home begins to fill with these people who all feel that they have a part to play in the child's last hours. The reality, we are told, is that the parents are left comforting the deeply distressed professionals and making tea, rather than focussing on the needs of themselves and their child.

Such well-meaning but misdirected care is the result of a communication barrier between groups. Whilst we recognize that working with young children does involve emotional commitment on the part of the professional, difficult as it may be, there are times when we must relinquish care to other groups by effectively communicating and collaborating. Case-conferencing is one of the better ways of ensuring that each professional group is aware of its boundaries and responsibilities when more than one group is involved in the care of the child. It is not only applicable to child protection practices, but also to a range of other situations. The presence of the parents (and the presence of the child, if appropriate) should be encouraged at these discussions, and they should be listened to. Care co-ordination through the role of key workers is a further example. This initiative, which started in 1999, aims to reduce the difficulties that parents face when trying to negotiate their way through the range of services to access support (see Chapter 12).

The National Service Framework for Children, Young People and Maternity Services (DH/DfES, 2004) emphasizes the need for good communication and collaboration, and will form useful sets of standards to reduce barriers within and between professional groups. This, alongside the establishment of early years partnerships, requiring local authorities to draw up Early Years Development and Childcare Plans from 1998 onwards, has set a strategic perspective on child care provision. The *Children Act* (2004) has been underpinned by the philosophy that early co-ordinated intervention has a positive impact on children's lives and has put in place a strategic framework for collaboration over future years. The Children Act ensures the integration of service planning, service commissioning and service delivery of mainstream health, education and family support facilities.

Effective communication and collaboration is thus vitally important in competent professional practice, and should form a major part of any training programme for early years professionals. As already mentioned, it is not something which is easy to accomplish, although it is perhaps true to say that some people appear to find it easier than others.

UNDERSTANDING DEVELOPMENT

A second theme which underlies the competent care of children relates to an understanding and knowledge of child development and those factors which influence such development. Professionals working with children must be aware of how children develop physically, psychologically, emotionally and socially, and several chapters within this book are devoted entirely to these aspects because we recognize the importance of this knowledge base.

Understanding development involves three distinct components which have been brought to the attention of the reader. First, there is the knowledge of normal patterns and sequences of growth and development. Such knowledge can be acquired in a number of ways, although we consider that the most effective way of learning about growth and development must always involve a combination of theory and integrated practice. A very simple example in relation to cognitive development and Piaget's theory of conservation is to ask students to try out some of the simpler experiments, such as manipulating rows of different-coloured buttons or rolling equally sized pieces of plasticine into different shapes, with children of different ages. Students are usually entranced by the children who fail to conserve, and delighted by the responses of those who can!

The second component which is integral to the above discussion is observation, which was introduced in Chapter 1 and revisited in later chapters. Observation is an essential part of the role of all early years practitioners, and is vital for the acquisition of our knowledge of growth and development. Students who are new to the study of early childhood may occasionally feel that they already have a very well-developed sense of observation, and indeed some do. The majority, however, find that in reality their skills require considerable refinement, and are pleased with the wealth of data that their developed skill offers. As with gaining knowledge of developmental processes, the student can learn a great deal about the skill of observation by watching children at play. Froebel (in Murray and Brown Smith, 1922) made much of observation of children and of the benefits for the student of studying the child's own powers of observation, saying 'become a learner with the child' (p. 101). Clutton Brock (in Murray and Brown Smith, 1922) wrote on a similar theme, but cautioned that when children observe, they do so in a different way to adults, because adults cannot observe without being influenced by other, interfering, events. He wrote that:

> 'The child feels ... delight among spring flowers; we can all remember how we felt it in the first apprehension of some new beauty of the universe ... most of us remember too the indifference of our elders. They were not considering the lilies of the field; they did not want us to get our feet wet among them ... parents and nurses (and teachers) have ... to be aware that the child, when he forgets himself in the beauty of the world, is passing through a sacred experience which will enrich and glorify the whole of his life. Children, because they are not engaged in the struggle for life, are more capable of this aesthetic self-forgetfulness.'
>
> (Murray and Brown Smith, 1922, p. 95)

The third component which is important for understanding growth and development, and which is integral to the other two components mentioned above, is assessment. Assessment, along with observation, was introduced to the reader in Chapter 1, and we have returned to it continually. Working with children during the early years is not a static process, but usually involves helping, enabling and facilitating the child to progress. In order to do this effectively, the practitioner – using his or her knowledge of growth and development and powers of observation – must engage in a process of assessment so that the child can be enabled in an appropriate and meaningful way. This principle is true in almost every setting, whether it be choosing an appropriate activity for a group of pre-school children in a nursery, or working with an individual child with learning disabilities on an early support programme (see Chapter 12). Assessment is also a fundamental part of the role and training of all early years practitioners, including teachers, nurses, midwives, health visitors, psychologists and social workers.

As with our other two components, learning assessment skills must involve practice as well as theory, so that students can apply their knowledge in a meaningful way.

THE FAMILY

The third theme which permeates this book is the role of the family in childhood, which was introduced in Chapter 2 and revisited in other chapters, particularly in Chapters 5 and 9.

Early years practitioners may *only* work with the child as part of a family. For example, health visitors, social workers and midwives rarely, if ever, work with individual children in isolation from the family. Other practitioners, such as teachers and nursery nurses, may consider children to be their 'primary' clients, but realize that the child is part of a family which will influence the development, behaviour and personality of the child. In recognition of this, most organizations encourage parental participation in pre-school and school educational activities, in healthcare, in child protection work, etc. The important message which we wish to bring to the attention of the reader is that it is not practicable to work with a child without considering the family context, because children do not grow up in vacuums, but are part of a living, interacting group that is far more influential upon the child's development than any other facet of childhood.

The family, above all others, will know the child and appreciate his or her uniqueness. They will be skilled in providing care and will understand the child's behaviour patterns. They may also hold the key which enables the practitioner to understand the individual child. To study a child outside the context of his or her family, or without at least acknowledging the power and influence of the family, is both narrow and mechanistic – and does not capture the true essence of childhood.

Sameroff (1989) discusses the concept of *codes* which influence behaviour within the family and, consequentially, the behaviour of the child. The first type of code he discusses is the *cultural code,* which organizes a society's child-rearing system and regulates 'the fit between individuals and the social system' (p. 25), so that individuals can fulfil an acceptable role within society. The second type of code is the *family code,* which determines behaviour within the family system and produces individuals who fulfil an acceptable role within the family. The third type of code is the *individual parent's code,* which originates from his or her own past experiences of family code. In other words, parents bring to the new family their own experiences of belonging to a different family, which will influence the interaction within the new family. This can clearly be a positive influence, but it can equally well be a negative one. Sameroff (1989) also discusses regulations within society and the family which are different to the parental styles described in Chapter 5, but are certainly not disconnected from them. Sameroff (p. 26) writes that, 'It is important to recognise the parent as a major regulating agency of child development, but it is equally important to recognise that parental behaviour is itself embedded in regulatory contexts.'

Regulations within the family include *macroregulations*, which provide the rules for a society and dictate the expected behaviour of individuals within each culture. *Miniregulations* are a second level of regulation, and regulate behaviour within the family. For example, miniregulations will operate in terms of how a family will discipline children, and how the family may view activities such as play and learning. The third type of regulation is *microregulations*, which Sameroff describes as 'momentary interactions between child and caregiver' (Sameroff, 1989, p. 28). For example, a parent may make a seemingly insignificant gesture, such as the slight raising of an eyebrow, which the child will recognize as displeasure, but of which a stranger will be unaware.

Codes and regulations will clearly influence the child's development as well as the way in which they behave outside the family, their attitudes, values, beliefs and aims. If, as professionals in early years settings, we wish to view parents as equal partners, we must be aware of factors within the family which can influence the child, so that we can work with the parents.

HOLISM

The final and probably strongest theme which underpins this entire book is that of holism, which was first brought to the attention of the reader in the introductory chapter. We have strongly advocated the notion that each practitioner must work within an holistic framework, even though he or she may come to work with the child and family in a very specialized way. If our work has a purpose, and we wish to be successful in our work, we must focus upon the whole child. For example, consider a teacher who is working with a child on a particular subject, but who ignores the signs that indicate that the child is clearly distressed and anxious. If the child's distress is not managed, he or she is unlikely to learn from the teacher, because we know that anxiety is a barrier to learning. Far better that the teacher spends time trying to find out why the child is distressed, before instigating appropriate intervention.

Holism also involves recognition that the child is part of a family, a culture and a society, as we have discussed in the preceding section. Failure to recognize the child as part of a larger network will result in his or her experiences of life not being utilized to their full potential. Children learn best by being active, by discussing their thoughts and feelings in a variety of situations, and by experimenting with their newly acquired skills. Learning does not only occur in the nursery or classroom, but also takes place within the family, where the child is able to consolidate and experiment in his or her natural world (see Chapter 7).

Our first theme of communication and collaboration is also a fundamental part of holism. As we have stated before, we come to the study of early childhood from a particular perspective or specialism. Childhood, however, is so complex that the child will form relationships and interact with a number of practitioners. Some children – particularly those with a long-term illness or disability – are likely to interact with more practitioners than others. The important point to make here is that each practitioner should have a knowledge of the roles and responsibilities of the other professionals, and should communicate and collaborate effectively in order to break down actual or potential barriers which could be harmful to the well-being of the child and his or her family.

Finally, our aim in writing this book was to bring together professionals from a variety of backgrounds to write about aspects of our shared interest, namely children during the early years. Each writer has brought to the debate a specialist slant, but each has also considered the child within our holistic framework. We hope you have enjoyed it!

REFERENCES

Corby, B (1995): Interprofessional co-operation and interagency co-ordination. In Wilson, K and James, A (eds), *The Child Protection Handbook*. London: Ballière Tindall, pp. 211–226.

Department of Health (2003): *National Service Framework for Children. Part 1: Standards for Hospital Services*. London: DoH.

Department of Health/Department for Education and Skills (2004): *National Service Framework for Children, Young People and Maternity Services*. London: DoH.

Murray, ER and Brown Smith, H (1922): *The Child under Eight*. London: Edward Arnold.

Sameroff, AJ (1989): Principles of development and psychopathology. In Sameroff, AJ and Emde, RN (eds), *Relationship Disturbances in Early Childhood: a Developmental Approach*. New York: Basic Books, pp. 17–32.

WEBSITES

Children Act 2004 – www.legislation.hmso.gov.uk/acts/acts2004/20040031.htm
Department for Education and Skills – www.dfes.gov.uk

INDEX

Abuse, *see* Child abuse
Academic achievement 119, 248, 253
    emotional literacy and 60
    father involvement and 88
    PSE education as lesser priority 58
Academic study of early childhood, *see* Early
    childhood studies
Access (for research) 18
Accidents 46–7, 181, 246–7, 249
Accommodation (in learning) 101, 102, 109
Acheson Report 28, 248, 249
Acts of Parliament, *see under* Legislation
Adaptation, learning through 101–2
Adolescence
    mental health problems 58
    teenage pregnancy 29–30
Adult Attachment Interview 87
Aesthetic needs 46, 47
Affective development, *see* Personal, social and
    emotional (PSE) development
AIDS, *see* HIV/AIDS
Alcohol
    child abuse survivors 95
    effect on fetus 28
Anonymity (in research) 10, 19
Antenatal care 27, 31, 32, 49
Antiretroviral therapy 271
Antisocial behaviour 58, 88, 119
Anxiety 252
Art, children in 168
Asian background/communities
    child nutrition 51, 52, 250
    see also Bangladesh; China
Assent (to research) 291, 292–3
Assessment
    disabled children 228, 230
    Foundation Stage Profile 155
    key skill 302
    Key Stage One 158
    special educational needs 234
    understanding development 301–2
    see also Observation of children
Assimilation 101, 102, 109
Associationism 4
Asthma 26, 252, 262
Attachment 59, 63–4
    Adult Attachment Interview 87

at 6 months *vs* 4 years 46, 47
false–belief task 64
love and belonging needs 46, 47
mother–child relationship 85–7
play 109
social understanding 64, 70, 71
socialization by 12 months 67
types of attachment 86–7
Attainment targets 157
Attunement (infant-carer) 66–7, 69, 124
Autism-spectrum disorders 64, 235, 250

Baby blues (three-day blues) 33
Band Aid 280
Bangladesh
    son preference 273
    street children 277
    weaning ceremony 50
Barnardos 245
BCG vaccination 246
Behavioural codes/regulations 302–3
Behavioural domain skills 61
Behavioural problems
    extent of 58
    poverty and 181
    pre-school socialization and 69
    school-aged children 252
    see also Antisocial behaviour; Autism-spectrum
        disorders; Crime; Special educational
        needs (SEN)
Behaviourism 4, 101, 105
Belonging, as need of child 46–7
Bernard van Leer Foundation (BVLF) 119
Biological theories of play 107–9
Birth asphyxia 272, 274
Black service users
    experience of 238
    see also Cultural aspects; Ethnicity
Blindness 273
Blood spot screening 42
Bottle-feeding 88, 102, 273, *see also*
    Breast-feeding
'Bounty bag' 50
Breast from Birth Charts (Child Growth
    Foundation) 48
Breastfeeding 48–9, 102, 169–70, 273–4
Bright Futures 252

Bristol Royal Infirmary inquiry 190
Bureaucracy 246

Care
    UNICEF definition 117
    see also Child care; Early childhood education
        and care (ECEC)
Carers
    abuse by 220, 221, 228
    disabled children 228, 236
    division of labour within home 178–9
    see also Child care; Child care policy; Parents
Casa Alianza (Guatemala street project) 278
Case conferences 300
Catholic Action for Street Children (Ghana) 278
Centile charts (growth) 43–5, 48
Cerebral palsy 24, 234, 251, 261
Changing Childbirth 32
Charitable organizations 197–8, 245
Check-lists 14–15
Chewing, and speech 49
Child abuse
    abusive process 204
    concept of significant harm 206
    defining 204, 206
    delay in revealing 207
    extent 209–10
    Fred and Rosemary West 79, 95
    guidance for professionals 211
    Inquiry Reports 204–5, 300
    misuse of adult power 220
    poverty and 181
    public concern 204
    within family 207
    see also Emotional abuse; Physical abuse;
        Sexual abuse
Child benefit 191
Child care
    drop-in provision 198
    family provision 176
    lone-parent families 82
    male partners 88, 176, 178–9
    working parents and demand 196–7
    see also Early childhood education and care;
        Nursery education
Child care policy
    administrative centralization 187
    child-centred 188
    diversity and inclusion 188
    historical viewpoint 186–7
    'less eligibility' principle 186
    local authority responsibility 188
    workhouse testing 186
Child development 37, 118
    assessment
        educational 151–2, 155, 158
        research 10–18
    Denver Development Screening test 38
    developmental scales 38
    factors influencing 38, 41

friendship role 93
health promotion and optimal 248
health visitor 47
importance of understanding 301–2
knowledge of normal 301
Maslow's hierarchy of needs 46–7, 63
milestones 38, 39–40
physical
    antenatal 27, 31, 32, 49
    growth 42–5, 48
    postnatal care 32–4, 48
    preconceptual care 29, 31–2
    see also Language; Learning; Personal, social
        and emotional (PSE) competence;
        Relationships; Screening
Child health
    geographic variation 249
    historical attitudes 245–6
    holism and integration 253
    inequalities 28, 248, 249
    long-term needs 250–3
    media role 244, 249
    poverty and 248–9
    promotion
        optimal development 248
        public health role 248
        in schools 248
    screening 41–5
    service provision
        history of 245–6
        'postcode lottery of care' 237, 247
        preventative services 246
    socio-economic factors 249
    see also Early childhood services
Child labour 166, 168, 245
Child maltreatment, *see* Child abuse
Child neglect 211–13, 213
    contributory factors 81, 211, 212
    definition 211
    effects 94
    emotional 212, 214–15
    examples 211
    therapeutic contract 212, 213
    see also Child abuse; Emotional neglect
Child pornography 270
Child Poverty Action Group 198
Child prostitution 207, 277
Child protection
    Children Acts (1989, 2004) 204, 205, 222
    disabled children 236
    family privacy/intervention 20
    government response to Laming Inquiry 205
    multidisciplinary approach 221–2
    professional challenges 203
    public expectation 203–4
Child Protection Registers 205, 206–8, 213
Child tax credit 191
Child/childhood, defining xi–xii, 165–6
Childhood depression 57, 62, 70, 94–5, 252
    see also Mental health

Childminders 177, 195, 196
Children Act 1989/2004, *see* Legislation
Children Living in Long-Stay Hospitals 227
Children in need
    assessment for services 230, 234
    disabled children 230
    see also Child health, service provision; Early
        childhood services
Children's Commission for England 205
Children's Commissioner 194, 258
Children's NHS Trusts 205, 248, 253, 258
Children's rights
    4Ps approach to 192–3
    childhood stereotyping 193
    competence of child 193
    empowerment of child 193–4
    ideology of family and 192
    participatory view 193
    protectionist view 193
    reality of poverty and 194
    in social policy 185
        constructionist *vs* realist perspective
            192
        increased importance 188, 192
    see also UN Convention on the Rights of
        the Child
China
    'barefoot doctors' and maternal
        mortality 272
    female infanticide 273
Chomsky's language theory 105
Chromosomal abnormalities 26, 27
Chronic illness
    community-based care 261
    see also Ill child, with long-term needs
Citizenship training 249
Codes, behavioural 302
Cognitive development
    language acquisition 105–6
    learning process 101–2
    play 108, 109–10
Cognitive domain skills 61
Cognitive-behavioural intervention 65
Collaborative care xi, 298–300
Comenius, Joan Amos (1592–1670) (early
    childhood pioneer) viii
Communication
    barriers to 299–300
    diagnosis and disclosure 230–2
    flexibility of human 103
    holistic approach xi, 103
    ill child 264
    inter-professional 298–300
    meta- 111, 112
    preverbal 66–7
    social understanding 64
    with disabled child 236
    see also Language; Speech
Community
    collaboration between schools and 145

Community care
    child with long-term needs 250–1
    children's nursing service 251, 260–1
    disabled child 226, 228–30
    promotion of health 248
Competence of child 193
Confidentiality 10, 19, 264
Congenital abnormalities 24, 26, 28, 29, 42
Conscience, development of 67
Consent (to research) 18, 292–3
    informed consent 19
Conservation, Piaget's theory of 301
Constructivism (interactionism) 5–6
    see also Social constructivism
Convention on the Rights of the Child, *see* UN
    Convention on the Rights of the Child
Corporal punishment 220
Crime, juvenile 58
Critical reading skills 287
Cultural factors
    attitudes towards children xii
    child development 38, 102
    codes of behaviour 302
    early childhood education and care 125–6
    learning theory 103
    nutrition of pre-school child 52
    play 105, 106, 107, 113
Cultural relativism xiii, 1, 17
Curriculum
    Curriculum Framework for Children 3–5
        (Scotland) 143
    Early childhood education and care guidelines
        130–2
    Excellence and Enjoyment 47
    hidden 154
    received 154
    spiral 103
    see also Foundation stage (4–5 years),
        curriculum; National Curriculum
        (England)
Cystic fibrosis 42, 261

*Dakar Framework for Action–Education for All:
    Meeting our Collective Commitments, The*
    276
Data collection 289
Day care 64, 69, 176–177, *see also* Child care
Deafness 235
Death
    accidental 249
    birth asphyxia 274
    child abuse 204–5, 222
    poverty and 248
    sudden infant 26, 49, 249
    see also Dying child
Debt (developing countries) 281
Declarations of the Rights of the Child 270, *see also*
    UN Convention on the Rights of the Child
Delinquency 58, 119
Dental health 248

Denver Development Screening test 38
Depression
    childhood 57, 62, 70, 94–5, 252
    postnatal 33
    see also Mental health problems
Desirable outcomes curriculum 143
Developing countries
    child labour 166
    child morbidity 273–4, 275
    child mortality 271–3
    debt 281
    definition 268–9
    disabled child 274–5
    education 276–8
    food and hunger 280–1
    health 270–5
    life expectancy 271–2
    political instability and war 279
    street children 277, 278
    wealth 281
    see also UN Convention on the Rights of the
        Child
Developmental milestones 38–40
Developmental scales 38
Developmentally appropriate practice (DAP)
        131–2, 145
Diabetes mellitus 26, 28, 261
Diaries 16
Diarrhoeal diseases 271, 273
Diet, see Nutrition
Diphtheria 246
Directors of Children's Services 258
Disability
    discrimination and stereotyping 227–8, 231
    legislation promoting inclusion 228–30
    medical vs social model 227–8, 229, 231
Disability and advocacy movements 228
Disabled children 226–43
    assessment and service provision 228, 230
    barriers to inclusion 226, 237
    child protection 236
    community-based care 250–1
    congenital abnormalities 24
    developing countries 274
    diagnosis and disclosure 230–3
    early school years 234–5
    education provision 228
    educator's attitudes 127, 149
    equality of opportunity 126
    institutional care 226, 227
    legislative changes 228–30
    mainstream education 226, 251
    move towards inclusion 226, 227–30, 251
    multiprofessional approach 235, 251
    number 226
    play 234, 237
    pre-school years 233–4
    and preventative health services 246
    right of assessment 228
    UN Convention on the Rights of the Child 230
    see also Special educational needs (SEN)

Disadvantaged children
    benefits of Early childhood education and
        care 119
    obesity in 250
    SureStart 31, 120–1, 124, 145, 189, 191, 234, 248
    see also Poverty; Socio-economic factors
Discourse analysis 165
Discrimination
    in classroom 126–7, 149
    disabled people 227, 228, 231
    and OECD ix
Dissociation 218
Domestic violence 181
Down syndrome 27
Drugs, teratogenic effect 28
Dying child
    approach to 252–3, 300
    formal education 252

Early childhood education and care (ECEC)
    age of formal teaching 143–4
    aims 118
    attachment theory 63–4
    benefits 118–20
    consensus framework 123–4
    cultural understanding 125–6
    ecological model 127
    educator–child interaction 128–30
    equality of opportunity 126–7
    evaluation 133–4
    holistic approach x–xi, 123, 124, 127
    inclusion 125–7, 149
    integrated/multiprofessional approach 124
    knowledge and skills 127–8
    learning activities 130–2
        contextually appropriate practice 131–2,
            145, 148
        curriculum guidelines widespread 130
        developmentally appropriate practice 131, 145
        English foundation stage curriculum 130
        Laever's experiential model 131
        Reggio Emilia 130
        Te Whariki 130
    partnership with families 132–3
    quality 120–3, 133–4
        children's views 123, 134
        Early Childhood Environment Rating Scale
            121–2, 134
        Excellence in Early Childhood framework 122
        experiential education 120
        OECD's Starting Strong report 121
        SureStart 120–1
    reflective practice 134
    respect 124–5
    right to free part-time 195
    service provision 195–7
    training and development 147
    UN approach to ix–x
    warmth of relationships 125
Early Childhood Environmental Rating Scale
        (ECES-R, ECERS-E) 121–2, 134

Early childhood services 185
   Children Act (2004) 205
   disabled child 228, 229
   early years partnerships 194
   employment-led reforms in child care 196–7
   empowerment 194
   improved co-ordination 194, 205–6
   voluntary services 197–8
   welfare care and 197
   see also Child care policy; Early childhood
      education and care
Early childhood studies
   childhood as social construct xii
   cultural relativism xii, xiii
   description xi–xiii
   early childhood pioneers viii–x
   ethical issues 18–19
   family as context for 302
   history of childhood xii–xiii, 168–9
   holistic perspective 164, 297
   multidisciplinary, integrated 3
   personal agenda 297
   reasons for studying xiii–xiv, 297
   theoretical perspectives 4–6
   value principles 1–3
Early Excellence Centres/Programmes x, 233–4
Early learning goals 130–1, 143, 150–1
Early school pathway
   assessment of child 155
   classroom environment 154
   first days in school 148–9
   fostering independence 154
   foundation stage curriculum 151–4
   Foundation Stage Profile 155
   key stages 142
   learning activities 152–4
   legislative requirements 144
   multiprofessional working 147–8
   outdoor environment 154–5
   role of parents 145–6
   socio-cultural context 146–8
   starting age 141–2
   wider team in classroom 146–7
Early Support Programme for Children 0–3
   (disabled pre-schoolers) x, 233
Early Years Development and Childcare
   Partnerships x, 123, 124, 194, 300
ECEC, see Early childhood education and care
Education
   attempts to define 117
   developing world 276–8
   effect of poverty 181
   health promotion and success of 253
   impact of illness 264–5
   Laever's model of experiential 120, 121, 125,
      131, 134
   principle of inclusion in mainstream 251
   as right of child 276–8
   see also Early childhood education and
      care (ECEC)
Education Action Zones 234

Educator–child interactions 128–30
Effective Provision of Pre-School Education
      (EPPE) study 121–2
Embryonic phase 24–5
Emotional abuse
   definition 213, 214
   effects 94
   examples 213–14
   identifying 214
   long-term legacy 215
   and neglect 214–15
   parental factors 215
   therapeutic intervention 215–16
Emotional development
   empathy 65, 67, 68
   intelligence/literacy 58, 61
   pro-social development 58, 65–6
   see also Attachment; Family; Personal, social and
      emotional (PSE) development; Relationships
Emotional domain skills 61
Emotional neglect 212, 214–15
   emotional abuse compared 214–15
   long-term effects 215
   parental inadequacy 211, 215
   see also Child neglect
Empathy
   development of 65, 67, 68
   see also Emotional development
Empiricism 4, 101
Empowerment
   black client and service delivery 238
   care of sick children 194
   patient in NHS 249
End Child Poverty (charity) 82
Enlightenment 168
Equilibration 101, 102
Ethical issues
   observation of child 18–19
   post-war codes of ethics 292
   research 290–3
'Ethnic cleansing' 279
Ethnicity
   black service users' experience 238
   disability 232
   early childhood education and care 126
   parenting style 82
   poverty 191
   and weaning 50, 51
Ethology 85
Evaluation 133–4
Event sampling 13–14
Every Child Matters 205, 258
   Next Steps 258
Evolutionary psychology 85
Excellence in Early Childhood (EECL) 122
Excellence and Enjoyment: A Strategy for Primary
      Schools 47, 144
Excellence For All Children 251, 253
Excellence in Schools 233
Expert patient programme 263
Eyesight testing 247

Failure to thrive 211
False–belief task ('theory of mind' test) 64
Family
    chaotic-rigid 83
    child-centred 181
    codes 302–3
    conjugal 172
    connected-separated 83
    context for childhood studies 302
    defining 170–2
    disabled child 233, 237
    division of labour 178–9
    dysfunctional 62, 84
    enmeshed-disengaged 83
    extended 170, 172, 175
    functions 170–1, 181
    holistic approach x, 132–3, 134, 297, 303
    ideology of 79, 192
    ill child
        coping behaviour and outcome 264
        and empowerment of 262–4
        minimizing impact of 264–5
    kinship links 175–6
    lone-parent 52, 82–3, 172–5, 191, 192
    multi- 173, 174
    nuclear 169, 170, 172, 173, 176, 178
    parents and schools 145–6
    reconstituted/blended 172
    regulations within 303
    residence 170
    social policy 185–6, 192, 196–7
    structural functionalism 164
    structures 84, 170, 172–6
    symmetrical 178
    understanding of their child 302
    unit 79
    well-balanced and adjusted 83–4
    women oppressed by 178
    women working in 177–8
    work-life balance 196–7
    working in partnership 132–3
Family planning clinic 31
Family relationships
    diversity 79
    dysfunctional 84
    parenting education 81–2
    parenting style 79–81
    significance 79
    structures 83
    well-balanced 83
Family Resources Survey 2002–3 226
Family structures
    adaptability 83
    cohesion 83
    Olsen model 84, 170, 172–6
Famine 280
Fantasy 110
Father–child relationship
    absent father 88
    benefits for child 88–9

involvement 87–8
    play 88
    sex-role development 89
    sibling relationships 89–92
Favouritism–hostility hypothesis 92
Feeding, see Nutrition
Feelings
    pre-school teaching about 60
    see also Emotional development
Feminism 164
    gender role education 166
    view of childhood 166
    women oppressed by family 178
Fetal alcohol syndrome 28
Fetal development 25–6
Field notes 16
Five-year Strategy for Children and Learners 144
Fluid intake 52
Folic acid supplement 29
Food
    global distribution 280
    see also Nutrition
Food in Schools Programme 54
Foreign debt 281
Foundation stage (4–5 years) x, 142
    curriculum x, 130, 143–4, 158, 195–6
    early learning goals 130–1, 143, 150–1
    planning 151–4
    preparation for National Curriculum 130–1, 150
    stepping stones 130–1, 150–1, 155
Foundation Stage Profile 155
Foundation stage unit 143
Frame analysis 112
Framework for Action on Values Education in Early
        Childhood (UNESCO) 127
Freud, Sigmund 78
Friendships
    benefits 93–4, 113
    children's views 123
    identifying 92
    impact of illness 264, 265
    number 92
    popularity 94
    pro-social development 66
    same-sex 68, 93
    similarities 93–4
    see also Peer relationships
Froebel, Frederick (1782–1852) (early childhood
        pioneer) viii–ix, 111, 118, 145, 288, 301
From Birth to Five: Children's Developmental
        Progress (M. Sheridan) 38
Fruit scheme 54

Games 110
GATT (General Agreement on Tariffs and Trade)
        280
Geldorf, Sir Bob (singer and social campaigner)
        170, 280
Gender differentiation
    early socialization 70

play 67–8
pro-social milestone 66
sex-role development 89
General Agreement on Tariffs and Trade
    (GATT) 280
General practitioner (GP)
    growth monitoring 43, 45
    health centres 190
    ill child 260, 261
    weaning 50
Genetic abnormalities 26, 27
    see also Sickle cell anaemia
Genetic counselling 31
Genetic influences 5
    child development 38
    cognitive processes 101
German measles (rubella) 26, 31
Gestation 24–6, see also Pregnancy
Ghana, street children 278
Grammar, universal 105
Grant Consortium project 61
Great Ormond Street Hospital (London) 245
Green revolution 280
Grief model 232
Gross national income (GNI) per capita 269
Growth charts, monitoring 42–5, 48
Guatamalan 'Casa Alianza' street child project 278

Health
    developing countries 270–5
    as emotive subject 244
    inequalities in UK 189
    WHO definition 24
    see also Child health; Ill child
Health Action Zones 189
Health care policy
    health inequalities 189
    NHS Act (1948) 188–9
    risks of ill health and 189
    role of parents 190–1
    see also Health promotion
Health centre 42, 190
Health Promoting Schools Programme 248
Health promotion
    at school 248
    optimal child development 248
    overview of strategies 189–90
    preventative services 246
    public health role 248
    screening 41–5
Health Survey for England, on obesity 250
Health visitor 166, 169, 190, 246
    breastfeeding 48
    child development 47
    children with long-term needs 251
    early problem detection 247
    growth monitoring 43, 45
    ill child 260
    weaning 50
Hearing screening 41–2, 247

Hierarchy of needs, Maslow's 46–7, 63
HIPC (Heavily Indebted Poor Countries)
    initiative 281
History of childhood
    19th century 168–9
    economic contribution 168
    Enlightenment 168
    industrialization xii, 168, 169
    medieval period xii, 167
HIV/AIDS
    child morbidity 250, 274
    stigma associated 274
    UN Rights of the Child 2
    virus transmission 287
    WHO antiretroviral therapy 271
Holistic approach
    child protection services 205–6, 211
    child within social context x, 297, 303
    communication and collaboration 303
    early childhood education and care 117–18,
        120, 128, 132–3, 134
    early childhood services provision 194
    early school pathway and 147, 152, 154, 159
    family x, 132–3, 234, 297, 303
    play, language and learning 99–100, 111–13
    principles of holism x–xi, 297
    PSE development 58
    see also Integrated services; Multidisciplinary
        approach; Partnership
Home Start 197
Hospital care
    admission vignette 284–7
    children's responses 284, 285–7
    history of 246
    ill child 250, 260–1, 264–5
    shift towards primary care 247–8
Household 171, 172
Housework 69, 178–9
Human development index (HDI) 269
Humanistic psychology 62–3
Hygiene and toileting 46
Hygienist movement xiii

Ill child
    confidentiality 264
    coping behaviour and outcome 264
    empowerment 264
    hospital-based care 257, 264–5
    local children's clinical networks 261–2
    NSF for Children 258, 259, 261
        Standard 6, 260–1, 265, 266
    shift towards community care 260–1
    unmet needs 47
        with long-term needs
        care plan 252
        invasive treatment 252
        minimizing impact on family 264–5
    see also specific illnesses; Disabled child; Dying
        child
Immunization, see Vaccination

Inclusion 88, 149, 156, 195
    mainstream education 226, 228–9, 234, 235, 251
Industrialization
    children during xii, 168, 169, 245
    nuclear family 176
Infant babbling 67, 105
Infant feeding 48–9, 273
Infant health
    genetic screening 27
    low birth weight 28
    maternal age 27
    maternal health 26–7
    mortality
        health inequalities 189
        historical aspects 16
    parental lifestyle 27–9
    strategies to optimize 29–34, 49
Infant mortality rate (IMR) 181, 246, 272–3
Infanticide 167, 273
Infectious diseases 48–9, 190, 246, 271, 273
    vaccination 31, 36, 190, 247
    see also specific illnesses
Institutionalization 226, 227
Integrated services 3, 123, 194
    child health 253
    child with long-term needs 251, 252
    Children Act (2004) emphasis 147, 239
    and family in early education 132–3, 134
    holistic development of child xi
    multiprofessional working 147
    principle of integration x, xi
    professional requirements 147
    social policy 195–7, 248
    SureStart emphasis on 191
Intelligence
    emotional 57, 58, 59–60
    interpersonal concept of multiple 57, 59
    see also Personal, social and emotional (PSE)
        competence
Intelligence quotient (IQ) 88
Interactionism, see Constructivism
1904 Interdepartmental Committee on Physical
        Deterioration 245
International Bank for Reconstruction and
        Development (World Bank) 269, 281
International Monetary Fund (IMF) 281
Involvement, Laevers' concept of 120, 131, 132,
        134, 135
IQ (intelligence quotient) 57, 88
Iron deficiency 49–50

James Bulger case 165

Keeping Children Safe 205
Kennedy Report (children's heart surgery) 257
Key Stage One (KS1) 130, 142, 143–4
    assessment prior to 155
    description 156, 157
    National Literacy/Numeracy Strategies 157, 158
    planning within 158

standard attainment tasks 159
transition to 155–6
Key workers 300
Kinship 50, 171, 172, see also Family

Laever's model of experiential education 120,
        121, 125, 131, 134
Laming Inquiry (death of Victoria Climbié) 221,
        257–8
    key recommendations 205
Language
    infant babbling 67, 105
    interpretation in research 290
    role in learning 104–5
    see also Learning theories; Play, language and
        learning; Speech
Language acquisition device (LAD) 105
Language acquisition support system (LASS) 106
Language acquisition theories
    cognitive 105
    integration in multiple domains 106
    learning or behaviourist 10
    linguistic determinism 104
    nativist 105
    social interactionism 106
Lay referral system 260
Lead members for children 258
Learning activities
    appropriate and challenging 130, 132
    early childhood education and care
        contextually appropriate practice 131–2,
            145, 148
        curriculum guidelines 130
        developmentally appropriate practice 131, 145
        English foundation stage curriculum 130
        Laever's experiential model 131
        Reggio Emilia 130
        Te Whariki 130
    early school pathway 152–4
    importance of 'talk' 128–9
    involvement 120, 131, 132, 134, 135
Learning difficulties
    inclusive practice 229, 235
    see also Special educational needs (SEN)
Learning support assistants 146
Learning theories
    constructivist view 101–2
    empiricist view 101
    nativist view 101
    nature–nurture debate 4, 5, 101
    role of language 104–5
    scaffolding 103
    schemas 101–2
    social interactionist 105
Legislation
    Carers and Disabled Children Act (2000) 228
    Children Act (1989) 185, 198, 238
        child protection 204, 205, 222
        consent to research 293
        disabled child 228, 229–30

Children Act (2004) x, 124, 181, 204, 205,
        222, 258
    education 146, 147, 159, 194
    integrated services 147, 159, 194, 198, 239, 300
    social policy 185, 190, 193, 194, 198
Coal Mines Act (1845) 245
Community Care Act (1990) 190
Disability Discrimination Act (1995) 228
Education Act (1887, 1906) 245
Education Act (1944) 142, 234
Education Act (1981) 234
Education Act (1987) 187–8
Education Act (2002) 143, 195–6
Education Acts (1993, 1996) 234
Education of Handicapped Children Act
        (1970) 234
Education Reform Act (1988) 142, 196
Factory Act (1844, 1850, 1853) 168
Factory Act (1901) 245
Mines Act (1842) 168
National Health Service Act (1948) 188–9, 190
New Poor Law (1834) 186
NHS Act (1948) 188–9, 190
Notification of Births Act (1907) 169
Poor Law Amendment Act (1889) 187
Poor Law Report (1934) 186
Public Health Act (1947) 188
Special Educational Needs and Disability Act
        (2002) 228
Ten Hours Act (1945) 245
    see also Rights of the child; UN Convention on
        the Rights of the Child
'Less eligibility' 186
Life expectancy 271–2
Linguistic determinism 104
Literacy
    emotional 60
    narrative approaches 112
    rates 276
    see also Personal, social and emotional (PSE)
        competence
Literacy–play research 112–13
Literature, critical reading 287
Local authorities
    child care services 188
    disabled child 228, 229, 230
    early childhood services 194, 300
    see also Local education authorities (LEAs)
Local children's clinical network
    description 261–2
    family-centred care 262–3
Local education authorities (LEAs)
    director of children's services 258
    holistic approach to early childhood education
        and care 124
    lead members 258
    legislative obligations 144–5
    school starting age 141
Lone-parent families 52, 82–3, 172–5, 191, 192
Low birth weight 28

McMillan, Margaret and Rachel ix, xiii
Marxism
    child services 169
    description 164
    role of family 178
    view of childhood 166
Maslow's hierarchy of needs 46–7, 63
Maternal bonding 86
Maternity services 32, 49
Means-testing 191
Measles 271, 275
Measles, mumps and rubella (MMR)
        immunization 190, 244
Media
    child health concerns 244, 249
    child protection 204, 205
    child-rearing influenced 169, 170, 190
Medieval period 168
Men
    division of labour within home 176–8
    see also Father–child relationship; Parents
Mental health
    child abuse survivors 94, 218
    father figure and 88
    health inequalities 248
    parental 62, 65, 66, 67, 70, 211, 212
    personal, social and emotional development
        58, 66
    pro-social development 70
    school nurse promotion 249
    school-aged children 252
    self-esteem 63
    socio-economic factors 58, 82, 181, 852
    see also Childhood depression
Mentalizing ability 70
Metacommunication 111, 112
Metarepresentation 112
Midwife 32, 48, 49, 190
'Mind-blindness' 64
'Mind-reading' 64, see also Social
        understanding
Minister for Children, Young People and Families
        x, 258
MMR (measles, mumps and rubella)
        immunization 190, 244
Morbidity 189, 190, 274–5
    HIV/AIDS related 150, 274
Mortality
    developed/developing countries 270–1
    health inequalities 189
    historical view 16
    infant 181, 246, 272–3
Mother
    bonding with infant 86
    death during childbirth 272
    false–belief task and pretend play 64
    infant health and care of 26–8
    postnatal coping strategies 33
Mother–baby friendly city (Quezon, Philippines)
        272

Mother–child relationship
    attachment theory 63, 85–7
    categories 86–7
    object permanence and fear of strangers 67
    other relationships 87
    sex role development 89
    sibling relationships 89–92
Multidisciplinary approach
    child health problems 42
    child with multiple needs 251
    child protection 221–2
    disabled children 234, 237–9
    early childhood education 147–8
    holistic approach x–xi, 297, 303–4
    multiprofessional working 147
    severely insecure children 63
    UNESCO model 3
Music 47

Narrative report 10–11
National Child Development Study 88
National Curriculum (England)
    attainment targets and league tables 196
    children as 'products' 166
    criticisms of 157
    foundation stage 131, 143
    introduction of 196
    key stages 142
    learning areas 130–1
    literacy/numeracy strategies 150, 157, 158
    personal, social and health education 156, 249
    programmes of study 157
    role of 156
    school curriculum based 156–7
    see also Key Stage One
National Health Service (NHS)
    clinical governance scores 249
    NHS Act (1948) 188–9, 190
    patient/client empowerment 249
    shift towards primary care 247–8
    star ratings 249
    see also Hospital care; Primary care
National Healthy Schools Standard 248
National Institute for Clinical Excellence (NICE) 32
National Literacy/Numeracy Strategies 150, 157, 158
National Report on Services for Disabled Children 238
National Service Frameworks (NSFs)
    aims of 258
    relevance to children 258, 259
National Service Framework for Children, Young People and Maternity Services (2004) x, 185, 189
    child health promotion 247
    child protection 204, 205, 207, 222
    description 190, 259
    diagnosis and disclosure 231
    empowerment 193–4
    exemplar of asthma 262

hospital services 246
ill child 258, 259, 260–1
    Standard 6, 260–1, 265, 266
integrated services 194, 205, 239, 300
local children's clinical network 261–2
maternity care 32
National Society for the Prevention of Cruelty to Children (NSPCC) 198
    extent of child abuse 207, 209, 211, 222
Nativism 4
    language acquisition 105
    learning 101
Nature–nuture debate 4, 5
    language acquisition 103–4
    learning 101
Needs of child
    at 6 month vs 4 years 45–7
    Maslow's hierarchy of 46–7, 63
    security of attachment 46, 47
Neonate, see Newborn
New Deal for Communities 31
New Zealand 168
    Te Whariki early years curriculum 130
Newborn (neonate)
    attachment theory 85–6
    father/mother involvement 88
    screening 32, 42
    strategies for health 29–34
NSPCC, see National Society for the Prevention of Cruelty to Children
Nuchal translucency screening 27
Nursery education 148, 177, 195, 251–2, 286
    attachment theory 47
    Early childhood education and care 117–140
    family–educator partnership 132–3, 134
    foundation stage curriculum 143
    increase in private 196
    McMillan sisters' philosophy ix
    Marxist view 166
    Ofsted inspection 134
    social policy, 195–6
Nursery nurses xiv, 48, 146, 149, 247
Nutrition
    at 6 months vs 4 years 45
    breast/bottle feeding 48–9, 102, 169–70, 273–4
    child development 38
    developing countries 273, 280–1
    food groups 53, 54
    hierarchy of needs 45, 46, 47
    maternal 28
    pre-school child 51–3
    school children 53–4, 249, 250
    sub- 53
    vegetarians 50, 51, 52–3
    weaning 49–51

Obesity 53–4, 248–9
Object permanence 67, 85
Observation of children
    data analysis 16–18

ethical issues 18–19
incidental 8
intentional 8
key skill 301
long-term 9
planning foundation stage 151–2
reasons for 6–7, 301
in research 288, 289
techniques 10–16
theory applied to data 17–18
triggered 8
understanding development 301
what might be observed 9–10, 301
Observer effects 289
Office for Standards in Education (Ofsted) 144,
    195–6, 205–6
early childhood education and care/nursery
    education 134
Foundation Stage Profile 155
Olsen model of family structure 84, 170, 172–6
Operant conditioning 101
Oral rehydration therapy 271, 273
Organization for Economic Co-operation and
    Development (OECD), education ix,
    117, 121
Otitis media 263
Out-of-school activities 177, 198
Owen, Robert (1771–1858) viii

Parent and toddler groups 197
Parenting style
authoritarian 80
authoritative 80–1
children outcome 80–1
demandingness 80
education 81–2
factors affecting 82–3
and neglect 81
permissive 80
pro-social development 65
responsiveness 80
uninvolved 81
Parents
attachment issues 87
behavioural codes 302
child nutrition 28, 53
child protection and involvement 204
collaboration with schools 145
consent to research 291, 292–3
diagnosis and disclosure 230–3
disabled children 230–2, 233, 235, 236, 237
dismissive 87
family–educator collaboration 132–3, 134,
    145–6
first days at school 148
as health carers 260
healthcare decisions and media 190
hospital admission of child 284, 285–7
influences on baby's health
    antenatal care 32

parental factors 26–9
postnatal period 32–4
preconceptual care 29, 31–2
socio-economic factors 29, 34
SureStart 31
lone 52, 82–3, 172–5, 191, 192
mental health problems 62, 65, 66, 67, 70
parenting education 81–2
physical abuse 220, 221
preoccupied 87
school nurse and 249
security of attachment 46, 47
working, and child care 197
see also Families
Partnership
child health and education 253
disabled children and their families 234, 237–9
family–educator 132–3 134, 145–6
parents and schools 145
schools and communities 145
wider team in classroom 146–7
see also Integrated services; Multidisciplinary
    approach
Peek-a-boo game 110
Peer relationships 69, 113
pro-social development and 66
social behaviour skills and 61
see also Friendships
Perinatal period
child morbidity and mortality 272, 274
screening 246
Personal skills (self-science) 60–2
Personal, social and emotional (PSE)
    competence
attachment 63–4
dysfunctional systems 62
emotional literacy 59–60
friendship role 93
overview of 59
pro-social development 65–6
self-discrepancy theory 62–3
self-esteem 62–3
skills approach 60–2
social understanding 64–5
Personal, social and emotional (PSE)
    development
first 8 months 66–7
12 months 67
18 to 36 months 67–9
36 to 48-plus months 80–1
delinquency and crime 57
holistic approach 58
perspective taking 70
scaffolding 69
social understanding 70
within foundation stage 151
Personal, social and health education (PSHE)
    156, 249
Pharmacists 50
Phenylketonuria screening 42

Physical abuse
  contributory factors 221
  deaths from 205, 209
  definition 220
  effects 94, 220–1
  examples 220
  historical view xii
Physical activity 54, 156, 159, 250
Physical development, *see under* Child
    development
Physical growth, *see* Growth
Plan-do-review 151
Planning, foundation stage 151–4
Plato (427–347 BC) 118, viii
Platt Report 260
Play
  6 months *vs* 4 years 46
  'as if' play 108, 112
  characteristics 107
  collective symbols 110
  cultural issues 105, 106, 107, 113
  defining 106–7
  disabled children 234, 237
  emotional containment 108
  games 110
  gender differentiation 67–8
  hospital admission 287
  as learning activity 128
  'other reference' 109
  practice 109, 112
  pretend 64, 67, 70, 110, 111
  recreation and relaxation 108
  role-playing 70, 111
  rules 110, 111
  sensorimotor 109
  sequential combinations 109
  symbolic 67, 109
  theories 107–11
  UN Convention on the Rights of the
      Child 128
  value of play 3
  wish fulfilment 112
  zone of proximal development 110
Play, language and learning
  holistic approach 99–100, 111–13
  interplay of 111–13
  value of play 3
  see also Language; Learning; Relationships
Play–literacy approach 112
Play theories
  classical/modern 107
  evolutionary/biological 107–9
  practice 107
  psychoanalytic, psychotherapeutic 108
  recapitulation 108
  socio-cognitive 108–11
  socio-dramatic 109–10
  socio-economic 108
  socio-emotional 108, 109, 110, 112
Play therapy 108–9

Playgroups 195, 197, 251
  change in provision 177
  early problem recognition 247
  first days at school 148
  hospital admission 286
  see also Early childhood education and care
      (ECEC)
Pointing 102–3
Poliomyelitis 246
Political instability 29
Post-modernism 5
Post-traumatic stress disorder (PTSD) 94, 95, 218
Postcode lottery of care 237, 247
Postnatal care 32–4, 48
Postnatal depression 33
Poverty 47, 119, 197
  behavioural problems 181
  child abuse 211
  definition 179
  early childhood 197
  effects 181
  ethnic groups 191
  government's antipoverty strategy x, 191–2,
      197
  health inequalities 189, 248
  lone-parent families 175, 191
  mental health 58, 82
  number of children 175, 179–80, 191, 194, 248
  parenting style 82
  pre-school nutrition 53
  social exclusion 191
  UN Agenda for Development (1997) 278
  UN Rights of the Child 2
  weaning 50
  welfare care 197
Practice nurse 247, 251, 260
Pre-school child
  attachment theory 63
  education of disabled and SEN 233–4
  emotional literacy 60
  nutrition 51–3
  see also Early childhood education and care
      (ECEC); Nursery education
Preconceptual care 29, 31–2
Pregnancy
  antenatal care 27, 31, 32, 49
  fetal development 24–6, 28
  postnatal care 32–4, 48
  preconceptual care 29, 31–2
  teenage 29–30
Premature baby 33, 261
Preventative health services, 246, *see also*
      Screening
Primary Care Trusts (PCTs) 48, 263
Primary health care 188, 247–8
Primary schools
  changes to school day 159
  future developments 159
  multiprofessional workforce 159
  nursery classes 195

Pro-social development 59, 65–6
  gender differentiation 70–1
Pro-social reflex 66
Programmes of study 157
Prostitution 207, 270
4Ps approach to children's rights 192–3
PSE, see Personal, social and emotional
  development
Psychoanalytic/psychotherapeutic approach to
  play 108
Psychological abuse 214
Public health
  aims 248
  co-ordinated approach 248
  definition 248
  health inequalities and poverty 248–9
  school nurse 249

Qualifications and Curriculum Authority (QCA)
  143, 144, 149
Quality
  defining 120
  see also Early childhood education and care
    (ECEC), quality
Quality Protects 206

Racism 82, 127, 149
Rating scales 289
Rationalism 4
Recapitulation theory of play 108
Reception year 143, 148, 195
  assessment 155
  foundation stage curriculum 150–1
  planning foundation stage 'journey' 151–5
  transition to Key Stage One 155–6
Record-keeping 299
Reflective practice 134
Reggio Emilia (Italy) 122–3, 127, 130
Regulations, family 303
Relationships
  abusive 94–5
  early, and PSE 58
  false–belief task and 64
  father involvement and later 88
  friendships 92–4
  play, learning and language 113
  primary 87
  similarity 93
  see also Attachment theory; Child abuse;
    Family; Father–child relationship;
    Mother–child relationship
Religious factors 50, 52
  see also Cultural factors; Ethnicity
  Research
  child's language 290
  consent 18, 292–3
  critical reading skills 287
  data collection 289
  ethical implications 290–3
    consent 291, 292–3

governance framework 291
  invasiveness 291
  therapeutic/non-therapeutic 291–2
functions 285
general principles 288
hospital admission 284–7
importance 285
interviews 290
post-war ethical codes 292
practice informed by knowledge 285–7
sampling 11–14, 288–9
small-scale studies 290
see also Observation
Research Governance Framework 291
Respite care 251
Rickets 52
Rights of the child, see UN Convention on the
  Rights of the Child
Role-playing 70, 111
Rolling planning process 151–2
Rubella (German measles) 26, 31
Rumbold Report 195
Rwanda, mass rape of women 279

Safeguarding Children 205
Safety needs of child 46–7
Salutogenesis (promotion of well-being) 248
Sampling 11–14, 288–9
Save the Children (charity) 197
Saving Lives 248
Scaffolding 69, 103, 113, 129
Schemas 101–2, 112
School
  behavioural problems 58
  child with long-term needs 251
  communities and 145
  disabled pupils 228
  emotional and behavioural problems 252
  first days at 148–9
  health promotion 248, 249, 252
  inclusive practice 226, 228–9, 234,
    235, 251
  integration vs segregation debate 235
  legislative requirements 144–5, 228-9
  managerial skills 147
  mental health problems 58
  nutrition 53–4, 249, 250
  obesity and 250
  physical activity 54
  seriously ill/dying children 252
  socio-cultural context 145–8
  special educational needs provision 251–2
  starting age 141–2
  valuing diversity 124–7, 149
  wider team in classroom 146–7
  working with parents 145–6
School curriculum 156–7, see also Foundation
  stage (4–5 years); Key Stage One; National
  Curriculum (England)
School health service 169, 249

School meals 54, 249, 250
School nurse 166, 246, 247, 249, 251
School performance tables 155, 196
Screening
    development 246
    eyesight 247
    hearing 41–2, 247
    neonatal 32, 42
    routine, broad-based 246, 247
    targeted 247
Script theory 112
Security
    friendship and 93
    hierarchy of needs 46–7
    see also Attachment
Self
    actual vs ideal 63
    ought 3
Self-actualization 46, 47, 63
Self-awareness 64
Self-discrepancy theory 62–3
Self-esteem 46
    development of 47, 63
    friendship 93
    importance of 63
    obesity 54
    popularity and high self-worth 94
Self-science (personal skills) 60–2
Self/other (autonomy/connectedness) 61, 71
Separation protest 85
Serial monogamy 172
Sex education 29
Sex role development 88, see also Gender
        differentiation
Sexism 127
Sexual abuse
    collecting evidence 216, 217
    definition 216
    delay in seeking help 207
    effects 94–5, 217–18
    examples 216
    exploitation 207
    flashbacks 218
    grooming of child 218
    healing process 219
    normal sexual interest 217
    overt/covert 216
    post-traumatic stress disorder 218
    prostitution 207
    stigma of label 217
    within family 207
Sexually transmitted diseases 217
Siblings
    attachment to mother 90
    benefit of having 90
    disabled child 233, 237
    false–belief task 64
    family selection of 92
    favouritism–hostility hypothesis 92
    parental treatment 90–2

same-sex 90
second child 89–90
social understanding 70
Sick child, see Dying child; Ill child
Sickle cell disorders 42, 250
Significant harm 206
Single-parent families 52, 82–3, 172–5, 191, 192
Skin-to-skin touching 86
Smiling 67, 85
Social comparison 93
Social competence
    'effectiveness in interaction' 61
    emotional literacy and 60
    Grant Consortium Project 61
    see also Personal, social and emotional (PSE)
        competence
Social constructivism
    defining 165
    learning theory 101–2
    literacy–play 112
    overview 5–6
    Reggio Emilia's approach 122
Social development, see Attachment; Family;
        Friendships; Personal, social and
        emotional (PSE) development;
        Socialization
Social interactionism
    description 164
    language acquisition 105, 106
    learning process 102
    view of childhood 166
    view of education 117
Social learning 85
Social policy 185–202, 298
    child's rights and interests 188, 192
    education 195–7
    family 185–6, 192, 196–7
    child care services 186–8, 195–7
    health care foundations 188–91
    integrated services 194, 195–7, 248
    nursery education 195–6
    reducing child poverty 191–2
    voluntary services 197–8
    welfare care 197
Social power 238
Social security system 191–2
Social services
    historical independence 246
    integration with other services 253
    social worker 47, 230, 251
Social understanding (theory of mind) 59, 61,
        64–5, 66, 70
Social worker 47, 230, 251
Socialization
    gender differentiation 66
    impact on PSE
        at 8 months 67
        at 12 months 67
        at 18–36 months 69
        36 to 48 months 70–1

pro-social development 65
    relationships 78
Socio-cognitive approach, to play 108, 110–11
Socio-economic factors
    child development 38
    childhood depression 62
    health of newborn baby 29, 34
    health status of child 29, 248–9
    mental health problems 58
    parenting style 82
    weaning 50
Socio-emotional play 109, 110
Sociological perspectives 164–7
    child in the family 170–6
    child in history 167–70
    child-centred family 181
    family structures 172–6
    family functioning 176–9
    poverty and family 179–81
    sociology defined 163
    types of 164–5
    working women 176–8
Special Educational Needs Code of Practice
        234, 251
Special educational needs (SEN)
    assessment 155, 234–5
    early childhood education and care 126
    emotional and behavioural difficulties 252
    inclusion in mainstream education 234,
        251–2
    integration vs segregation debate 235
    legislation 234–5
    number of children 226, 234, 251–2
    special schools 235, 250, 252
    statement 226, 234
    see also Disabled children
Speech
    chewing and 49
    cognitive restructuring 105
    egocentric 104, 105
    infant babbling 67, 105
    internal/overt 105
    over-socialized 105
    see also Language; Learning theories
Spiral curriculum 103
Split age classes 41–3
Standard attainment tasks (SATS) 159, 166
Standardized testing, criticisms 103
Starting Strong 121
STEP (Systematic Training for Effective
        Parenting) 81–2
Stepping stones 130–1, 150–1, 155
Stereotyping
    'beautiful is good' 94
    children's learning of 126, 149
    children's rights 193
    disabled people 227, 231
Strange situation procedure 86–7
Strangers, fear of 67
Street children 245, 277, 278

Structural functionalism 164
    child services 169
    education 164
    family 170–1
    view of children 166
Study of Pedagogical Effectiveness (J. Moyle)
        127, 128
Sudden infant death 26, 49, 249
Suicide attempts 94, 95
Summer play schemes 198
SureStart x, 31, 120–1, 124, 145, 189, 234, 248

Tanzania, foreign debt cancellation 281
Tax credits 191
Te Whariki (New Zealand) early years
        curriculum 130
Teachers
    attachment theory 63–4
    children with long-term needs 251
    curriculum guidance document 151
    foundation stage journey 151–4
    inclusion in schools 149
    managerial skills 147
    multidisciplinary nature of work 147–8
    ultimate responsibility 148
Teaching assistants 146, 149
Teenage pregnancy 29–30
Teratogens 28
Terminally ill children, see Dying children
Theory of mind ('mind-reading', social
        understanding), see Social understanding
Thinking
    sustained shared, 129–30
    see also Learning; Thought
Third World, see Developing countries
Thought
    enactive/iconic/symbolic 103
    relationship with language 104–5
    verbal 105
    see also Learning
Three-day blues (baby blues) 33
Time sampling 11–13
Tobacco use 26, 28, 31, 32, 191, 271
Together from the Start x, 233
Tuberculosis 246

United Nations (UN)
    Agenda for Development (1997) 278
    human development index 269
    Millennium Development Goals 276
UN Convention on the Rights of the Child 2, 269
    10 objectives ix, 2
    abuse and exploitation 271
    children's views of quality in ECEC 123
    consent in research 19
    definition of child 165
    disabled child 230, 271, 275
    discrimination 279
    education and care 117, 276–8
    employment 278

UN Convention on the Rights of the Child (*Cont.*)
    guiding principles ix, 2, 230
    health 191, 270, 270–5
    history of 270
    life expectancy 271
    play 31, 128
    political instability and war 276–8
    ratification ix, 270
    self-identity 279
    standard of living 278
UN Education, Scientific and Cultural
        Organisation (UNESCO) 277, 278
    cost-benefit of early years' investment ix
    global model of childhood values 1–2, 3, 127
    view of early childhood education 117–118, xi
UN International Children's Emergency Fund
        (UNICEF)
    aid during war 279
    definition of care 117
    education 276
    infant mortality 273
Underfeeding 45

Vaccination 31, 46, 190, 244, 246, 247
Valuing People 229
Vegans, vegetarianism 50, 51, 52–3
Verbatim reporting 15–16
Victoria Climbié Inquiry, *see* Laming Inquiry
    (death of Victoria Climbié)
Vitamin A deficiency-related blindness 273
Vitamin D deficiency 52
Voluntary services 197–8, 245

'Walking bus' 54
War 279
Water fluoridation 249
Wealth
    developing countries 281
    see also Poverty; Socio-economic factors

Weaning 49–51
Welfare care 197
Well-being, promotion 248
West, Fred and Rosemary (child abuse) 79, 95
*What To Do If You're Worried A Child Is Being
    Abused* 211
Wish fulfilment, play as 112
Wolfenden Report 197
Women
    feminist views 164, 166, 178
    labour division within home 178–9
    in workplace 176–8
    see also Mother–child relationship; Parents
Work
    child health and future employment 253
    employment-led reforms of child care 196–7
    family-work balance, and social policy 196–7
    labour division within home 178–9
    women in 176–8
Workfare (welfare-to-work) 197
Workhouse 186, 187, 245
Working tax credit 191
World Bank, *see* International Bank for
    Reconstruction and Development
World Declaration on Education for All
    (UNICEF) 276
World Health Organization (WHO)
    antiretroviral therapy initiative 271
    definition of health 24
    Global Strategy on Infant and Young Child
        Feeding 273
    Health Promoting Schools Programme 248
    maternity care 272–3
    rehabilitation services for disabled 274
    weaning 49

Zone of proximal (next) development (ZPD)
    103, 110, 129, 132, 152